Parkinson's Disease: A Growing Concern

Parkinson's Disease:
A Growing Concern

Editor: Helena Shelton

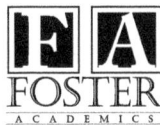

FA
FOSTER
ACADEMICS

www.fosteracademics.com

www.fosteracademics.com

FA
FOSTER
ACADEMICS

Cataloging-in-Publication Data

Parkinson's disease : a growing concern / edited by Helena Shelton.
    p. cm.
Includes bibliographical references and index.
ISBN 978-1-63242-716-8
1. Parkinson's disease. 2. Brain--Diseases. I. Shelton, Helena.
RC382 .P37 2019
616.833--dc23

Foster Academics,
118-35 Queens Blvd., Suite 400,
Forest Hills, NY 11375, USA

ISBN 978-1-63242-716-8 (Hardback)

Contents

Preface

Parkinson's disease is a neurodegenerative disorder affecting the central nervous system, with gradually deteriorating motor abilities. After Alzheimer's disease, it is the second most common neurodegenerative disorder. Hallucinations or delusions occur in 50% of the cases with Parkinson's disease, and may indicate the start of dementia. There is no cure for Parkinson's disease, but various treatment pathways aimed at providing relief such as surgery, physical treatment and medications are available to improve quality of life. Typically, antiparkinson medications such as levodopa with dopamine agonists are prescribed for patients in the initial stages of the disease. Lesional and deep brain stimulation surgery is performed on those for whom medications fail. This book covers in detail some existing theories and innovative concepts revolving around Parkinson's disease. Its objective is to give a general view of the different clinical aspects of this disease. A number of latest researches have been included in this book to keep the readers up-to-date with the global concepts in this area of study.

The researches compiled throughout the book are authentic and of high quality, combining several disciplines and from very diverse regions from around the world. Drawing on the contributions of many researchers from diverse countries, the book's objective is to provide the readers with the latest achievements in the area of research. This book will surely be a source of knowledge to all interested and researching the field.

In the end, I would like to express my deep sense of gratitude to all the authors for meeting the set deadlines in completing and submitting their research chapters. I would also like to thank the publisher for the support offered to us throughout the course of the book. Finally, I extend my sincere thanks to my family for being a constant source of inspiration and encouragement.

Editor

Pharmacotherapeutic Challenges in Parkinson's Disease Inpatients

Unax Lertxundi, Rafael Hernández,
Saioa Domingo-Echaburu,
Javier Peral-Aguirregoitia and Juan Medrano

Abstract

During the natural history of Parkinson's disease (PD), many patients require hospital admission for medical or surgical problems other than the motor features of PD. Therefore, they are often admitted to non-neurological wards where the staff is unfamiliar with PD management. Among the issues related to hospitalization in patients with PD, drug-related problems such as inappropriate levodopa timing of administration, the use of contraindicated, centrally acting antidopaminergic drugs and anticholinergic burden remain among the most troublesome.

Keywords: Parkinson's disease, antidopaminergic, levodopa, inappropriate prescription, antipsychotic

1. Introduction

Parkinson's disease (PD) is a chronic, progressive neurodegenerative disease known to occur primarily from middle age to later in life [1]. The frequency of PD varies depending on the diagnostic criteria, study population, and is estimated to be 0.3% of the entire population, about 1–2% in people over 60–65 years [1] and 3–5% in people 85 years and older [2, 3]. It is a common progressive and disabling neurological disorder characterized by the degeneration of several different neuronal populations that lead to the cardinal features of PD, which are tremor, bradykinesia, rigidity and postural instability [4].

During the natural history of the disease, many patients require hospital admission for medical or surgical problems other than the motor features of PD. As a consequence, they are often admitted to non-neurological wards where staff is unfamiliar with PD management, as it is generally managed in the outpatient setting [5, 6]. The problems and complications faced by PD patients while in hospital have urged specialists to develop specific guidelines [7]. Among the issues related to hospitalization in PD patients, drug-related problems remain amongst the most troublesome [8, 9]. In this chapter we will review some of them, such as inappropriate levodopa timing administration, centrally acting antidopaminergic drug administration and anticholinergic burden.

2. Inappropriate inpatient levodopa administration

Management of medication regimens increases in complexity as PD progresses, frequently leading to prescriptions taken six or more times per day. Besides, dosing intervals are specific to each individual patient. Although adequate anti-PD medication management is essential during hospital admissions (regarding drugs, dosages and specific dosage schedules), its management is frequently described as suboptimal, leading to adverse clinical sequelae.

One of the first studies about the problem came from a retrospective study of patients with PD hospitalized in the United Kingdom [10]. In that report, an alarming percentage of patients admitted to the hospital had critical medications stopped or omitted. Even more worryingly, of these around 60% experienced significant adverse effects, including the need to transfer a patient to the intensive care unit. In another study carried out in surgical wards of a Scottish hospital, three out of four hospitalized patients with PD did not receive their medications on time or had had doses entirely omitted [11]. In the same line, in a small study we conducted in Alto Deba hospital (in the Basque Country, Spain) we found that chronic anti-PD prescription was omitted in 12/73 admissions [12].

In a survey of National Parkinson Foundation Center, the majority of the participating centers were not confident that medication schedules were adhered to during hospital stays, perhaps because the importance of medication timing in PD was not well understood by hospital staff [13]. Again, from a patient perspective, a survey carried out by a Dutch team showed that incorrect medication distribution contributed to intrahospital deterioration [14].

The same Dutch team published a prospective study that showed that medication error was the most important risk factor for deterioration [15]. More recently, a cross-sectional chart review carried out in 339 consecutive hospital encounters from 212 PD subjects in Florida has shown that patients who had delayed administration or missed at least one dose stayed longer [16].

Skelly et al. [17], in a study carried out in the Royal Derby Hospital in the United Kingdom (National Parkinson Foundation Centre of Excellence for Parkinson's Disease), reported that 2.5% of all doses were not administered because the drug was not available on time. It has to be remarked that this happened in a ward specially designed to treat patients with PD, with an enhanced stock of anti-PD medications [17]. We consider that this problem is likely to be aggravated in other non-specialized wards and especially in smaller hospitals.

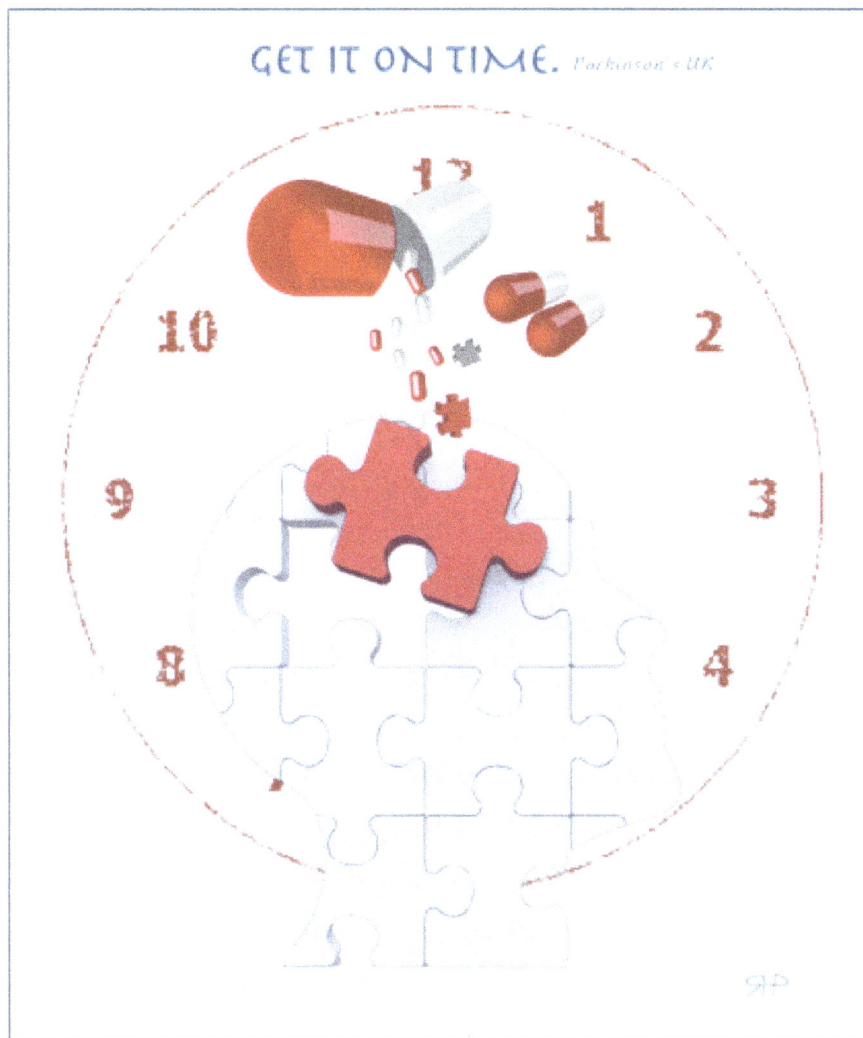

Figure 1. The importance of on-time levodopa administration.

To counteract this difficulty, Parkinson's United Kingdom "**Get it on time campaign**" [18], (**Figure 1**) among others [19], advices that all commercially available antiparkinsonian drugs should be timely available in all hospital wards. Given the data described previously, we find this unfeasible, especially in small hospitals where the availability of all the anti-PD drugs would certainly result in the expiration of many of these drugs before they could be used. May be a reasonable solution can be found in Skelly et al.'s own final considerations: *"The available stock was not used as flexibly as we had hoped: e.g. doses of modified release medications were omitted rather than a temporary switch to available standard release drugs."*

The Institute for Safe Medication Practices (ISMP) has recently issued a generic recommendation that, whereas undoubtedly helpful, will result insufficient. Their recommendation specifically states *"avoiding non-formulary delays ensuring that your formulary provides common*

PD medications and doses so that drug administration is not delayed while the pharmacy obtains non-formulary medications" [20]. Based on the available data, we have recently proposed an algorithm to prevent drug omissions and delays [21] using the equivalent dosages proposed by Tomlinson et al. [22] (**Table 1**).

Drug	Conversion Factor
Immediate release levodopa	1
Controlled release levodopa	0.75
Entacapone*	LD 0.33
Tolcapone*	LD 0.5
Duodopa®	1.11
Pramipexole	100
Ropirinole	20
Rotigotine	30
Selegiline	10
Rasagiline	100
Amantadine	1
Apomorphine	10
Bromocriptine	10

*To calculate the total LED for COMT inhibitors (entacapone and tolcapone), the total levodopa (including controlled release levodopa if COMT inhibitor is given simultaneously) amount should be calculated and then multiplied by the appropriate value. For Stalevo®, the levodopa and COMT inhibitor should be split and calculated separately.

Table 1. Conversion factors to calculate levodopa equivalent dose (LED) adapted from ref [22].

In **Figure 2**, we provide an example for how the algorithm could be applied to prevent an omission.

Nevertheless, if a PD patient must be kept *Nil per Os (NPO)*, thus interfering with the patient's unique schedule of medication administration, a neurologist or Neurology team should oversee the medication regimen change to avoid complications, using alternatives such as intradermal rotigotin or subcutaneous apomorphine [23]. In the same study mentioned above, 88% of admissions (227/257) were some dosage was not administered because of "oral intolerance" or NPO status, no alternative drug was used. In four hospitals, no patient received an alternative drug.

Paraphrasing Magdalinou *"PD medications should be regarded as important as insulin is for diabetics"* [10]. We completely agree. It is about time we take the appropriate measures to minimize the problem.

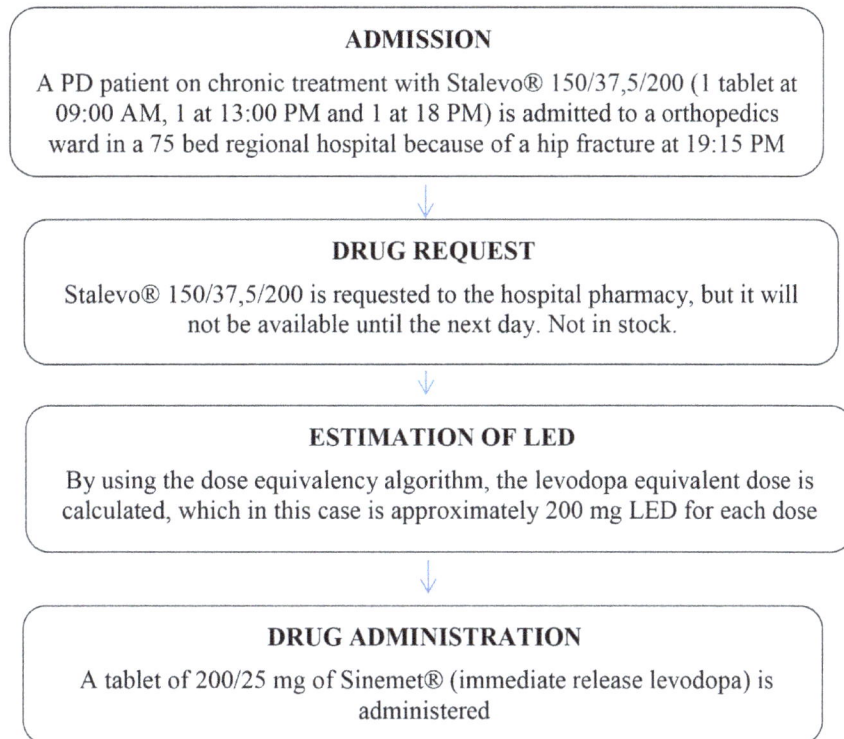

ADMISSION

A PD patient on chronic treatment with Stalevo® 150/37,5/200 (1 tablet at 09:00 AM, 1 at 13:00 PM and 1 at 18 PM) is admitted to a orthopedics ward in a 75 bed regional hospital because of a hip fracture at 19:15 PM

↓

DRUG REQUEST

Stalevo® 150/37,5/200 is requested to the hospital pharmacy, but it will not be available until the next day. Not in stock.

↓

ESTIMATION OF LED

By using the dose equivalency algorithm, the levodopa equivalent dose is calculated, which in this case is approximately 200 mg LED for each dose

↓

DRUG ADMINISTRATION

A tablet of 200/25 mg of Sinemet® (immediate release levodopa) is administered

---

Figure 2. Theoretical example of the algorithm application.

3. Central-acting antidopaminergic administration

Not only anti-PD drugs like levodopa should be taken into account when patients are admitted to hospital. Some drugs are considered inappropriate in PD, since in the same way as dopaminergic drug omissions, they can worsen motor functioning. This is the case with central-acting dopamine antagonists.

While PD has traditionally been considered a motor system disorder, it is nowadays recognized to be a complex condition with diverse clinical features that include neuropsychiatric and many other non-motor symptoms. Researchers are increasingly attending to and characterizing the non-motor symptoms of the disease such as depression, apathy, dementia and psychosis.

3.1. Psychosis

Although patients with both parkinsonism and dementia commonly experience spontaneous visual hallucinations, delusions and paranoia even in the absence of medications for the motor dysfunction, the introduction of dopaminergic therapies frequently triggers or exacerbates the underlying propensity to psychosis in patients who have PD dementia. Correctable infectious, toxic and metabolic etiologies (delirium) must be ruled out. If symptoms persist, antiparkinsonian drugs should be slowly reduced, which usually results in a worsening of the parkinsonian features that may be poorly tolerated. When these measures fail, therapy with antipsychotic drugs might be needed [24–26].

Almost all antipsychotic drugs are known to produce PD exacerbation. Clozapine is the only antipsychotic that has level I evidence to support its use in these patients [26]. Nevertheless, quetiapine is frequently considered the first-line choice for treating psychotic symptoms in PD (e.g., by the American Academy of Neurology), and it is usually reported as the most frequently used [27]. The rest of antipsychotic agents, especially high potency drugs such as haloperidol, are considered inappropriate in PD. In the same line, and as PD disease usually affects old people (aged >65 years), the most frequently used tools employing explicit criteria to detect potentially inappropriate prescriptions in older patients (Beers and STOPP-START) criteria consider inappropriate all antipsychotics other than clozapine or quetiapine [28, 29]. We were surprised to find aripiprazole included as one of the least-problematic antipsychotic therapies for PD psychosis, at the same level as quetiapine and clozapine in the last version of the Beers criteria. Despite its promising receptorial profile, preliminary experience with aripiprazole shows a discouraging safety and efficacy profile in individuals with PD, who represent the most stringent test of a drug's potential for inducing parkinsonism. In this sense, severe worsening of motor function has been reported, with one individual requiring parenteral fluid substitution and another requiring nasogastric tube feeding [30]. In light of the evidence mentioned above and considering the widespread use of the Beers criteria, we believe including aripiprazole in the same category as clozapine and quetiapine for the treatment of PD psychosis could do more harm than good [31].

Delirium, or acute confusional state, has been reported as very prevalent in PD inpatients, and being involved in as many as a quarter of admissions [32, 33]. Dementia, which mainly affects patients with advanced disease, constitutes a known risk factor for delirium. As pointed out before, correctable infectious, toxic and metabolic etiologies should be ruled out before considering antipsychotic treatment. Sadly, many times haloperidol is prescribed in our setting to treat "agitation" in patients, either with PD or not.

3.2. Nausea and vomiting

Nausea and vomiting, which are common adverse effects of anti-PD medications (levodopa and dopamine agonists), might require treatment with antiemetic drugs. Metoclopramide and other centrally acting antiemetics are contraindicated in PD patients because they block dopaminergic receptors in the nigrostriatal area, generating deleterious motor effects [26]. Some cases of metoclopramide-associated encephalopathy have even been reported [34, 35].

On the other side, domperidone has traditionally been considered as the gold standard, since it does not readily cross the blood-brain barrier [26]. Nevertheless, its cardiac safety has been put into question recently [36, 37].

3.3. Hiccups

Hiccups are starting to be considered one more "non-motor" symptom of PD [38]. A study evaluated the presence of hiccups in 90 PD patients and 100 age-matched controls, finding that hiccups were more frequent in PD patients than in healthy controls. Interestingly, chlorpromazine (a "typical" antipsychotic formally contraindicated in PD) is usually used to treat incoercible hiccups.

Whatever the reason for they were prescribed, centrally acting antidopaminergic drugs have shown to generate deleterious effects in PD inpatients. The study carried out in Florida, which was mentioned above [16], showed that contraindicated dopamine blocking agent's administration (which occurred in 23% of the cases) was significantly related to an increased length of stay (8,2 vs 3,5 days)(**Figure 3**).

In conclusion, avoiding drugs known to exacerbate motor symptoms should be a priority. Clozapine and quetiapine should be preferred among antipsychotics [9]. Regarding antiemetic use, low dose of domperidone seems reasonable.

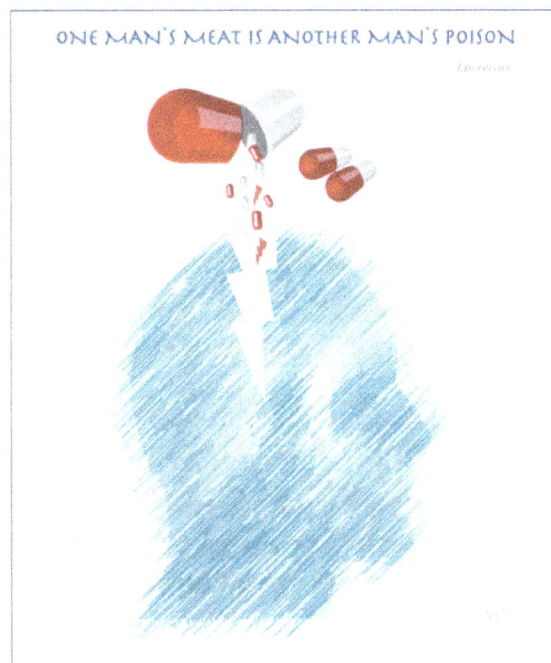

ONE MAN'S MEAT IS ANOTHER MAN'S POISON

Figure 3. Deleterous effects of antidopaminergics in Parkinson's Disease.

4. Anticholinergic burden in PD inpatients

Anticholinergic toxicity is often the consequence of the cumulative burden of multiple medications and metabolites rather than a result of the action of a single drug [39]. Thus, treatment of comorbidities (e.g., bladder control problems, psychosis and depression) with drugs with anticholinergic properties could contribute to aggravate the problem. Indeed, the most frequently used tools employing explicit criteria to detect potentially inappropriate prescriptions in the elderly dedicate a specific section to anticholinergic drug use [28, 29]. Drugs with anticholinergic activity can lead to adverse reactions in the central nervous system such as cognitive disturbance, especially in elderly people, so extreme caution is required when using them in people with previously known cognitive dysfunction. In this sense, dementia has a prevalence of 80–90% in the most advanced phases of PD [25, 27]. Besides, using anticholinergics in patients on cholinesterase inhibitors (which are the treatment of dementia in PD) could limit their beneficial effect due to a pharmacodynamic interaction [28]. Further, peripheral anticholinergic side effects, including tachycardia, constipation, urinary retention and blurred vision, should also be considered because they may lead to serious morbidity, especially in PD patients who frequently present with autonomic dysfunction.

Anticholinergics like trihexyphenidil, biperiden and benztropine have remained one of the available antiparkinsonian drugs in the antiparkinsonian armamentarium. But considering the potential risks, it is easier to understand why nowadays anticholinergics are hardly used to treat PD, with the exception of severe tremor in younger patients without cognitive dysfunction [40].

In a recent study on PD patients admitted to acute care hospitals in the Basque Health care system, we found that anticholinergic burden was relatively high and arose from drugs prescribed to treat non-motor symptoms and other comorbidities rather than the motor symptoms of the disease [41]. Interestingly, the total number of drugs and cholinesterase drug prescriptions were independently associated with anticholinergic drug use whatever the scale administered (the study was performed using four different scales to measure anticholinergic burden).

As described above, anticholinergic toxicity is often the result of the cumulative burden of multiple medications. For that purpose, many drug lists have been designed to measure the total anticholinergic burden, but they substantially differ both in which drugs are included and in the anticholinergic activity assigned to each compound [42]. Moreover, some drugs with undoubted anticholinergic properties (such as biperiden, solifenacin, trospium and fesoterodine) that were prescribed to some inpatients had to be discarded in this study as these compounds do not appear in any of the published lists [43], including the list providing a systematic review of the literature, which in our opinion is the most complete so far [44]. Thus, developing a credible, consistent, periodically updated screening tool to measure anticholinergic burden should be a priority, in order to avoid confusion in the future [45].

In definitive, potential anticholinergic toxicity should be kept in mind by clinicians, especially in those elderly patients suffering from cognitive dysfunction. Alternative drugs that lack anticholinergic activity should be used when possible.

In conclusion, all professionals involved in healthcare should pay attention to the specific pharmacotherapeutic challenges faced by PD patients in acute care hospitals. Efforts should be made to administer each levodopa dose on time. Drugs with central antidopaminergic activity like haloperidol and metoclopramide should be avoided. And finally, using alternative drugs without antimuscarinic properties when possible seems a reasonable option.

Author details

Unax Lertxundi[1*], Rafael Hernández[2], Saioa Domingo-Echaburu[3],
Javier Peral-Aguirregoitia[4] and Juan Medrano[5]

*Address all correspondence to: Unaxlertxundietxebarria@osakidetza.net

1 Pharmacy Service, Araba's Mental Health Network, Vitoria-Gasteiz, Spain

2 Internal Medicine, Araba's Mental Health Network, Vitoria-Gasteiz, Spain

3 Pharmacy Service, Alto Deba's Integrated Health Organization, Arrasate, Spain

4 Pharmacy Service, Galdakao-Usansolo Hospital, Galdakao, Spain

5 Psychiatry Service, Bizkaia's Mental Health Network, Portugalete, Spain

References

[1] De Lau LM, Breteler MM. Epidemiology of Parkinson's disease. Lancet Neurol. 2006; 5: 525-535.

[2] Alves G, Forsaa EB, Pedersen KF, et al. Epidemiology of Parkinson's disease. J Neurol. 2008; 255 (Suppl 5): 18-32.

[3] De Rijk MC, Tzourio C, Breteler MM, et al. Prevalence of parkinsonism and Parkinson's disease in Europe: the EUROPARKINSON Collaborative Study. European Community Concerted Action on the Epidemiology of Parkinson's disease. J Neurol Neurosurg Psychiatry. 1997; 62: 10.

[4] Chou KL. Clinical manifestations of Parkinson disease. Available from: http://www.uptodate.com/contents/clinical-manifestations-of-parkinson-disease?source=search_result&search=parkinson+disease&selectedTitle=1~150 [Accessed: 02/16/2016].

[5] Hassan A, Wu SS, Scmhidt P, et al, NPF-QII Investigators. High rates and the risk factors for emergency room visits and hospitalization in Parkinson's disease. Parkinsonism Relat Disord. 2013; 19: 949-954.

[6] Temlett JA, Thompson PD. Reasons for admission to hospital for Parkinson's disease. Intern Med J. 2006; 36: 524-526.

[7] Aminoff MJ, Christine CW, Friedman JH, et al. National Parkinson Foundation Working Group on Hospitalization in Parkinson's disease. Management of the

hospitalized patient with Parkinson's disease: current state of the field and need for guidelines. Parkinsonism Relat Disord. 2011; 17: 139-145.

[8] Wood LD, Neumiller JJ, Setter SM, et al. Clinical review of treatment options for select nonmotor symptoms of Parkinson's disease. Am J Geriatr Pharmacother. 2010; 8: 294-315.

[9] Lertxundi U, Domingo-Echaburu S, Irigoyen I, et al. Challenges in the pharmacotherapeutic management of the hospitalised patient with Parkinson's disease. Rev Neurol. 2014; 58: 353-364.

[10] Magdalinou KN, Martin A, Kessel B. Prescribing medications in Parkinson's disease (PD) patients during acute admissions to a District General Hospital. Parkinsonism Relat Disord. 2007; 13: 539-540.

[11] Derry CP, Shah KJ, Caie L, et al. Medication management in people with Parkinson's disease during surgical admissions. Postgrad Med J. 2010; 86: 334-337.

[12] Domingo-Echaburu S, Lertxundi U, Gonzalo-Olazabal E, et al. Inappropriate antidopaminergic drug use in Parkinson's disease inpatients. Cur Drug Ther. 2012; 7: 164-169.

[13] Chou KL, Zamudio J, Schmidt P, et al. Hospitalization in Parkinson's disease: a survey of National Parkinson Foundation Centers. Parkinsonism Relat Disord. 2011; 17: 440-445.

[14] Gerlach OH, Broen MP, van Domburg PH, et al. Deterioration of Parkinson's disease during hospitalization: survey of 684 patients. BMC Neurol. 2012; 12: 13.

[15] Gerlach OH, Broen MP, Weber WE. Motor outcomes during hospitalization in Parkinson's disease patients: a prospective study. Parkinsonism Relat Disord. 2013; 19: 737-741.

[16] Martínez-Ramírez D, Giugni JC, Little CS, et al. Missing dosages and neuroleptic usage may prolong length of stay in hospitalized Parkinson's disease patients. PLoS One. 2015;10: e0124356.

[17] Skelly R, Brown L, Fakis A, et al. Does a specialist unit improve outcomes for hospitalized patients with Parkinson's disease? Parkinsonism Relat Disord. 2014; 20: 1242-1247.

[18] Parkinson's UK. "Get It on Time" campaign. Available from: www.parkinsons.org.uk [Accessed 2015/04/28].

[19] Aware in Care Campaign. National Parkinson Foundation. Available from: http://www.awareincare.org. [Accessed 2015/04/28].

[20] Cohen M, Smetzer L. ISMP medication error report analysis delayed administration and contraindicated drugs place hospitalized Parkinson's disease patients at risk. Hosp Pharm. 2015; 50: 559-563.

[21] Lertxundi U, Isla A, Solinís MA, Domingo-Echaburu S, et al. A proposal to prevent omissions and delays of antiparkinsonian drug administration in hospitals. Neurohospitalist. 2015; 5: 53-54.

[22] Tomlinson CL, Stowe R, Patel S, et al. Systematic review of levodopa dose equivalency reporting in Parkinson's disease. Mov Disord. 2010; 25: 2649-2653.

[23] Brennan KA, Genever RW. Managing Parkinson's disease during surgery. BMJ. 2010; 341: c5718.

[24] Domingo-Echaburu S. Antipsychotic use in Parkinson's disease. In: Lertxundi U, Hernández R, Medrano J, eds. Psychopharmacolical Issues in Geriatrics. Bentham Science; 2015. pp. 273-286.

[25] Friedman JH. Parkinson disease psychosis: update. Behav Neurol. 2013; 27: 469-477.

[26] Lertxundi U, Peral J, Mora O, et al. Antidopaminergic therapy for managing comorbidities in patients with Parkinson's disease. Am J Health Syst Pharm. 2008; 65: 414-419.

[27] Weintraub D, Chen P, Ignacio RV, et al. Patterns and trends in antipsychotic prescribing for Parkinson's disease psychosis. Arch Neurol. 2011; 68: 899-904.

[28] American Geriatrics Society 2015. Beers Criteria Update Expert Panel. American Geriatrics Society 2015 updated beers criteria for potentially inappropriate medication use in older adults. J Am Geriatr Soc. 2015; 63: 2227-2246.

[29] O'Mahony D, O'Sullivan D, Byrne S, et al. STOPP/START criteria for potentially inappropriate prescribing in older people: version 2. Age Ageing. 2015; 44: 213-218.

[30] Lertxundi U, Isla A, Solinís MA, et al. Adverse reactions to antipsychotics in Parkinson's disease: an analysis of the Spanish Pharmacovigilance Database. Clin Neuropharmacol. 2015; 38: 69-84.

[31] Lertxundi U, Domingo-Echaburu R, Peral-Aguirregoitia J, et al. Beers 2015 criteria. Aripiprazole in Parkinson´s disease. J Am Geriatr Soc. 2016. in press.

[32] Lubomski M, Rushworth RL, Tisch S. Hospitalisation and comorbidities in Parkinson's disease: a large Australian retrospective study. J Neurol Neurosurg Psychiatry. 2015; 86: 324-330.

[33] Boorsma M, Joling KJ, Frijters DH, et al. The prevalence, incidence and risk factors for delirium in Dutch nursing homes and residential care homes. Int J Geriatr Psychiatry. 2012; 27: 709-15.

[34] Messerschmidt KA, Johnson BR, Khan MA. Encephalopathy associated with metoclopramide use in a patient with Parkinson's disease. Am J Health Syst Pharm. 2012; 69: 1303-1306.

[35] Robottom BJ, Shulman LM, Anderson KE, et al. Metoclopramide-induced encephalopathy in Parkinson's disease. South Med J. 2010; 103: 178-180.

[36] Spanish Agency for Medicines and Health Products. Domperidone and cardiac risk: restrictions on authorization conditions. 2014. Nota informativa 4-2014. Available from http://www.aemps.gob.es/informa/notasInformativas/medicamentosUsoHumano/seguridad/2014/docs/NI-MUH_FV_04-2014-domperidona.pdf [Accessed: 2015/10/29].

[37] Lertxundi U, Domingo-Echaburu S, Soraluce A, et al. Domperidone in Parkinson's disease: a perilous arrythmogenic or the gold standard? Curr Drug Saf. 2013; 8: 63-68.

[38] Miwa H, Kondo T. Hiccups in Parkinson's disease: an overlooked non-motor symptom? Parkinsonism Relat Disord. 2010; 16: 249-251.

[39] Hernández R, Gómez de Segura A, Medrano J, et al. Potentially inappropriate medication in elderly. In: Lertxundi U, Hernández R, Medrano J. eds. Psychopharmacological Issues in Geriatrics, Bentham Science; 2015, pp. 65-96.

[40] Goetz CG, Pal G. Initial management of Parkinson's disease. BMJ. 2014; 349: g6258.

[41] Lertxundi U, Isla A, Solinis MA, et al. Anticholinergic burden in Parkinson's disease inpatients. Eur J Clin Pharmacol. 2015; 71: 1271-1277.

[42] Lertxundi U, Domingo-Echaburu S, Hernandez R, et al. Expert-based drug lists to measure anticholinergic burden: similar names, different results. Psychogeriatrics. 2013; 13: 17-24.

[43] Lertxundi U, Domingo-Echaburu S, Ruiz-Osante B, et al. Comments on Duran et al.'s systematic review of anticholinergic risk scales (EJCP 2DOI 10.1007/s00228-013-1499-3). Eur J Clin Pharmacol. 2013; 69: 1729.

[44] Durán CE, Azermai M, Vander Stichele RH. Systematic review of anticholinergic risk scales in older adults. Eur J Clin Pharmacol. 2013; 69: 1485-1496.

[45] Lertxundi U, Domingo-Echaburu S, Hernandez R, et al. Confusion on anticholinergic burden measurement. J Am Geriatr Soc. 2015; 63: 1054.

2

Cell-Based Therapies for Parkinson's Disease: Preclinical and Clinical Perspectives

Andrea R. Di Sebastiano, Michael D. Staudt,
Simon M. Benoit, Hu Xu, Matthew O. Hebb and
Susanne Schmid

Abstract

Parkinson's Disease (PD) is a highly prevalent neurodegenerative disease that affects millions of people globally and remains without definitive treatment. There have been many recent advances in cell-based therapy to replace lost neural circuitry and provide chronic biological sources of therapeutic agents to disease-affected brain regions. Early neural transplantation studies highlighted the challenges of immune rejection, graft integration, and the need for renewable, autologous graft sources. Neurotrophic factors (NTFs) offer a potential class of cytoprotective agents that may complement dopamine (DA) replacement and cell-based therapies in PD. In fact, chronic NTF delivery may be an integral goal of cell transplantation in PD, with ideal grafts consisting of autologous drug (e.g., DA, NTF)-producing cells capable of integration and function in the host brain. This chapter outlines the past and recent preclinical and clinical advances in cell-based and NTF therapies as promising and integrated approaches for the treatment of PD.

Keywords: transplantation, tissue graft, stem cells, pluripotent cells, autologous cells, dopamine replacement, neurotrophic factors

1. Introduction

Parkinson's disease (PD) is the second most common neurodegenerative disorder, following Alzheimer's disease. In the developed world, the prevalence of PD is approximately 0.3% of the population and 1% of those over 60 years of age [1]. Hallmarks of PD include degeneration of dopamine (DA) neurons in the substantia nigra (SN) and of dopaminergic nerve terminals in the striatum, as well as the formation of Lewy bodies containing alpha-synuclein [2–4]. However, PD also has widespread effects on neurons and nonneuronal cells throughout the nervous system [4].

Motor symptoms of PD include bradykinesia (i.e. slowness of movement), rigidity, and rest tremor. These motor symptoms are often seen with postural and gait instability, sleep disorders, sensory dysfunction, neuropsychiatric conditions, and dysautonomia [5]. Nonmotor symptoms of PD include dementia, depression, gastrointestinal, or sexual dysfunction and are managed accordingly. Current therapies for PD aim to improve symptomology, but unfortunately there are no disease modifying treatments. Recent preclinical studies have provided promising leads for the development of potential new therapies to restore or preserve neurological function in patients with PD. As the pathophysiology of PD has become better understood, efforts are expanding to augment or replace the degenerated neural circuitry using cell-based therapies. The goal of this chapter is to discuss past and current approaches to cell-based therapies in PD, including studies to replace lost dopaminergic cells through neural grafting, and the potential of neurotrophic factors (NTFs) to promote DA neuron survival.

2. Current therapies

2.1. Medical therapies

The use of levodopa is the mainstay of PD treatment, and it is usually administered together with a decarboxylase inhibitor, carbidopa. Levodopa can cross the blood-brain barrier, whereas DA and carbidopa cannot. Carbidopa therefore prevents the peripheral conversion of levodopa to DA, allowing for higher doses in the central nervous system. Identified in the 1960s, levodopa was the first medication demonstrated to provide a significant clinical and mortality benefit in the treatment of PD [6]. However, long-term use of levodopa can lead to loss of therapeutic effect, dyskinesia, and neuropsychiatric complications, likely due to the progressive loss of DA neurons and increasing off-target effects of DA ([7], for review see [8]). Levodopa is converted by catechol-O-methyl transferase (COMT) to an inert metabolite [9]; as such, COMT inhibitors may be administered to prevent peripheral metabolism and increase levodopa availability to the brain. The use of selective monoamine oxidase B (MAO-B) inhibitors was initially thought to be neuroprotective and has since been used in symptom control [10] as monotherapy in early PD, as well as an adjunct treatment to levodopa [11]. Cholinergic, adrenergic, glutamatergic, and serotonergic drugs are also being used for treating PD symptoms that do not respond to DA treatment or for treating levodopa-induced side effects. All medical therapies only provide partial and temporal relief of symptoms and are not disease modifying [8].

2.2. Standard surgical therapies

Prior to the advent of levodopa therapy, ablative therapies were used in the control of motor symptoms. Pallidotomy and thalamotomy were used in the symptomatic control of rigidity and tremor, respectively [12,13]. Pallidotomy has been demonstrated to provide sustained improvement for tremor, rigidity, bradykinesia, and drug-induced dyskinesias, compared with medical therapy [14]. In the past decades, deep brain stimulation (DBS) has become the standard of surgical care for PD owing to the versatility of stimulator programming, and the avoidance of creating a permanent surgical lesion [15]. The two primary targets of DBS are the internal globus pallidus (GPi) and subthalamic nucleus (STN). DBS improves motor symptoms and often permits a reduction of medication dose and associated side effects, but does not slow or halt progression of the disease [16].

3. Burgeoning therapies for PD

3.1. Cell-based therapies

As PD is characterized by the loss of dopaminergic nigrostriatal neurons, cell-based therapies initially focused on the potential to replace these neurons and replenish DA supply in the striatum using fetal mesencephalic neural grafts. More recently, studies have included the transplantation of induced pluripotent stem cells (iPSCs), reprogrammed somatic cells or induced neural progenitor cells (iNPCs).

3.2. Fetal transplantation

3.2.1. Preclinical studies

Early PD transplantation studies involved grafting of fetal ventral mesencephalic (fVM) tissue into the anterior chamber of the rat eye [17]. These studies identified the optimal developmental stage of the neural tissue to be used to promote DA neuron survival and outgrowth [17]. The first graft transplantation studies in a unilaterally lesioned 6-hydroxydopamine (6-OHDA) PD rat model examined the effects of solid grafts of fetal adrenal medullary or fVM tissue implanted into the lateral ventricle or preformed cavities adjacent to the striatum and reported reduced amphetamine-induced rotation behavior [18]. Subsequent studies showed that grafting cell suspensions of fVM tissue from 14- to 15-day-old rat fetuses into the striatum of 6-OHDA rats also reduced amphetamine-induced rotation behavior [19]. Follow-up studies used fVM tissue from 9- to 19-week-old human fetuses. These implants reduced and even reversed motor asymmetry in unilaterally lesioned 6-OHDA rats [20].

3.2.2. Clinical studies

In 1987, solid graft adrenal medullary transplants were implanted in the head of the caudate in two patients and produced significant clinical improvement, including reduced tremor [21]. Unfortunately, follow-up studies showed only modest clinical effect, with concerns regarding efficacy and safety of this technique. Many patients suffered major postsurgical complications and psychiatric problems, thus this transplant approach was abandoned. Subsequent open label studies in six human patients utilized human fVM tissue from 6- to 8-week-old fetuses grafted into the caudate and putamen, demonstrating overall clinical improvement and normal DA signaling seen by ^{18}F-Fluorodopa (^{18}F-FDOPA) uptake in Positron Emission Tomography (PET) imaging [22–24]. Two patients in this study continued to demonstrate clinical improvement 20 years later [25]. In a subsequent open label study nigral grafts from 6- to 7-week-old embryos were implanted into the caudate and putamen of seven PD patients [26,27]. Significant improvement in the activities of daily living was noted after 12 months, in both "on" and "off" states. The dose of levodopa could be reduced by an average of 39%. Four patients reported an "important difference in their daily lives," two patients reported improvement in "some respects," and one patient did not improve. Other open label studies with a small number of patients also showed mostly beneficial effects ([28–31], reviewed in [32]).

A randomized double-blind controlled trial (RDBCT) enlisted 34 patients that underwent transplantation of fetal mesencephalic tissue into the putamen or sham surgery. The patients showed limited clinical improvement, despite graft survival and significant reinnervation of the striatum as confirmed by PET and at autopsy. Interestingly, patients with less severe motor dysfunction showed significant clinical improvement, suggesting this technique may have produced some degree of neuroprotection. Furthermore, graft-induced dyskinesias were observed in over half of the patients [33]. Interestingly, these patients underwent a 2- and 4-year follow-up RDBCT that demonstrated clinical improvement regardless of the age of the patient, which was accompanied by significantly increased ^{18}F-FDOPA uptake in the putamen [34]. Another RDBCT had 40 patients with advanced PD undergo transplantation. When results were normalized according to age, patients under the age of 60 showed significant clinical improvement, as measured with the Unified Parkinson's Disease Rating Scale (UPDRS) and Schwab and England score, while those over the age of 60 did not [35]. Clinical improvement was correlated with increased ^{18}F-FDOPA uptake in 85% of patients with a transplant and postmortem examination confirmed dopaminergic cell survival and fibre outgrowth; however, 15% of patients developed graft-induced dyskinesias or dystonia [35].

To more accurately assess the potential of fetal grafts, a new European study has been designed to optimize and control for patient selection, tissue composition, tissue placement, and trial design. TRANSEURO is an open label multicenter trial to define the feasibility and efficacy of human fetal ventral mesencephalic grafts in patients with PD (https://clinicaltrials.gov/ct2/show/NCT01898390). The primary outcome measure of this study is the change in motor UPDRS scores in the absence of PD medications at 3 years posttransplantation. It is hoped that this new trial will shed light on the true potential of dopaminergic allografts for PD treatment.

The use of human fVM tissue, however, is complicated by ethical issues and difficulty in obtaining human tissue. Strategies are being developed that involve expansion of fVM tissue and its dopaminergic neuroblasts [36], and other cell sources are also being investigated for cell-based treatment of PD.

3.3. Native human stem cells

3.3.1. Preclinical studies

Human embryonic stem cells (hESCs) were first isolated from the inner cell mass of blastocysts. These cells demonstrate pluripotency and have been shown to differentiate into neural cells, including neurons, astrocytes, and oligodendrocytes [37,38]. hESCs may prove useful to avoid the technical concerns associated with the use of fetal tissue. hESCs have been shown to differentiate into midbrain DA neurons, and injection of these cells in 6-OHDA lesioned rats [39] and 1-methyl-4-phenyl-1,2,3,6-tetrahydropyridine (MPTP)-lesioned monkeys [40] leads to significantly improved motor function in both models. However, the development of clinical applications using these cells has been slowed by various biological and social factors, including the potential for immune rejection and tumor formation, as well as ethical and political opposition [41].

Alternative stem cell sources have been investigated for differentiation into a neural lineage, in particular mesenchymal stem cells (MSCs) from bone marrow, umbilical cord blood, dental pulp, and adipose tissue [42]. Autologous MSCs are favorable due to their availability, potential for differentiation, and the absence of ethical issues associated with hESCs. In addition, MSCs have been demonstrated to exert regenerative and neuroprotective effects in a number of animal PD models potentially, due to endogenous NTF expression. MSCs have been shown to differentiate into dopaminergic cells that express tyrosine hydroxylase [43]. Implantation of these differentiated MSCs into the striatum of 6-OHDA mice led to significant behavioral improvement, with striatal graft cells confirmed at postmortem analysis [43].

3.3.2. Clinical studies

There is currently very limited clinical data on the efficacy of hESCs in PD. An initial clinical study in seven PD patients demonstrated that transplantation of autologous bone-marrow-derived MSCs was safe and feasible with no serious adverse side effects. Unfortunately, no clinical efficacy was observed, potentially due to the small number of patients and uncontrolled nature of the trial [44].

3.4. Induced pluripotent stem cells

3.4.1. Preclinical studies

With the discovery that somatic cells, such as fibroblasts, can be reprogrammed to a pluripotent state by viral delivery of four transcription factors, Oct4, Sox2, Klf4, and cMyc [45,46], studies have focused on the potential of these induced pluripotent stem cells (iPSCs) to improve current cell-based therapies for treatment of many degenerative medical conditions, including PD. Compared with fetal grafting and hESC cells, iPSCs provide increased accessibility as well as ethical advantages. These cells can differentiate into many different cell types including cardiomyocytes [47], hepatocytes [48], oligodendrocytes [49], glia, and neuronal subtypes [50]. Murine iPSCs have also been shown to be reprogrammed into dopaminergic neurons that express the transcription factors Nurr1, Pitx3 and tyrosine hydroxylase and demonstrate electrophysiological properties of DA neurons [51]. Subsequent studies demonstrated successful differentiation of dopaminergic neurons from both established human iPSC lines and patient-derived somatic cells [52,53].

In all of these studies, iPSC-derived DA cells demonstrated expression of key dopaminergic markers and electrophysiological properties of DA neurons. Furthermore, these DA cells were successfully incorporated into a 6-OHDA rat model of PD, leading to significantly reduced motor asymmetry [52]. Most recently, primate-derived iPSCs were successfully transplanted back into the putamen of MPTP lesioned monkeys; these autografts led to significant motor improvements, and postmortem analysis showed graft survival and outgrowth into the transplanted putamen [54]. Despite promising results in preclinical studies, several factors have provided road blocks to utilization of these cells in humans, including use of viruses to modify cells and risk of tumorigenicity [55].

3.4.2. Clinical studies

The first pilot study in humans was performed in Japan in 2014, and utilized iPSC-derived autologous pigmented retinal epithelial cells for treatment of macular degeneration. Transplantation in the first patient was completed without adverse effects; however, long-term follow-up is necessary [56]. Unfortunately, iPSCs derived from fibroblasts of a second patient were discovered to have genetic mutations, including three single-nucleotide variations and three copy-number variants, prompting suspension of the trial [57]. Studies are now focusing on use of allogenic partially matched donor cells from the Center for iPS Cell Research and Application, an iPSC bank, for treatment of macular degeneration [57]. There is also potential to transform fibroblasts directly into neurons (iN cells) or dopamine cells (iDA cells) using specific transcription factors: Ascl1, Brn2, Mrt1l, without or with Lmx1a and FoxA2, respectively [58–60]; however, this technology still needs to be tested in preclinical models.

3.5. Autologous brain-derived progenitor cells (BDPCs)

Recently, the safety and feasibility of performing small volume brain biopsies has been demonstrated in PD patients undergoing DBS surgery [61]. These tissue specimens yield an expandable cell population that expresses several NTFs known to be highly protective against PD neurodegeneration, including glial-derived neurotrophic factor (GDNF), brain-derived neurotrophic factor (BDNF), and cerebral dopamine neurotrophic factor (CDNF) [61]. The cultures yield large numbers (i.e. 10^7) of cells with limited capacity for self-renewal. These cells, called BDPCs, also show expression of progenitor and neural markers including nestin, Olig1, and GalC. Colocalization of neural and oligodendroglial markers suggests these BDPCs may be grafted into the host brain to integrate as autologous glia [61]. A patient-derived cellular source of neuroprotective agents, reimplanted into the host brain, may confer long-lasting therapeutic benefit in PD patients. Preclinical studies on the potential for these BDPCs to be used as an autologous cell-based therapy for PD are currently underway.

4. Neurotrophic factors

Neurotrophic factors (NTFs) are being intensively evaluated as therapeutic agents for PD owing to their known roles in neuronal survival, differentiation, and plasticity. Additionally, NTF deficiency has been associated with PD and replacement or enhancement of NTF signaling confers neuronal protection in both in vitro and in vivo preclinical PD models [62]. These secreted proteins regulate vital biological programs in the developing and adult nervous systems and are currently the most potent cytoprotective agents known against PD-related degeneration in the brain [63]. The NTF families include (1) glial-derived neurotrophic factor (GDNF) family of ligands (GFL), (2) neurotrophins, (3) neuropoietic cytokines (neurokines), and (4) cerebral DA neurotrophic factor (CDNF)/mesencephalic astrocyte-derived neurotrophic factor family (MANF). To date, GDNF and other GFL members have received the most attention in development of potential new clinical therapies for PD [64].

4.1. GDNF family of ligands

GDNF was the first member of the GDNF family of ligands (GFL) to be discovered. Other members include neurturin (NRTN), persephin (PSPN), and artemin (ARTN). GFLs are important for cell survival, neurite outgrowth, cell differentiation, and cell migration [65].

4.1.1. Preclinical studies

Application of GDNF to rat ventral mesencephalic cultures increased survival, neurite length, and differentiation of DA neurons [66]. GDNF also reduced apoptosis and enhanced cell survival in cultures derived from monkey, porcine, and human mesencephalic tissues [67]. These effects extend to promote differentiation and protection of dopaminergic neurons against 6-OHDA and MPTP neurotoxins [65]. Numerous in vivo studies have demonstrated therapeutic effects of GDNF in the 6-OHDA rat model of PD; the infusion of recombinant GDNF significantly increased DA neuron survival in both the SN and ventral tegmental area and improved parkinsonian symptomology, including motor impairments and amphetamine-induced rotational behavior [68–71]. GDNF has also been shown to be neuroprotective in the MPTP mouse model of PD [72,73]. Studies in nonhuman primates have demonstrated that intracerebral administration of GDNF in MPTP-treated rhesus monkeys results in significant improvements in bradykinesia, rigidity, and postural instability, as well as increased DA levels in the midbrain, globus pallidus, and SN [74].

4.1.2. Clinical studies

Based on the success of using GDNF in preclinical models of PD, GDNF has now been studied in four clinical trials via infusion into the ventricular system or putamen [75]. The first RDBCT compared effects of intracerebroventricular administration of recombinant methionyl human GDNF (r-metHuGDNF, Liatermin®; Amgen) in escalating doses or placebo in 50 PD patients over a period of 8 months. No significant improvement in "on" and "off" total and motor UPDRS was seen in patients treated with GDNF. Adverse effects included paresthesias, nausea, and vomiting. A follow-up open label study in 16 of these patients for 20 months showed no additional improvement in PD symptomology. It was felt that the adverse effects resulted from off-target GDNF influence and the lack of therapeutic benefit from an inability of GDNF to diffuse into the parenchyma from the ventricular source [76].

A subsequent open label study that enrolled 5 PD patients investigated the effects of intra-parenchymal delivery of GDNF via implanted catheters in the dorsal putamen (unilateral in one patient; bilaterally in four patients) and connected to an extracranial pump system [77]. After one year, there were no serious clinical side effects, a 39% improvement in the off-medication UPDRS motor scores and a 61% improvement in the activities of daily living (ADL) subscore. Medication-induced dyskinesias were considerably reduced and (PET) scans of ^{18}F-FDOPA uptake showed a significant 28% increase in putamen DA storage after 18 months [78]. In a follow-up report, the group described one of the patients with bilateral GDNF infusions who had received treatment for 39 months, then was followed clinically and with PET for another 36 months. The UPDRS motor and ADL scores "off" medication remained im-proved by 74% and 76%, respectively, levodopa usage ceased after a year, and at 36 months post-GDNF cessation, the ^{18}F-FDOPA uptake remained 29% higher in the posterior putamen [79]. Another group led a second open label study that enrolled 10 patients treated unilater-ally with intraputamenal GDNF [80]. A significant increase in total and motor UPDRS scores was observed after 24 weeks, but benefit was lost with cessation of treatment. These positive outcomes spurred a second multicenter, placebo-controlled trial in which 34 PD patients were randomized to receive bilateral intraputamenal GDNF (15 µg/putamen/day; a dose lower than that of the previous studies) or placebo via continuous infusion. At 6 months, there was no significant treatment benefit reflected in the "off" UPDRS motor scores; however, a 32.5% increase in putamenal ^{18}F-FDOPA uptake was observed in the GDNF-treated cohort [81]. The disparate outcomes of these studies may reflect differences in study design, cohort size, drug dosage, and/or delivery systems. The r-metHuGDNF manufacturing company subsequently withdrew the agent on the grounds of safety concerns regarding production of neutralizing antibodies in several patients and related cerebellar injuries in animal studies, although no such injuries were reported in human trials. Efforts are now underway to evaluate adeno-associated virus (AAV)-mediated GDNF in an open label phase I for patients with advanced PD (https://www.clinicaltrials.gov/ct2/show/NCT01621581).

4.2. Neurturin

4.2.1. Preclinical studies

Neurturin (NTRN) shares 40% sequence homology with GDNF [82] and has been shown to promote survival of DA neurons in the nigrostriatal system [82–84]. In vitro, NTRN leads to neurite outgrowth in cultured spinal motor neurons and protects against glutamate toxicity. Early studies infusing NTRN directly into the SN was shown to be neuroprotective against 6-OHDA toxicity, while striatal infusion improved behavioral parameters of DA neuronal function in rats [83,85]. In MPTP-lesioned monkeys, intraputamenal infusion of NTRN led to significant improvement in parkinsonian deficits as well as increased DA metabolite levels in the globus pallidus [86]. CERE-120, an (AAV) vector expressing NTRN, has also shown potential therapeutic benefit in preclinical studies [87]. When MPTP-lesioned monkeys were given CERE-120 into the striatum, motor symptoms were improved and loss of DA neurons was reduced [88]. After one year follow-up, no toxic adverse effects were observed [89].

4.2.2. Clinical studies

A Phase 1 open-label clinical trial demonstrated safety, tolerability, and potential therapeutic benefit in PD patients after one year [90]. A subsequent RDBCT enrolled 58 patients to receive AAV2-NTRN bilaterally into the putamen or sham surgery. The primary endpoint was change from baseline to 12 months in the UPDRS motor score in the off state, and no significant difference was found between patients treated with AAV2-NTRN compared with control individuals. Three of 38 patients in the AAV2-NTRN group and two of 20 in the sham surgery group developed tumors, with uncertain relations to the actual treatment [91]. Postmortem analysis of two patients revealed that, unlike the animal studies, putamenal AAV-NTRN injections did not confer adequate retrograde labeling of neurons in the SN [92]. This deficiency in axonal transport of AAV-NTRN to the SN was addressed in a phase 1 safety study that enrolled six patients who received bilateral dual injections into the putamen and SN [93]. Two-year follow-up suggested that the procedures were well-tolerated and no serious adverse effects were reported. A second phase 2 RDBCT was then conducted, enrolling 51 patients to receive bilateral putamen and SN AAV-NTRN (https://clinicaltrials.gov/ct2/show/ NCT00985517). In 2013, it was announced that the trial did not demonstrate statistically significant improvement in patient UPDRS scores after 15–24 months of follow-up. However, a more robust response to CERE-120 was observed in PD patients treated within 5 years of diagnosis, and no safety concerns were raised. There was a marked placebo effect as the control patients and the CERE-120 treated patients both improved significantly following surgery. Long-term observational studies of the participants are planned to assess delayed clinical effect (http://www.prnewswire.com/news-releases/ceregene-reports-data-from-parkinsons-disease-phase-2b-study-203803541.html).

4.3. Preclinical studies with other neurotrophic factors

4.3.1. Persephin/artemin

Persephin (PSPN) shows approximately 40% sequence homology to GDNF and NTRN [94]. PSPN promotes survival of cultured ventral midbrain dopaminergic neurons as well as motor neurons and prevents their degeneration after 6-OHDA toxicity [94]. PSPN-overexpressing neural stem cells grafted into the striatum prevented loss of DA neurons and led to behavioral improvements in 6-OHDA lesioned rats [95]. Artemin (ARTN) promotes survival of DA neurons in culture [96] and also protects against DA neuron degeneration in the striatum following neurotoxic doses of methamphetamine [97]. Although early preclinical studies have shown therapeutic benefit of both PSPN and ARTN, more studies are necessary before these NTFs can be tested in a clinical setting.

4.3.2. BDNF

Brain-derived neurotrophic factor (BDNF) is an essential regulator of neuronal differentiation and plasticity. It has been suggested that alterations in BDNF expression may be responsible for the development of neurodegenerative disorders [98]. Postmortem studies of PD patients have demonstrated that BDNF levels are reduced in the substantia nigra pars compacta as a result of decreased transcription of the BDNF gene [99]. Another study reported that only 10% of melanized neurons in the substantia nigra of PD patients were immunoreactive for BDNF expression, compared with 65% in healthy controls [100]. Serum BDNF levels have also been shown to correlate with a loss of striatal DA transporter binding in PD patients, suggesting an influence on striatal neurodegeneration [101]. Animal studies have demonstrated that BDNF antisense oligonucleotide infusion in rats produces a Parkinsonian phenotype [102], and BDNF knockout mice have reduced dopaminergic neurons in the substantia nigra [103]. BDNF promotes *in vitro* survival and differentiation of human and rat embryonic dopaminergic neurons, and it has protective effects against various toxins including 6-OHDA and MPTP [99]. In a nonhuman primate model of PD, intrathecal BDNF infusion resulted in milder PD symptoms and less neuronal cell loss in the substantia nigra [104]. To date, there are no clinical studies evaluating the efficacy of BDNF therapy in human PD, likely due to the logistical challenges of CNS drug delivery and dosing, as BDNF has poor blood-brain barrier penetration if administered parenterally, and intrathecal or intraventricular delivery results in poor penetration of the brain parenchyma [105].

4.3.3. CDNF/MANF

Mesencephalic astrocyte-derived neurotrophic factor (MANF) was first discovered in 2003 and was shown to be selectively neuroprotective for dopaminergic neurons [106]. Later, cerebral DA neurotrophic factor (CDNF) was discovered as a homologue of MANF with 59% sequence homology [107]. CDNF has been shown to be neuroprotective to DA neurons and intrastriatal injection of CDNF or AAV-CDNF reduces degeneration of DA neurons and parkinsonian behavior in rats and increases TH levels in the striatum and SN [107–110]. Interestingly, intranigral infusion of a combination of both CDNF and MANF via lentiviral mediated delivery reduced amphetamine-induced rotational behavior and increased striatal TH-fibers and TH-positive neurons in the substantia nigra [111]. Intranigral CDNF alone also improved behavior and increased TH fibers in the striatum, but both to a lesser extent than with CDNF/MANF together, and did not protect against TH neuronal loss in the SN [111]. Intra-nigral MANF alone did not affect behavior or striatal TH fibers, but did protect against SN neuronal loss [111]. Results of these studies suggest that combined delivery of CDNF/MANF may be more effective than single NTFs and may be a more effective potential therapeutic treatment for PD, although neither NTF has been tested in a clinical setting.

5. Conclusions

There remains a critical need for new therapies to delay or prevent the progression of PD. As discussed in this chapter, cell-based therapies may provide a promising therapeutic benefit to

PD patients. NTFs offer a potential class of cytoprotective agents that complement DA replacement and cell-based therapies in PD, with ideal grafts consisting of immunologically inert cells that continuously produce and release these agents in the host brain. Further development and refinement of these potential therapies is essential to develop personalized care for PD patients.

Author details

Andrea R. Di Sebastiano[1], Michael D. Staudt[1], Simon M. Benoit[1], Hu Xu[1], Matthew O. Hebb[1,2] and Susanne Schmid[2*]

*Address all correspondence to: Susanne.schmid@schulich.uwo.ca

1 Clinical Neurological Sciences, Schulich School of Medicine & Dentistry, University of Western Ontario, London, ON, Canada

2 Anatomy & Cell Biology, Schulich School of Medicine & Dentistry, University of Western Ontario, London, ON, Canada

References

[1] de Lau, L.M. and M.M. Breteler, Epidemiology of Parkinson's disease. Lancet Neurol, 2006. 5(6): pp. 525–35.

[2] Spillantini, M.G., et al., Alpha-synuclein in Lewy bodies. Nature, 1997. 388(6645): pp. 839–40.

[3] Damier, P., New aspects in the pathophysiology of dyskinesia. Salpetriere Deep Brain Stimulation Group. Adv Neurol, 1999. 80: pp. 611–7.

[4] Dickson, D.W., Parkinson's disease and parkinsonism: neuropathology. Cold Spring Harb Perspect Med, 2012. 2(8).

[5] Massano, J. and K.P. Bhatia, Clinical approach to Parkinson's disease: features, diagnosis, and principles of management. Cold Spring Harb Perspect Med, 2012. 2(6): p. a008870.

[6] Cotzias, G.C., M.H. Van Woert, and L.M. Schiffer, Aromatic amino acids and modification of parkinsonism. N Engl J Med, 1967. 276(7): pp. 374–9.

[7] Marsden, C.D. and J.D. Parkes, "On-off" effects in patients with Parkinson's disease on chronic levodopa therapy. Lancet, 1976. 1(7954): pp. 292–6.

[8] Lotia, M. and J. Jankovic, New and emerging medical therapies in Parkinson's disease. Expert Opin Pharmacother, 2016: pp. 1–15.

[9] Nutt, J.G. and J.H. Fellman, Pharmacokinetics of levodopa. Clin Neuropharmacol, 1984. 7(1): pp. 35–49.

[10] Parkinson Study, G., Effects of tocopherol and deprenyl on the progression of disability in early Parkinson's disease. N Engl J Med, 1993. 328(3): pp. 176–83.

[11] Stern, M.B., et al., Double-blind, randomized, controlled trial of rasagiline as monotherapy in early Parkinson's disease patients. Mov Disord, 2004. 19(8): pp. 916–23.

[12] Spiegel, E.A., H.T. Wycis, and H.W. Baird, 3rd, Long-range effects of electropallidoansotomy in extrapyramidal and convulsive disorders. Neurology, 1958. 8(10): pp. 734–40.

[13] Hassler, R. and T. Riechert, [Indications and localization of stereotactic brain operations]. Nervenarzt, 1954. 25(11): pp. 441–7.

[14] Vitek, J.L., et al., Randomized trial of pallidotomy versus medical therapy for Parkinson's disease. Ann Neurol, 2003. 53(5): pp. 558–69.

[15] Munhoz, R.P., A. Cerasa, and M.S. Okun, Surgical treatment of dyskinesia in Parkinson's disease. Front Neurol, 2014. 5: pp. 65.

[16] Deep-Brain Stimulation for Parkinson's Disease Study, G., Deep-brain stimulation of the subthalamic nucleus or the pars interna of the globus pallidus in Parkinson's disease. N Engl J Med, 2001. 345(13): pp. 956–63.

[17] Olson, L. and A. Seiger, Development and growth of immature monoamine neurons in rat and man in situ and following intraocular transplantation in the rat. Brain Res, 1973. 62(2): pp. 353–60.

[18] Freed, W.J., et al., Transplanted adrenal chromaffin cells in rat brain reduce lesion-induced rotational behaviour. Nature, 1981. 292(5821): pp. 351–2.

[19] Brundin, P., et al., The rotating 6-hydroxydopamine-lesioned mouse as a model for assessing functional effects of neuronal grafting. Brain Res, 1986. 366(1–2): pp. 346–9.

[20] Brundin, P., et al., Behavioural effects of human fetal dopamine neurons grafted in a rat model of Parkinson's disease. Exp Brain Res, 1986. 65(1): pp. 235–40.

[21] Madrazo, I., et al., Open microsurgical autograft of adrenal medulla to the right caudate nucleus in two patients with intractable Parkinson's disease. N Engl J Med, 1987. 316(14): pp. 831–4.

[22] Lindvall, O., et al., Grafts of fetal dopamine neurons survive and improve motor function in Parkinson's disease. Science, 1990. 247(4942): pp. 574–7.

[23] Lindvall, O., et al., Human fetal dopamine neurons grafted into the striatum in two patients with severe Parkinson's disease. A detailed account of methodology and a 6-month follow-up. Arch Neurol, 1989. 46(6): pp. 615–31.

[24] Lindvall, O., et al., Transplantation of fetal dopamine neurons in Parkinson's disease: one-year clinical and neurophysiological observations in two patients with putaminal implants. Ann Neurol, 1992. 31(2): pp. 155–65.

[25] Kefalopoulou, Z., et al., Long-term clinical outcome of fetal cell transplantation for Parkinson disease: two case reports. JAMA Neurol, 2014. 71(1): pp. 83–7.

[26] Freed, C.R., et al., Survival of implanted fetal dopamine cells and neurologic improvement 12 to 46 months after transplantation for Parkinson's disease. N Engl J Med, 1992. 327(22): pp. 1549–55.

[27] Freed, C.R., et al., Transplantation of human fetal dopamine cells for Parkinson's disease. Results at 1 year. Arch Neurol, 1990. 47(5): pp. 505–12.

[28] Spencer, D.D., et al., Unilateral transplantation of human fetal mesencephalic tissue into the caudate nucleus of patients with Parkinson's disease. N Engl J Med, 1992. 327(22): pp. 1541–8.

[29] Peschanski, M., et al., Bilateral motor improvement and alteration of L-dopa effect in two patients with Parkinson's disease following intrastriatal transplantation of foetal ventral mesencephalon. Brain, 1994. 117 (Pt 3): pp. 487–99.

[30] Widner, H., et al., Bilateral fetal mesencephalic grafting in two patients with parkinsonism induced by 1-methyl-4-phenyl-1,2,3,6-tetrahydropyridine (MPTP). N Engl J Med, 1992. 327(22): pp. 1556–63.

[31] Freeman, T.B., et al., Bilateral fetal nigral transplantation into the postcommissural putamen in Parkinson's disease. Ann Neurol, 1995. 38(3): pp. 379–88.

[32] Olanow, C.W., J.H. Kordower, and T.B. Freeman, Fetal nigral transplantation as a therapy for Parkinson's disease. Trends Neurosci, 1996. 19(3): pp. 102–9.

[33] Olanow, C.W., et al., A double-blind controlled trial of bilateral fetal nigral transplantation in Parkinson's disease. Ann Neurol, 2003. 54(3): pp. 403–14.

[34] Ma, Y., et al., Dopamine cell implantation in Parkinson's disease: long-term clinical and (18)F-FDOPA PET outcomes. J Nucl Med, 2010. 51(1): pp. 7–15.

[35] Freed, C.R., et al., Transplantation of embryonic dopamine neurons for severe Parkinson's disease. N Engl J Med, 2001. 344(10): pp. 710–9.

[36] Ribeiro, D., et al., Efficient expansion and dopaminergic differentiation of human fetal ventral midbrain neural stem cells by midbrain morphogens. Neurobiol Dis, 2013. 49: pp. 118–27.

[37] Thomson, J.A., et al., Embryonic stem cell lines derived from human blastocysts. Science, 1998. 282(5391): pp. 1145–7.

[38] Barberi, T., et al., Neural subtype specification of fertilization and nuclear transfer embryonic stem cells and application in parkinsonian mice. Nat Biotechnol, 2003. 21(10): pp. 1200–7.

[39] Roy, N.S., et al., Functional engraftment of human ES cell-derived dopaminergic neurons enriched by coculture with telomerase-immortalized midbrain astrocytes. Nat Med, 2006. 12(11): pp. 1259–68.

[40] Takagi, Y., et al., Dopaminergic neurons generated from monkey embryonic stem cells function in a Parkinson primate model. J Clin Invest, 2005. 115(1): pp. 102–9.

[41] Cooper, O., M. Parmar, and O. Isacson, Characterization and criteria of embryonic stem and induced pluripotent stem cells for a dopamine replacement therapy. Prog Brain Res, 2012. 200: pp. 265–76.

[42] Glavaski-Joksimovic, A. and M.C. Bohn, Mesenchymal stem cells and neuroregeneration in Parkinson's disease. Exp Neurol, 2013. 247: pp. 25–38.

[43] Offen, D., et al., Intrastriatal transplantation of mouse bone marrow-derived stem cells improves motor behavior in a mouse model of Parkinson's disease. J Neural Transm Suppl, 2007(72): pp. 133–43.

[44] Venkataramana, N.K., et al., Open-labeled study of unilateral autologous bone-marrow-derived mesenchymal stem cell transplantation in Parkinson's disease. Transl Res, 2010. 155(2): pp. 62–70.

[45] Takahashi, K. and S. Yamanaka, Induction of pluripotent stem cells from mouse embryonic and adult fibroblast cultures by defined factors. Cell, 2006. 126(4): pp. 663 76.

[46] Takahashi, K., et al., Induction of pluripotent stem cells from adult human fibroblasts by defined factors. Cell, 2007. 131(5): pp. 861–72.

[47] Kuzmenkin, A., et al., Functional characterization of cardiomyocytes derived from murine induced pluripotent stem cells in vitro. FASEB J, 2009. 23(12): pp. 4168–80.

[48] Espejel, S., et al., Induced pluripotent stem cell-derived hepatocytes have the functional and proliferative capabilities needed for liver regeneration in mice. J Clin Invest, 2010. 120(9): pp. 3120–6.

[49] Czepiel, M., et al., Differentiation of induced pluripotent stem cells into functional oligodendrocytes. Glia, 2011. 59(6): pp. 882–92.

[50] Hu, B.Y., et al., Neural differentiation of human induced pluripotent stem cells follows developmental principles but with variable potency. Proc Natl Acad Sci U S A, 2010. 107(9): pp. 4335–40.

[51] Wernig, M., et al., Neurons derived from reprogrammed fibroblasts functionally integrate into the fetal brain and improve symptoms of rats with Parkinson's disease. Proc Natl Acad Sci U S A, 2008. 105(15): pp. 5856–61.

[52] Hargus, G., et al., Differentiated Parkinson patient-derived induced pluripotent stem cells grow in the adult rodent brain and reduce motor asymmetry in Parkinsonian rats. Proc Natl Acad Sci U S A, 2010. 107(36): pp. 15921–6.

[53] Swistowski, A., et al., Efficient generation of functional dopaminergic neurons from human induced pluripotent stem cells under defined conditions. Stem Cells, 2010. 28(10): pp. 1893–904.

[54] Hallett, P.J., et al., Successful function of autologous iPSC-derived dopamine neurons following transplantation in a non-human primate model of Parkinson's disease. Cell Stem Cell, 2015. 16(3): pp. 269–74.

[55] Momcilovic, O., et al., Genome wide profiling of dopaminergic neurons derived from human embryonic and induced pluripotent stem cells. Stem Cells Dev, 2014. 23(4): pp. 406–20.

[56] Reardon, S. and D. Cyranoski, Japan stem-cell trial stirs envy. Nature, 2014. 513(7518): pp. 287–8.

[57] Garber, K., RIKEN suspends first clinical trial involving induced pluripotent stem cells. Nat Biotechnol, 2015. 33(9): pp. 890–1.

[58] Pang, Z.P., et al., Induction of human neuronal cells by defined transcription factors. Nature, 2011. 476(7359): pp. 220–3.

[59] Pfisterer, U., et al., Direct conversion of human fibroblasts to dopaminergic neurons. Proc Natl Acad Sci U S A, 2011. 108(25): pp. 10343–8.

[60] Chanda, S., et al., Generation of induced neuronal cells by the single reprogramming factor ASCL1. Stem Cell Rep, 2014. 3(2): pp. 282–96.

[61] Xu, H., et al., Neurotrophic factor expression in expandable cell populations from brain samples in living patients with Parkinson's disease. FASEB J, 2013. 27(10): pp. 4157–68.

[62] Rangasamy, S.B., et al., Neurotrophic factor therapy for Parkinson's disease. Prog Brain Res, 2010. 184: pp. 237–64.

[63] Kordower, J.H. and A. Bjorklund, Trophic factor gene therapy for Parkinson's disease. Mov Disord, 2013. 28(1): pp. 96–109.

[64] Rodrigues, T.M., et al., Challenges and promises in the development of neurotrophic factor-based therapies for Parkinson's disease. Drugs Aging, 2014. 31(4): pp. 239–61.

[65] Airaksinen, M.S. and M. Saarma, The GDNF family: signalling, biological functions and therapeutic value. Nat Rev Neurosci, 2002. 3(5): pp. 383–94.

[66] Lin, L.F., et al., GDNF: a glial cell line-derived neurotrophic factor for midbrain dopaminergic neurons. Science, 1993. 260(5111): pp. 1130–2.

[67] Meyer, M., et al., Improved survival of embryonic porcine dopaminergic neurons in coculture with a conditionally immortalized GDNF-producing hippocampal cell line. Exp Neurol, 2000. 164(1): pp. 82–93.

[68] Beck, K.D., et al., GDNF induces a dystonia-like state in neonatal rats and stimulates dopamine and serotonin synthesis. Neuron, 1996. 16(3): pp. 665–73.

[69] Bowenkamp, K.E., et al., Glial cell line-derived neurotrophic factor supports survival of injured midbrain dopaminergic neurons. J Comp Neurol, 1995. 355(4): pp. 479–89.

[70] Winkler, C., et al., Short-term GDNF treatment provides long-term rescue of lesioned nigral dopaminergic neurons in a rat model of Parkinson's disease. J Neurosci, 1996. 16(22): pp. 7206–15.

[71] Clarkson, E.D., W.M. Zawada, and C.R. Freed, GDNF improves survival and reduces apoptosis in human embryonic dopaminergic neurons in vitro. Cell Tissue Res, 1997. 289(2): pp. 207–10.

[72] Schober, A., et al., GDNF applied to the MPTP-lesioned nigrostriatal system requires TGF-beta for its neuroprotective action. Neurobiol Dis, 2007. 25(2): pp. 378–91.

[73] Chen, Y.H., et al., MPTP-induced deficits in striatal synaptic plasticity are prevented by glial cell line-derived neurotrophic factor expressed via an adeno-associated viral vector. FASEB J, 2008. 22(1): pp. 261–75.

[74] Gash, D.M., et al., Functional recovery in parkinsonian monkeys treated with GDNF. Nature, 1996. 380(6571): pp. 252–5.

[75] Aron, L. and R. Klein, Repairing the parkinsonian brain with neurotrophic factors. Trends Neurosci, 2011. 34(2): pp. 88–100.

[76] Nutt, J.G., et al., Randomized, double-blind trial of glial cell line-derived neurotrophic factor (GDNF) in PD. Neurology, 2003. 60(1): pp. 69–73.

[77] Gill, S.S., et al., Direct brain infusion of glial cell line-derived neurotrophic factor in Parkinson disease. Nat Med, 2003. 9(5): pp. 589–95.

[78] Patel, N.K., et al., Intraputamenal infusion of glial cell line-derived neurotrophic factor in PD: a two-year outcome study. Ann Neurol, 2005. 57(2): pp. 298–302.

[79] Patel, N.K., et al., Benefits of putaminal GDNF infusion in Parkinson disease are maintained after GDNF cessation. Neurology, 2013. 81(13): pp. 1176–8.

[80] Slevin, J.T., et al., Improvement of bilateral motor functions in patients with Parkinson disease through the unilateral intraputaminal infusion of glial cell line-derived neurotrophic factor. J Neurosurg, 2005. 102(2):pp. 216–22.

[81]   Lang, A.E., et al., Randomized controlled trial of intraputamenal glial cell line-derived neurotrophic factor infusion in Parkinson disease. Ann Neurol, 2006. 59(3): pp. 459–66.

[82]   Kotzbauer, P.T., et al., Neurturin, a relative of glial-cell-line-derived neurotrophic factor. Nature, 1996. 384(6608): pp. 467–70.

[83]   Horger, B.A., et al., Neurturin exerts potent actions on survival and function of midbrain dopaminergic neurons. J Neurosci, 1998. 18(13): pp. 4929–37.

[84]   Akerud, P., et al., Differential effects of glial cell line-derived neurotrophic factor and neurturin on developing and adult substantia nigra dopaminergic neurons. J Neurochem, 1999. 73(1): pp. 70–8.

[85]   Oiwa, Y., et al., Dopaminergic neuroprotection and regeneration by neurturin assessed by using behavioral, biochemical and histochemical measurements in a model of progressive Parkinson's disease. Brain Res, 2002. 947(2): pp. 271–83.

[86]   Grondin, R., et al., Intraputamenal infusion of exogenous neurturin protein restores motor and dopaminergic function in the globus pallidus of MPTP-lesioned rhesus monkeys. Cell Transplant, 2008. 17(4): pp. 373–81.

[87]   Gasmi, M., et al., AAV2-mediated delivery of human neurturin to the rat nigrostriatal system: long-term efficacy and tolerability of CERE-120 for Parkinson's disease. Neurobiol Dis, 2007. 27(1): pp. 67–76.

[88]   Kordower, J.H., et al., Delivery of neurturin by AAV2 (CERE-120)-mediated gene transfer provides structural and functional neuroprotection and neurorestoration in MPTP-treated monkeys. Ann Neurol, 2006. 60(6): pp. 706–15.

[89]   Herzog, C.D., et al., Expression, bioactivity, and safety 1 year after adeno-associated viral vector type 2-mediated delivery of neurturin to the monkey nigrostriatal system support cere-120 for Parkinson's disease. Neurosurgery, 2009. 64(4): pp. 602–12; discussion 612–3.

[90]   Marks, W.J., Jr., et al., Safety and tolerability of intraputaminal delivery of CERE-120 (adeno-associated virus serotype 2-neurturin) to patients with idiopathic Parkinson's disease: an open-label, phase I trial. Lancet Neurol, 2008. 7(5): pp. 400–8.

[91]   Marks, W.J., Jr., et al., Gene delivery of AAV2-neurturin for Parkinson's disease: a double-blind, randomised, controlled trial. Lancet Neurol, 2010. 9(12): pp. 1164–72.

[92]   Bartus, R.T., et al., Bioactivity of AAV2-neurturin gene therapy (CERE-120): differences between Parkinson's disease and nonhuman primate brains. Mov Disord, 2011. 26(1): pp. 27–36.

[93]   Bartus, R.T., et al., Safety/feasibility of targeting the substantia nigra with AAV2-neurturin in Parkinson patients. Neurology, 2013. 80(18): pp. 1698–701.

[94]   Milbrandt, J., et al., Persephin, a novel neurotrophic factor related to GDNF and neurturin. Neuron, 1998. 20(2): pp. 245–53.

[95]   Akerud, P., et al., Persephin-overexpressing neural stem cells regulate the function of nigral dopaminergic neurons and prevent their degeneration in a model of Parkinson's disease. Mol Cell Neurosci, 2002. 21(2): pp. 205–22.

[96]   Baloh, R.H., et al., Artemin, a novel member of the GDNF ligand family, supports peripheral and central neurons and signals through the GFRalpha3-RET receptor complex. Neuron, 1998. 21(6): pp. 1291–302.

[97]   Cass, W.A., et al., Protection by GDNF and other trophic factors against the dopamine-depleting effects of neurotoxic doses of methamphetamine. Ann N Y Acad Sci, 2006. 1074: pp. 272–81.

[98]   Zuccato, C. and E. Cattaneo, Brain-derived neurotrophic factor in neurodegenerative diseases. Nat Rev Neurol, 2009. 5(6): pp. 311–22.

[99]   Murer, M.G., Q. Yan, and R. Raisman-Vozari, Brain-derived neurotrophic factor in the control human brain, and in Alzheimer's disease and Parkinson's disease. Prog Neurobiol, 2001. 63(1): pp. 71–124.

[100] Parain, K., et al., Reduced expression of brain-derived neurotrophic factor protein in Parkinson's disease substantia nigra. Neuroreport, 1999. 10(3): pp. 557–61.

[101] Ziebell, M., et al., Striatal dopamine transporter binding correlates with serum BDNF levels in patients with striatal dopaminergic neurodegeneration. Neurobiol Aging, 2012. 33(2): pp. 428 e1–5.

[102] Porritt, M.J., P.E. Batchelor, and D.W. Howells, Inhibiting BDNF expression by antisense oligonucleotide infusion causes loss of nigral dopaminergic neurons. Exp Neurol, 2005. 192(1): pp. 226–34.

[103] Baquet, Z.C., P.C. Bickford, and K.R. Jones, Brain-derived neurotrophic factor is required for the establishment of the proper number of dopaminergic neurons in the substantia nigra pars compacta. J Neurosci, 2005. 25(26): pp. 6251–9.

[104] Tsukahara, T., et al., Effects of brain-derived neurotrophic factor on 1-methyl-4-phenyl-1,2,3,6-tetrahydropyridine-induced parkinsonism in monkeys. Neurosurgery, 1995. 37(4): pp. 733–9; discussion 739–41.

[105] Nagahara, A.H. and M.H. Tuszynski, Potential therapeutic uses of BDNF in neurological and psychiatric disorders. Nat Rev Drug Discov, 2011. 10(3): pp. 209–19.

[106] Petrova, P., et al., MANF: a new mesencephalic, astrocyte-derived neurotrophic factor with selectivity for dopaminergic neurons. J Mol Neurosci, 2003. 20(2): pp. 173–88.

[107] Lindholm, P., et al., Novel neurotrophic factor CDNF protects and rescues midbrain dopamine neurons in vivo. Nature, 2007. 448(7149): pp. 73–7.

[108] Voutilainen, M.H., et al., Chronic infusion of CDNF prevents 6-OHDA-induced deficits in a rat model of Parkinson's disease. Exp Neurol, 2011. 228(1): pp. 99–108.

[109] Back, S., et al., Gene therapy with AAV2-CDNF provides functional benefits in a rat model of Parkinson's disease. Brain Behav, 2013. 3(2): pp. 75–88.

[110] Ren, X., et al., AAV2-mediated striatum delivery of human CDNF prevents the deterioration of midbrain dopamine neurons in a 6-hydroxydopamine induced parkinsonian rat model. Exp Neurol, 2013. 248: pp. 148–56.

[111] Cordero-Llana, O., et al., Enhanced efficacy of the CDNF/MANF family by combined intranigral overexpression in the 6-OHDA rat model of Parkinson's disease. Mol Ther, 2015. 23(2): pp. 244–54.

3

Mucuna and Parkinson's Disease: Treatment with Natural Levodopa

Rafael González Maldonado

Abstract

Mucuna pruriens is a tropical bean containing large amounts of levodopa and is the most important natural remedy for Parkinson's disease. Famous neurologists have patented methods of extraction for its advantages over the synthetic forms, Sinemet and Madopar. This natural levodopa is less toxic and has a faster and more lasting effect and can delay the need for pharmaceuticals and combination therapies. Currently, there are many patients with Parkinson's disease who take *Mucuna* and spontaneously reduce the dose of conventional drugs and do so behind their doctors' backs. *Mucuna* should always be taken under medical supervision.

Keywords: *Mucuna pruriens*, Parkinson's disease, levodopa, natural, treatment, benefit, dyskinesia, conventional

1. Introduction

Mucuna pruriens is a species of bean that grows in the tropics. It is very rich in natural levodopa, which is better tolerated and more potent than the synthetic levodopa in Sinemet, Madopar, or Stalevo. *Mucuna* seed extract has been an effective treatment of Parkinson's disease (PD) in many patients. Scientific studies attest to it, and renowned neurologists have patented the specific techniques for extracting levodopa from this plant. They *relate to the use of Mucuna pruriens seeds for the preparation of a pharmaceutical composition for the treatment of Parkinson's disease to obtain a broader therapeutic window in L-Dopa therapy, to delay a need for combination therapy, to obtain an earlier onset and longer duration of L-Dopa efficacy, and to prevent or alleviate acute and chronic L-Dopa toxicity* [3, 44]."

Meanwhile, patients have recorded their positive experiences with *Mucuna*; they buy it online (no prescription needed) and use it in secrecy without consulting their neurologist. It is used without control, and if there are not more accidents, it is because it is relatively safe (although there are risks if misused), and most of the capsules sold contain very low doses, almost like a diet supplement. The formula at high concentrations is dangerous, especially when mixed with antiparkinsonian drugs. Neither the patients nor the doctors (most of them) have clear ideas about this plant, its ingredients (not only levodopa), the proportions in which it is absorbed, or how to manage it.

2. *Mucuna pruriens*: the plant

Mucuna pruriens is a kind of "hairy" or furry bean, native to Southeast Asia, especially the plains of India, but also widely distributed in tropical regions of Africa and the Americas (particularly in the Caribbean). The wide dissemination of the plant explains its variety of names, depending on the location: velvet beans, cowhage, itch bean, picapica, Fogareté, Kapikachu, sea bean, deer eyes, yerepe, Atmagupta, nescafe, and chiporazo. *Mucuna* is a legume (such as common beans, peas, lentils, peanuts) and the largest natural source of levodopa.

This annual plant grows as a climbing shrub with long tendrils that enable it to reach more than 15 feet in height. Young plants are almost completely covered by a diffuse orange hair that disappears as they age. It grows or is cultivated as fodder to enrich the soil (adding a lot of nitrogen) or for its medicinal qualities.

Mucuna is called "pruriens" because of the intense itching produced by their contact. The orange "hairs" of flowers and pods of *Mucuna pruriens* contain chemicals (including serotonin) that, when they come in contact with the skin, cause intense irritation and itching and sometimes very troublesome injury including allergies and severe swelling.

In India, *Mucuna* has been the main healing herb for three thousand years. All parts of the plant are used in more than 200 indigenous medicinal preparations. The seeds contain up to 7% levodopa, which is used in the treatment of Parkinson's disease. In the Ayurvedic medicine, velvet bean is recommended as an aphrodisiac, and studies have shown that its use causes a rise in testosterone levels, increased muscle mass and strength, and also improves coordination and attention.

Extract of *Mucuna* seed powder contains large amounts of levodopa and a little serotonin and nicotine along with other ingredients that are only partially known. In the treatment of Parkinson's disease, such extracts seem to be more effective and less toxic than the synthetic preparations [1].

3. *Mucuna*: therapeutic possibilities

The interest in *Mucuna* increased after 1937 when it was discovered that the variant contained large amounts of levodopa. However, this amino acid alone does not justify the many medical applications of this interesting plant.

In the treatment of Parkinson's disease, some results in groups of patients and in experimental animals show that, apart from natural levodopa, *Mucuna pruriens* has other ingredients that show outstanding features. It must contain other substances that improve the absorption of levodopa and metabolic efficiency, as explained below.

To date, 50 substances have been identified in the powder of its seeds [2]. Other still unidentified components must exist in *Mucuna*, such as portions or mixtures of alkaloids, proteins, peptides, polysaccharides, glycosides, glycoproteins, and several phytochemicals including tryptamine, alanine, arginine, glutathione, isoquinolone, mucunine, nicotine, prurienine, serotonin, tyrosine, etc., [3].

These substances, identified or not, confer special powers on *Mucuna*, perhaps boosting the levodopa or adding some kind of dopamine agonism and even extended its effects. We need to continue investigating them.

3.1. Strategies to enhance levodopa

Trials have been conducted in which *Mucuna* seeds are germinated in darkness or in different conditions of light and providing varied nutrients (oregano, proteins from fish, etc.). Results showed that by adding oregano to seeds germinated in darkness, *Mucuna* sprouts containing 33% more levodopa have been obtained [4]. Other researchers selected some cells from the ground and then grew them grow in a medium that allows nutrients to be supplied; in this way they have managed successfully to increase the concentration of levodopa [5, 6].

3.2. Beneficial effects of *Mucuna*

Mucuna is recommended in Ayurveda to treat more than 200 diseases—as a vital tonic, an aphrodisiac, a remedy to reduce stress, a good diuretic, etc.—and is also used against parasites, to control diabetes and lower cholesterol. And, of course, it is a treatment for *kampavata* (the equivalent of Parkinson's disease). Western science seems to confirm many of these effects. *Mucuna* improves libido, semen quality, etc., and even works against snake bites.

Mucuna increases the adaptation and regeneration of tissues in general and has been shown to increase growth hormone [7]. It has an anabolic effect and increases muscle mass; it also has antioxidant properties and favors the protective functions of the liver [8].

Diabetics and people with high cholesterol may benefit from *Mucuna* [9]. In rats it has been shown to lower cholesterol by 61%, and glucose was reduced by 39% [10]. *Mucuna* enhances the recovery of diabetic neuropathy induced in animals [11]. In humans it delays the onset of diabetic nephropathy.

Mucuna also protects the stomach to relieve gastric mucosal lesions induced experimentally in rats [12]. *Mucuna* contains prurienine which increases intestinal peristalsis and is a good remedy for constipation, so prevalent in Parkinson's disease patients. It usually enhances motility and gastric emptying, although some patients assert otherwise.

3.3. Aphrodisiac and antiepileptic

Mucuna increases libido, or sexual drive, in men and women due to its dopamine-inducing properties; dopamine is the substance of desire and profoundly influences all appetites. In male animals *Mucuna* raises testosterone levels and increases sexual activity [13]. In men with fertility problems, *Mucuna* clearly enhances sexual drive and power while improving the quality of the sperm: it increases the number of cells and also gives them greater mobility [14]. It is assumed that it acts on the hypothalamus-pituitary-gonadal axis.

Researchers can cause status epilepticus or catalepsy in experimental animals by various techniques: electroshock, pilocarpine, or Haloperidol. These improve if treated with velvet beans [15].

3.4. Snake poison antidote

This is not an exaggeration or a myth. *Mucuna* is a good antidote for snake bites, possibly by a direct effect on the venom, attributed to its glycoprotein antitrypsin content [16] but also because it is procoagulant and prevents cardiorespiratory depression induced by poison.

Specifically, *Mucuna* reduces mortality due to bites from the following snakes: Gariba viper (*Echis carinatus*), Viper Malaya, and spitting cobra (*Naja sputatrix*) [17].

3.5. Kampavata is Parkinson's disease

In India there were Parkinson's disease patients three thousand years before the birth of James Parkinson. These were diagnosed as *Kampavata*, a disease characterized by trembling (*Kampa* in Sanskrit). In Ayurveda this process was classified within the group of neurological disorders (*Vata Rogas*) [18, 19].

They obviously lacked Sinemet and Madopar but were treated naturally with levodopa, obtained by crushing *Mucuna* seeds, which they later diluted and administered as a beverage [20]. For thousands of years; this therapy has worked, these patients have improved and, above all, according to that we know, showed fewer side effects than people taking synthetic drugs.

3.6. The seeds are cooked in cow's milk

In an interesting clinical trial, 18 Parkinson's disease patients were treated according to the criteria of Ayurvedic medicine. They received a concoction of powder of *Mucuna pruriens* cooked in cow's milk along with other traditional plants (*Hyoscyamus reticulatus*, *Withania somnifera*, *Sida cordifolia*) [21].

The results found that this treatment improved rigidity and bradykinesia; tremor was diminished and cramps subsided; however, sialorrhea (drooling or excessive salivation) worsened. Later, the powder of plants which had been added to the milk was analyzed, and it was found that each dose used contains 200 mg of levodopa [21].

The Hindu *Mucuna* extract contains a small amount of levodopa that fails to justify the significant clinical improvement of parkinsonian symptoms. This suggests that in the *Mucuna*, there are other substances that enhance the role of levodopa (such as carbidopa, entacapone, or tolcapone) or other active ingredients with antiparkinsonian effects [20, 22, 23].

One important thing is guaranteed by Ayurveda: after thousands of years of using these plant extracts, thousands or millions of patients have continued to improve their symptoms without significant adverse effects.

4. *Mucuna* works better than Sinemet

In 1978, a publication by R.A. Vaidya in India stated that Parkinson's disease could be treated with extracts of a plant, *Mucuna pruriens*, which contains natural levodopa and is tolerated better than the synthetic version [24]. In the West the scientific writings that described improvement in parkinsonian symptoms after eating *Mucuna* or other beans appear between 1990 and 1994 [18, 25, 26]. These legumes could replace some of the conventional medications. There are some recipes from "Parkinsonian cuisine" that are based on beans [22, 27].

4.1. *Mucuna* seed powder

Scientific journals have begun publishing cases of improvement in patients after eating *Mucuna*. The Parkinson's Disease Study Group undertook a multicenter clinical study (in collaboration with several hospitals) with 60 patients, of which 26 took Sinemet before the test and the other 34 were "pharmacologically virgins" (they had never taken levodopa). All were treated for 12 weeks with powder from *Mucuna* seeds: an average of six bags, each containing 7.5 grams, equivalent to 250 mg of levodopa. In other words, each sachet contained the same amount of levodopa as a Sinemet 25/250 but without the carbidopa. Neurologists of four centers screened patients using the appropriate scales (UPDRS) and found considerable improvement that was statistically confirmed [28]. Thus, Ayurveda medicinal recipes have demonstrated their clinical effectiveness.

4.2. Zandopa: a medicine with *Mucuna*

This legume seems to work. Investigations gave evidence of this, and *Mucuna* seed powder (called HP-200) was marketed as a drug, under the brand name Zandopa [2]. It was first distributed in India and has been available in the United Kingdom since 2008. Now customers can buy it freely online without a prescription. It is important to be careful, however, because the levodopa dose is relatively high (250 mg per sachet) when combined with carbidopa or other antiparkinsonian drugs.

4.3. Improvement in mice doubles or triples

We can experimentally induce parkinsonism (unilateral or bilateral) in rodents via certain toxic substances. Used in these trials, levodopa from *Mucuna* has no side effects and produces an improvement that is double or triple that of the synthetic version [29].

In another experiment, animals ate extract of *Mucuna* for a year. They were then put down, and their neurotransmitters were measured in different areas of their brains. Interestingly, no changes were seen in the nigrostriatal pathway, but dopamine was significantly increased in the cerebral cortex [2]. This has two possible explanations: that natural levodopa is more potent or that *Mucuna* contains other beneficial chemicals.

4.4. Improvement in humans

This clinical study [1] complies with the strict requirements laid down by the most rigorous scientific methodology established by the Quality Committee of the American Academy of

Neurology [30]. This was a randomized, double-blind, crossover study which adhered to precise objectives and clearly defined protocols and was carried out by several independent observers.

They studied eight Parkinson's disease patients at (on average) 62 years of age, 12 years after diagnosis with a stage of progression of 3.5 on the Hoehn and Yahr scale. Prior to this test, they were treated with levodopa (572 mg mean value). In addition, patients were taking other previous associated drugs (amantadine, pergolide, ropinirole, pramipexole, or cabergoline) that remain unchanged. All had a rapid response to levodopa (1.5 to 4 hours) along with very disabling motor fluctuations during the morning.

Each subject was hospitalized three times (1 week apart) and went without any medication the night before the test. The next morning, at the same time, each received at random one of three combinations: one dose of 200 mg of levodopa with 50 mg of carbidopa (two tablets of Sinemet Plus) or two or four sachets of *Mucuna* (15 or 30 grams) equivalent to 500 or 1000 mg of natural levodopa (100 or 200 according to the conversion factors).

The results were clearly better in those who take two sachets of *Mucuna* extract: improvement in their symptoms occurred faster, their plasma levodopa levels were higher, and clinical efficacy was more durable. In addition, their dyskinesia was not worsened. The details follow.

4.5. "Citius, altius, fortius et durabilius"

The Olympic motto *faster, higher, stronger* can be applied to *Mucuna*, because, in comparison to Sinemet, it acts more rapidly (34 minutes instead of 68), produces a greater elevation of the plasma level of levodopa (110% higher), and appears to be stronger (the effectiveness of natural levodopa is double or triple that of the synthetic version). In addition, the improvement achieved is more durable (with *Mucuna* the "on" phase is prolonged 37 minutes longer than with Sinemet). Therefore, it can be described as *citius, altius, fortius… durabilius*.

4.6. Twice as effective

We have seen that the *Mucuna* seed extract naturally contains levodopa. If we quantify and compare it to the same dose of synthetic levodopa contained in tablets of Sinemet (or Madopar), we find that levodopa from *Mucuna* is approximately twice as powerful in controlling parkinsonian symptoms [31].

The efficacy of synthetic levodopa (without carbidopa) has been compared to that of natural levodopa (*Mucuna*) using rats with experimentally induced parkinsonism. The natural levodopa proved to be two times as effective at improving symptoms [32]. This test maintained the following proportions: 125 and 250 milligrams of synthetic levodopa were compared with the equivalent dose of natural levodopa (respectively, 2.5 and 5 grams of *Mucuna* powder 5%). Then the test was repeated, this time adding 50 mg of carbidopa to the two types of levodopa. Again, *Mucuna* proved to be more efficient.

4.7. The problem of volume

Mucuna is more effective, more rapid, and durable; however, to achieve a dose that will offer the same relief as Sinemet or Madopar, it would be necessary to prescribe large amounts of seed powder dissolved in liquid [24, 33]. The need to consume seed powder several times a day would soon overwhelm the patient, and the treatment would be abandoned as too cumbersome.

The solution to the problem can be found in concentrated extracts. This allows for the presentation of *Mucuna* in tablets or capsules, facilitating the application of different doses of the product and making it easy to manage daily consumption of *Mucuna* in the amounts deemed necessary. There is another choice that requires the cooperation of the neurologist: *Mucuna* could be used in association with carbidopa to achieve greater efficiency with less seed powder.

4.8. *Mucuna* with carbidopa

The first trials that compared the effects of Sinemet with *Mucuna* required six or seven daily sachets of powdered seeds. This can be maintained for a few days but becomes quite cumbersome with time. Actually those studies were done to compare natural levodopa (*Mucuna*) to a synthetic combination of levodopa and carbidopa (i.e., the contents of Sinemet).

The solution seems simple: add carbidopa to *Mucuna*. This increases the efficiency of the natural levodopa contained therein and therefore eliminates the need to take large amounts of seed powder. We must be careful when capsules of concentrated extracts are used because the dose can be excessive when you consider that *Mucuna* is more effective than synthetic levodopa.

There are published trials in which *Mucuna* is administered in combination with carbidopa and is compared to Sinemet. Rats with experimentally induced hemi-parkinsonism were treated with powdered *Mucuna* seeds (2.5 and 5 g) associated with carbidopa (50 mg) and in contrast to other groups wherein the equivalent synthetic levodopa dose (125 and 250 mg) was also associated with carbidopa. *Mucuna*-carbidopa proved to be more than twice as effective as Sinemet, and this was found by measuring the rotation contralateral (on the injured side) of the animals in each group [32].

Very recently, a new trial was performed to investigate whether *Mucuna pruriens* (MP) may be used as alternative source of levodopa for indigent individuals with Parkinson's disease (PD) who cannot afford long-term therapy with marketed levodopa preparations. Eighteen patients were included in a double-blind, randomized, controlled, crossover study [34]. It shows that single-dose *Mucuna pruriens* intake met all noninferiority efficacy and safety outcome measures in comparison to dispersible levodopa/benserazide. Clinical effects of high-dose MP were similar to levodopa alone at the same dose, with a more favorable tolerability profile [34].

We know that the carbidopa in Sinemet prevents the peripheral side effects of levodopa (nausea, rapid heart rate) and enhances mobility. It appears that the carbidopa in *Mucuna* is even more effective: it decreases mild side effects and doubles or triples patients' strength [1].

4.9. Other advantages of *Mucuna*

Mucuna does not produce dyskinesia. A different study, this time in monkeys (with unilateral parkinsonism induced experimentally), produced very interesting results on the possibility of dyskinesias. One group was treated with Sinemet (levodopa and carbidopa), another with *Mucuna* plus carbidopa, and the third only with *Mucuna*. All the animals experienced an improvement in their symptoms. Dyskinesia was then assessed by the study of spontaneous activity in the substantia nigra. Larger dyskinesia appeared in the Sinemet group. In those treated with the combination of *Mucuna* and carbidopa, dyskinesia seemed more moderate. Interestingly, in those who had only taken *Mucuna*, no dyskinesia was found [35].

Long-term Mucuna without dyskinesia. A similar experiment was performed, but this time *Mucuna* treatment was continuous, extending for a year. It was done in rodents and compared *Mucuna* with Madopar. One group was treated with Madopar (levodopa and benserazide), another with *Mucuna* plus benserazide, and the third only with *Mucuna*. All were controlled for a year. The symptoms were alleviated in all groups, but the improvement was significantly higher in those who were treated with *Mucuna* plus benserazide.

To highlight the results of long-term use: after 1 year, major dyskinesia appeared in rats that had taken Madopar. Rodents treated with *Mucuna* plus benserazide had some minor dyskinesia while for animals that took only *Mucuna*, none at all [36]. Even more, in an experiment with different dyskinesias (those produced by neuroleptics like haloperidol), these repetitive movements improved when *Mucuna* was administered [37].

Mucuna is neuroprotective. It seems that natural levodopa from *Mucuna* (or the whole of the components in this legume) is nontoxic and even neuroprotective [38]. This has been demonstrated in mice (with experimentally induced parkinsonism) which were given synthetic levodopa or *Mucuna*. Those treated with *Mucuna* experienced an improvement in most of the symptoms. Also, when they were slaughtered 1 year later for brain analysis, it was found that the endogenous contents of levodopa, dopamine, norepinephrine, and serotonin in the *substantia nigra* were significantly restored [2].

In other studies with rodents, researchers agree that the extract of *Mucuna* clearly is neuroprotective compared to synthetic levodopa [39] or estrogen [40]. They believe that this is due to its antioxidant and chelating activity (processing of iron) and because it avoids mutagenic effects in DNA [41, 42].

Antioxidant and neuroprotective properties of *Mucuna* have also been shown in rodents that were previously damaged experimentally by nerve toxins such as paraquat. The results also highlighted the improvement in habits and cognitive functions of these animals [43].

Dosage does not increase over time! It sounds too good to be true: treatment with *Mucuna* does not produce dyskinesia; and it also improves secondary abnormal movements which occur with chronic synthetic levodopa therapy. One more thing, with *Mucuna* it would be not necessary to gradually increase the dose as time goes on, as is the case with those taking synthetic drugs.

Below, I transcribe literally the benefits of *Mucuna* extracts as reflected in the scientific foundations of the patent carried out by Van der Giessen, Olanow, Lees, and Wagner [3]: "Conventional L-Dopa therapy requires a gradual increase of the effective dose over time resulting of progression of disease and/or the neurotoxic effects of L-Dopa or dopamine with an increase of toxic reactions and, over time, the appearance of dyskinesia, increasing in severity with dose. In clinical experiences with *Mucuna pruriens* seed preparations, these negative phenomena have not been observed in that for the effective treatment of Parkinson's, the *dose of Mucuna pruriens derived L-Dopa remained relatively stable over longer periods of time, and in that dyskinesia, even in patients with pre-existing dyskinesia following long term therapy with conventional L-Dopa* preparations, appeared to be less in occurrence and severity..." [3].

After reading this, it seems strange that *Mucuna* is not yet dispensed in all pharmacies as a revolutionary drug.

4.10. atents of extracts of *Mucuna*

The proprietaries over certain techniques of *Mucuna* extracts—WO 2004039385-A2 [44] and US 7470441-B2 [3]—are very prestigious researchers. They have developed specific techniques to extract various substances from *Mucuna,* not only levodopa. As they have detailed, many of the ingredients are indicated "…for preventing, alleviating or treating neurological diseases," for general use as "a pharmaceutical combination for neuroprotection or neurostimulation," and, more specifically, "for the treatment of Parkinson's disease." They have left little to no chance.

4.11. Zandopa and a cocktail with *Mucuna*

The previously mentioned Zandopa brand from Zandu Laboratories, which owns the patent for *Mucuna* powder product known as HP-200, was used in important clinical trials [28, 45] and has been marketed for several years. Som C. Pruthi has patented [46] a combination from the Ayurveda tradition that mainly contains *Mucuna* (between 55 and 99%), together with *Piper longum* and *Zingiber officinale.* He described a woman diagnosed with Parkinson's disease at age 51 that did not tolerate conventional medicines. She took Pruthi's combination of *Mucuna* for 12 years. In this long period, it was found that progression of the disease was very slow and side effects were not detected.

4.12. An extra-concentrated extract

The drawback of *Mucuna* powder and primitive extracts is the large volume of legume one needs to consume in order to achieve sufficient blood levels of levodopa. This produces over-eating and gastrointestinal upset and causes many to abandon this therapy. To avoid this trouble, Manyam has patented a method [47] involving the removal of grease from the coty-ledons of the seeds. Using ethanol as a solvent, the concentrated extract is isolated and finally freeze-dried.

With this technique, it is possible to process 2.5 kilograms (over 5 pounds) of *Mucuna* powder, which is then reduced to just 46 grams (1.6 ounces). In this conversion the relative proportions of levodopa are maintained (or even increased). So the amount of vegetable to be ingested is reduced to less than 2%. In this way, it can be supplied as tablets, capsules, or syrup and even diluted for injection [47]. On the other hand, its efficacy has been demonstrated in vitro and in animals: when this concentrated extract is supplied to rats with "induced parkinsonism," their symptoms improve twice as much as the treatment with synthetic levodopa [32].

4.13. More benefits than conventional levodopa

The foundations of the patent, based on the references provided, reveal that, in relation to standard levodopa-carbidopa medications (Sinemet) or levodopa-benserazide (Madopar), the extracts of *Mucuna* have important advantages that confirm those listed in the previous chapter.

Mucuna has a wider therapeutic window: the range of dosage in which a drug can be used without causing toxic effects. That means that there is a large margin between the minimally effective dose of *Mucuna* and one that could cause damage in the body.

Patients get better sooner with it. Researchers gave patients a tablet of Sinemet, and they noticed the "on" effect after 54 minutes. But when they took *Mucuna*, they were already active after only 23–27 minutes [1]. In addition to being quick-acting, *Mucuna* (at a dose of 30 grams) has been found to be effective for longer durations: patients were still "on" for 204 minutes after taking the seed extract, beating Sinemet tablet by half an hour [1].

Neither acute nor chronic toxic effects have been described. Even with high doses of *Mucuna*, there were less adverse effects (nausea, abdominal discomfort) than in patients who received the equivalent of the conventional drugs [3]. Other long-term studies of *Mucuna* (in monkeys and rats) have shown that the dreaded dyskinesia and other symptoms associated with continuous treatment with levodopa are lower and in some cases even tend to improve [35, 36].

4.14. Other benefits of *Mucuna*

According to the application for the patent, *Mucuna* alone may suffice to relieve patients' symptoms for a period of time, and therefore combination therapy (levodopa plus agonists) can be delayed. Even more, these renowned specialists believe that *Mucuna* extracts may be useful in the treatment of multiple neurodegenerative processes: chorea, Parkinson's and Alzheimer's diseases, and vascular dementia [3]; further applications include many other metabolic disnutritional disorders and, systemic, endocrine and autoimmune disturbances (vitamin deficiency, lupus, demyelinating, etc.), as well as neurotoxic, ischemic, or traumatic injuries [44].

Anecdotally, a woman with white hair has been described that after 3 months of treatment with *Mucuna*, it turned back to black [50], "like when I was young," she said. This is food for thought: the threads connecting youth, dopamine, suffering, old age, stress, and gray hair [48, 49].

4.15. *Mucuna* is more than levodopa

The available data has shown that *Mucuna pruriens* has special properties that distinguish it from synthetic levodopa. These data provide a basis for the patent registered by Olanow and Lees (quoted *verbatim*): "the Mucuna pruriens formulation seems to possess potential advantages over existing commercially available synthetic L-Dopa formulations in that it combines a rapid onset of action with a comparable or longer duration of therapeutic response without increasing dyskinesias or acute LD toxicity in spite of much higher LD plasma levels…" [3].

Natural ingredients (known or unknown) combined with levodopa may contribute to improvement of parkinsonian symptoms and reduction of dyskinesia [44]. This opens up the anticipation of important therapeutic progress and the hope of further studies to confirm that extracts of *Mucuna* seeds are a safe and effective alternative [35]. Currently, patients who are using *Mucuna* under medical advice generally report a lowering of their doses of conventional drugs, and fewer side effects, in both the short and long terms.

5. Contraindications and warnings

Mucuna has some drawbacks. In principle, the levodopa itself (albeit with other natural ingredients that improve tolerance) shares many of the contraindications and precautions applicable to synthetic levodopa. These warnings are well known, and we will review some of them.

I want to begin by highlighting the main stumbling block to the beneficial use of *Mucuna*: ignorance on the part of the patient and lack of medical information. A physician should monitor treatment at all times.

5.1. Patients do not know what they are taking

A major obstacle to treatment with *Mucuna* is that patients don't have clear ideas about the drugs' intended purpose. They have heard of several cases where *Mucuna* worked well, but usually these observations have come to them from people without any scientific knowledge, from nonprofessional websites or from commercial information intended for product sales.

Mucuna is sold freely on the Internet, and many patients take it without medical supervision. Worse still, they engage in speculation based on bizarre opinions they encounter in the forums, and they absorb this erroneous information and therefore lack sufficient knowledge to use it appropriately. However, occasionally patients are right or are very close to the truth, but there is still a danger of misuse. At times patients take *Mucuna* simply because despair leads them to try anything.

5.2. Most doctors are skeptics

Many patients complain of the disdainful reaction they encounter when they ask their doctors about adding *Mucuna* to their treatment regimen. As it is an "unorthodox" therapy, it is perfectly understandable that the physician does not want to prescribe *Mucuna*: it is not part of the generally accepted body of treatments they are trained to manage. When a doctor decides to incorporate *Mucuna*, he faces new difficulties, particularly with patients treated with other drugs. This requires the additional effort of studying the situation and designing a strategy for each individual case.

On the other hand, we cannot allow patients to treat themselves in hiding. Therefore, it is desirable that as doctors, we have to educate ourselves about *Mucuna* so that we can choose to use it or not in a particular type of patient. One should never despise the unfamiliar. After studying the properties of *Mucuna* and weighing its advantages and disadvantages, we should decide on a rational basis whether it is beneficial, neutral, or inadvisable for a specific case.

If the patient perceives that we master the subject, he will entrust his care to us, rather than attempting to treat himself. That way, he will cooperate if we ban the *Mucuna* or recommend a gradual dosage pattern. We earn their trust when we have enough information and credibility.

5.3. Why are there no frequent major problems?

Mucuna is not a placebo but, rather, has important effects. However anyone can buy it without a prescription, and most are taking it without medical supervision. These patients are not sufficiently familiar with the properties of *Mucuna*; they do not know the side effects or complications that may arise; they do not take into account the interactions with other medications or the differences between individuals.

While this scenario suggests a public health issue, it fortunately does not usually cause serious problems. Why? I think that one reason is the safety of the components of *Mucuna*, which has been used for millennia in thousands or hundreds of thousands of patients in India without significant harmful effects. Another issue is that the products are sold often in small doses as a dietary supplement. That is not, however, always the case: there are some preparations with excessive doses especially when combined with carbidopa (in Sinemet, Madopar, or Stalevo), dopamine agonists, or other antiparkinsonian drugs. It is necessary to use extreme caution.

5.4. Contraindications of levodopa

Although better tolerated, *Mucuna* contains a natural form of levodopa. In theory it should share the same contraindications, interactions, and precautions of synthetic levodopa: It is contraindicated in children, pregnancy, and lactation (prolactin inhibition) and schizophrenia or psychosis. It should be used with caution (and is best avoided) in cases of a medium to severe degree of heart disease or diabetes. Do not take it with MAOIs or with ergot. Use caution (due to the additive effect) if the patient takes levodopa (Sinemet, Madopar), COMT inhibitors (Entacapone Stalevo), or dopamine agonists (rotigotine, pramipexole, ropinirole).

5.5. Side effects with levodopa

Mucuna should not be used in individuals with known allergy or hypersensitivity to *Mucuna pruriens* or components. There have been some side effects of *Mucuna*. In a study of patients with Parkinson's disease, a derivative of *Mucuna pruriens* caused minor adverse effects, which were mainly gastrointestinal in nature. Isolated cases of acute toxic psychosis have been reported [51] probably due to levodopa content. Therefore, as with Sinemet and Madopar, its use should be avoided in patients with psychosis or schizophrenia.

5.6. Specific warning about *Mucuna*

We assume that all contraindications, interactions, precautions, and side effects that we know about synthetic levodopa should be considered when taking levodopa from *Mucuna*.

Specific contraindications include thinning of the blood (anticoagulants), and care should be taken with antiplatelet and anti-inflammatory drugs because *Mucuna* increases clotting time. *Mucuna* should not merge with anticoagulants (Sintrom, Dabigatran, heparin, warfarin) or with antiplatelet drugs such as clopidogrel. Caution should be exercised, and the additive effect should be taken into account if it is associated with acetylsalicylic acid and nonsteroidal anti-inflammatory drugs (NSAIDs).

We should also be careful with antidiabetic medicines: *Mucuna* lowers glycemic index, and thus is to be considered a potential additive effect. Other interactions are possible, so always consult your regular doctor. On the one hand, it can be argued that *Mucuna* has been used for many centuries in India and has been available for several years online without a prescription, and yet serious problems have not been revealed. But that is just an observation.

Regarding Sinemet and Madopar, we have thousands of controlled studies, while publications on *Mucuna* are still scarce. One must therefore use greater caution when choosing *Mucuna*. While the future appears to be positive, we need the confirmation of more scientific studies.

6. Dosage and presentations

To use *Mucuna* correctly, the premise is to be clear about what you want: it is simply a legume that contains levodopa naturally. Synthetic levodopa usually used in pharmaceutical preparations may be replaced in whole or in part by the levodopa contained in *Mucuna*.

This sounds simple, but the point is that the dosages and concentrations can vary, so the guidelines must be individualized, and as we said, at present the patients (and even some doctors) lack sufficient information.

6.1. Before using *Mucuna*

It is essential to find a neurologist who is interested in *Mucuna* and who is adequately informed about this amazing plant and how it can influence the treatment of Parkinson's disease. You should confirm everything with him and not conceal any information that may affect the treatment of your disease.

6.2. A strategy to start using *Mucuna*

First of all, ask your neurologist who knows your case. He can tell you if you can be treated with *Mucuna* or not, based on your specific situation, based on the stage of your Parkinson's disease, and taking account other pathologies and conditions.

Secondly, your doctor will advise you on the purchase of the adequate formulation of *Mucuna* depending on the dose administered. It is prudent to start with low-dose tablets and subsequently increase gradually; there is always time to increase the dosage. Patience is key in the beginning: if you rush treatment for quick results, it is likely that you will experience some side effects which, although they are usually mild, can be bothersome. If the treatment proceeds too slowly on the other hand, you may think that the *Mucuna* is not working and give up.

Third, adjustment of the treatment: you almost always have to modify the dose and frequently have to remove some of the drugs previously prescribed (for Parkinson's disease or for your other pathologies).

6.3. Careful with mistakes in dosage

There is no proven effective dose for *Mucuna*. In clinical studies, some patients take 15 to 30 grams (half an ounce to one ounce) of *Mucuna* preparation orally for a week, but I discourage such quantities, which I consider too high.

Any medication (which *Mucuna* is) should be administered initially in small amounts, keeping in mind the particular case of the patient and the purpose of the treatment. Doses of 15 and 30 grams of *Mucuna* seed extract were used for a specific experiment, with strict medical checkups, knowing well the formulation of the product and its origin and taking into account many other factors.

The researchers work under controlled conditions: they select patients without contraindications and remove any incompatible drugs and other medications that may alter the absorption or metabolism of levodopa, etc. That is not what happens when a patient buys *Mucuna* just anywhere and self-medicates with little information and without medical supervision.

6.4. Be careful when buying *Mucuna*

A consumer may purchase capsules of 200 mg of levodopa with a 15% concentration or 800 mg tablets with a 50% concentration, and these are two completely different products. Sometimes patients have bought the product on eBay knowing nothing of their provider, and they receive a package whose content is not guaranteed and whose concentration is not safe. The patient then will then dilute the material in water without knowing how much to measure out. Always use *Mucuna* extracts that are dispensed by known, reliable suppliers. In the final chapter, we give a brief description of some of these.

6.5. Presentations

They are so widely available that the Internet is flooded with numerous commercial offers. In summary the presentations of *Mucuna* may be grouped into seven sections: (1) powder; (2) tinctures or concentrated extracts; (3) low-dose (15 to 30 mg of "real" natural levodopa) capsules or tablets, ideal to start taking *Mucuna*; (4) medium- or (5) high-dose capsules or tablets, (6) tincture or *Mucuna* drops, and (7) *Mucuna* mixed with other substances.

The classic presentation of *Mucuna*, the only one used in clinical trials, is powder from *Mucuna* seeds. It is very bothersome to prepare as the powder must be diluted in water or other liquid (not milk because it hinders absorption). It has a very unpleasant taste that laboratories try to hide by sweetening it. The great advantage is the ability to adjust the exact for smaller doses that are always recommended at the beginning. In countries (such as Spain) where it is more difficult to find capsules or tablets with small doses, one may start with *Mucuna* powder. There are many brands offered, but here I describe only the original, which is sent directly from India.

6.6. Zanpora HP-200

This drug was marketed in India after the publication of an innovative study in Parkinson's disease patients in which an average of six sachets (±3) of *Mucuna* seed powder (7.5 grams with levodopa 250 mg, i.e., 3.3%) were administered to each patient.

I would like to emphasize that this *Mucuna* levodopa dose is relatively high (1500 milligrams), especially for those who had never taken levodopa, and if combined with one or two tablets of Sinemet, there is an obvious risk of overdose. Other than those patients, there were no problems probably because this natural levodopa is not combined with carbidopa (as in Sinemet). In theory the levodopa from *Mucuna*, as it lacks carbidopa, should be removed rapidly from the blood, unless the plant contains other ingredients to avoid it.

After taking the *Mucuna* powder (dissolved in water), blood levels of levodopa behave similarly to those observed with the synthetic version of levodopa. The difference is that the maximum dose does not show as marked an effect [45] and clinical efficacy is similar or greater.

6.7. Common mistakes in prescribing Zandopa

Equivalences of Zandopa powder are administered to people who take only levodopa (without carbidopa), something which hardly occurs in the West, so that errors are very common.

According to the manufacturer, every measure of *Mucuna* powder (7.5 grams) is equivalent to 250 mg of synthetic levodopa. But this is only when the patient does not take carbidopa at all. However, almost all patients mix *Mucuna* powder with some Sinemet or Stalevo in which case it is necessary to assume that the carbidopa is working.

The equivalence for Zandopa is not clear to the uninitiated. If you follow the laboratory indications, you must give 30 grams of powder to replace the Sinemet 25/250 tablet (four small cups). This is the ratio that was used in the original study, but in practice it is too high and can cause side effects (nausea, vomiting, and malaise) so I do not recommend it. The dosage is individualized, and you have to start with small, adequately spaced doses. The laboratory has verified this and thus expressed it in the brochure, although not sufficiently emphasized.

7. *Mucuna* and conventional levodopa

Mucuna preparations usually sold online contain small amounts of levodopa. Furthermore, it is not combined with (carbidopa-like) "enhancers" and so has hardly any effect on symptoms.

As previously stated, in order to achieve the clinical effect of a tablet of Madopar or Sinemet, 1000 mg of levodopa *Mucuna* must be given. That would be like 4 scoops (30 g of seed powder) of Zandopa or nearly 17 capsules of other preparations providing 60 mg per dose. For example, a patient taking four daily tablets of Sinemet or Madopar who wants to switch to *Mucuna* alone would need 4000 mg natural levodopa daily, i.e., 120 mg of seed powder (a bottle of Zandopa contains 175 mg) or 66 capsules of Bonusan (60 mg levodopa each) or 40 capsules of Solbia (100 mg levodopa each). Few patients want to take on such a cost.

The problem is further complicated by the fact that the actual content of levodopa in many products sold online is lower than stated on the label [52].

7.1. Adding carbidopa to *Mucuna*

The synthetic levodopa in Sinemet is enhanced by carbidopa. This increases its clinical effectiveness and prevents peripheral side effects (nausea, tachycardia).

Carbidopa further improves the effects of *Mucuna*: it reduces the mild side effects and doubles or triples its effectiveness. This factor must be taken into account when a patient combines *Mucuna* and Sinemet (or Madopar or Stalevo): the carbidopa in these drugs also interacts with the natural levodopa in *Mucuna* by strengthening its clinical effects, and the dose should be greatly reduced.

And what happens when the patient does not take Sinemet or other drugs? Then *Mucuna* may be insufficient. These patients complain that *Mucuna* "does not do anything," and this is due to the fact that their decarboxylase is quickly removed from the blood, without allowing time for a sufficient amount to reach the brain.

The solution seems to be to add carbidopa, which in some countries is sold separately (as Lodosyn). When Lodosyn is not available, there is the option of taking half a tablet of Sinemet Plus (12.5 mg carbidopa) and subtract the amount of synthetic levodopa (50 mg), taking into account that it will now be more potent.

7.2. Enhancing levodopa

One inexpensive and clinically effective option is to use levodopa enhancers that are contained in conventional drugs. It is a good idea to mix the *Mucuna* seed powder with very low doses of Madopar (e.g., half a tablet in the morning and half at night). Thus, only 200 mg of synthetic levodopa is provided, but this has the advantage that there are 50 mg of benserazide included. This will greatly enhance the effectiveness of natural levodopa in the added *Mucuna*.

One can also add green tea; its polyphenols are inhibitors of decarboxylase (such as benserazide or carbidopa), further reinforcing the levodopa. The overall bioavailability of levodopa will be improved. In some patients a spectacular result has been obtained, as we have previously published [53, 54].

7.3. Risks of combining *Mucuna* and green tea

Green tea enhances the effect of beans in general and of *Mucuna* in particular. This effect can also be seen in patients taking Sinemet or Madopar: it is recommended that patients be aware of this phenomenon due to the increase in potency it can produce.

Carbidopa-like effect. There is something in green tea that acts like carbidopa. It contains polyphenols which inhibit dopa-decarboxylase [55], an action similar to that carried out by the carbidopa or benserazide contained in Sinemet or Madopar.

Entacapone-like effect. In addition, there is something that acts like entacapone in green tea. Polyphenol, epigallocatechin gallate (EGCG) promotes the entry into the brain of levodopa and prolongs its bioavailability in the bloodstream because it inhibits the COMT enzyme [56]. This action is similar to that of entacapone, namely, that beans mixed with green tea have Stalevo-like effects but with different proportions. Obviously, if you take levodopa (*Mucuna* or otherwise), its effectiveness will be reinforced, and this should be taken into account as there is risk of overdose. Always consult your doctor.

These "carbidopa-like" and "entacapone-like" effects can be seen with green tea, and they are independent of their other neuroprotective benefits [57] so the tea is recommended for many Parkinson's disease patients.

7.4. Complexities of adjusting *Mucuna*

As *Mucuna* seed powder does not contain carbidopa (theoretically), the clinical effectiveness of 1000 mg of natural is equivalent to a tablet of Sinemet 250/25 or of Madopar 200/50 (**Figure 1**).

7.5. *Mucuna*: the levodopa for the poor

In Africa and the Caribbean, I have seen Parkinson's disease patients in a very deteriorated state, who are not treated with levodopa because they are unable to afford Sinemet, Madopar, or Stalevo. Neither they nor their governments can bear this expense. Ironically in their countries, levodopa is everywhere; *Mucuna* grows spontaneously and spreads so fast that they even have to pull up it so it does not invade other crops.

The plant contains a large amount of levodopa, a treasure trove for those patients in the third world. Ailing inhabitants need this levodopa to live better and longer. It is outrageously unfair. A recent study [58] offered an option: the use of *Mucuna* levodopa is very accessible in countries that cannot afford Sinemet, Madopar, or Stalevo.

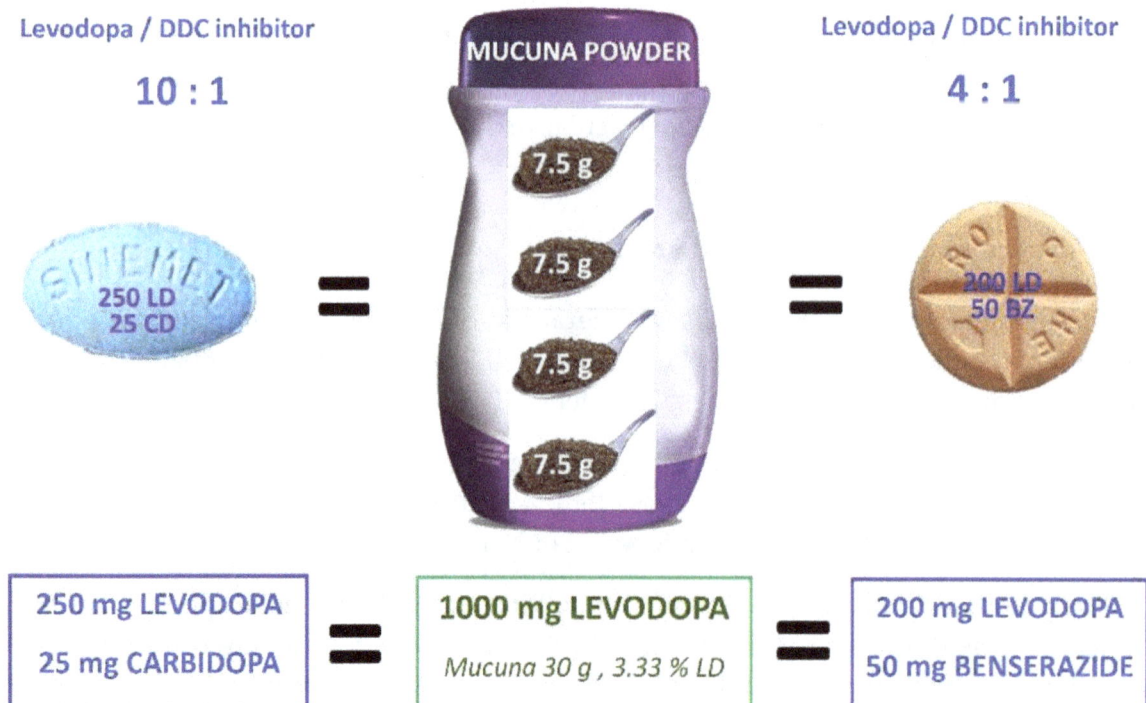

Figure 1. Clinical effectiveness of *Mucuna* compared with Sinemet and Madopar [54] (see text).

7.6. Neurologists in Ghana and Zambia

I applaud the laudable deeds of neurologists who have opened clinics for patients in Ghana and Zambia where they have already served over 100 patients. There they cannot prescribe Sinemet because it costs a prohibitive dollar and a half each day per patient; meanwhile *Mucuna pruriens* grows spontaneously all around them. With the collaboration of the local authorities, they began to systematically prepare seeds of *Mucuna* (harvesting 12 different types) cooking them first to eliminate antinutritive substances.

They administered *Mucuna* without special extraction methods, although they could not integrate carbidopa, and have obtained the first results: the levels of levodopa in the blood increase, demonstrating that it is being absorbed [58, 59]. Patients improved although the system is so primitive that they suffered some side effects such as nausea, dry mouth, and orthostatic hypotension [59].

The initiative of these pioneers of *Mucuna* treatment in Africa is promising. However, this situation must be regulated. Who could ever infringe on such an important humanitarian effort?

Studies of *Mucuna* in Parkinson's disease should be expanded. Inexpensive levodopa should be provided to patients with few resources in poor countries. It could be that doctors and patients of the West finally imitate the less fortunate.

Author details

Rafael González Maldonado

Address all correspondence to: info@neuroconsulta.com

Neuroconsulta, Granada, Spain

References

[1] Katzenschlager R et al. Mucuna pruriens in Parkinson's disease: A double blind clinical and pharmacological study. Journal of Neurology, Neurosurgery, and Psychiatry. 2004; **75**:1677

[2] Manyam BV, Dhanasekaran M, Hare TA. Effect of antiparkinson drug HP-200 (mucuna pruriens) on the central monoaminergic neurotransmitters. Phytotherapy Research. 2004; **18**:97-101

[3] Der Giessen RV, Olanow W, Lees A, Wagner H. Method for preparing *Mucuna pruriens* see extract. United States Patent, US 7,470,441 B2, Dec. 30, 2008

[4] Randhir R, Kwon YI, Shetty K. Improved health-relevant functionality in dark germinated mucuna pruriens sprouts by elicitation with peptide and phytochemical elicitors. Bioresource Technology. 2009;**100**:4507-4514

[5]   Raghavendra S et al. Enhanced production of L-DOPA in cell cultures of mucuna pruriens L. and mucuna prurita H. Natural Product Research. 2012;**26**:792-801

[6]   Aguilera Y et al. Changes in nonnutritional factors and antioxidant activity during germination of nonconventional legumes. Journal of Agricultural and Food Chemistry. 2013;**61**:8120-8125

[7]   Alleman RJ Jr et al. A blend of chlorophytum borivilianum and velvet bean increases serum growth hormone in exercise-trained men. Nutrition and Metabolic Insights. 2011;**4**:55-63

[8]   Obogwu MB, Akindele AJ, Adeyemi OO. Hepatoprotective and in vivo antioxidant activities of the hydroethanolic leaf extract of mucuna pruriens (Fabaceae) in antitubercular drugs and alcohol models. Chinese Journal of Natural Medicines. 2014;**12**:273-283

[9]   Majekodunmi SO et al. Evaluation of the anti-diabetic properties of mucuna pruriens seed extract. Asian Pacific Journal of Tropical Medicine. 2011;**4**:632-636

[10] Dharmarajan SK, Arumugam KM. Comparative evaluation of flavone from mucuna pruriens and coumarin from Ionidium suffruticosum for hypolipidemic activity in rats fed with high fat diet. Lipids in Health and Disease. 2012;**11**:126

[11] Grover JK, Rathi SS, Vats V. Amelioration of experimental diabetic neuropathy and gastropathy in rats following oral administration of plant (*Eugenia jambolana*). Indian Journal of Experimental Biology. 2002;**40**:273-276

[12] Golbabapour S et al. Acute toxicity and gastroprotective role of M. Pruriens in ethanol-induced gastric mucosal injuries in rats. BioMed Research International. 2013;**2013**:974185

[13] Suresh S, Prakash S. Effect of mucuna pruriens (Linn.) on sexual behavior and sperm parameters in streptozotocin-induced diabetic male rat. The Journal of Sexual Medicine. 2012;**9**:3066-3078

[14] Ahmad MK et al. Effect of mucuna pruriens on semen profile and biochemical parameters in seminal plasma of infertile men. Fertility and Sterility. 2008;**90**:627-635

[15] Champatisingh D et al. Anticataleptic and antiepileptic activity of ethanolic extract of leaves of mucuna pruriens: A study on role of dopaminergic system in epilepsy in albino rats. Indian Journal of Pharmacology. 2011;**43**:197-199

[16] Scirè A et al. The belonging of gpMuc, a glycoprotein from mucuna pruriens seeds, to the Kunitz-type trypsin inhibitor family explains its direct anti-snake venom activity. Phytomedicine. 2011;**18**:887-895

[17] Fung SY, Tan NH, Sim SM. Protective effects of mucuna pruriens seed extract pretreatment against cardiovascular and respiratory depressant effects of Calloselasma rhodostoma (Malayan pit viper) venom in rats. Tropical Biomedicine. 2010;**27**:366-372

[18] Manyam BV. Paralysis agitans and levodopa in "Ayurveda": Ancient Indian medical treatise. Movement Disorders. 1990;**5**:47-48

[19] Ovallath S, Deepa P. The history of parkinsonism: Descriptions in ancient Indian medical literature. Movement Disorders. 2013;**28**:566-568

[20] Manyam BV, Sánchez-Ramos JR. Traditional and complementary therapies in Parkinson's disease. Advances in Neurology. 1999;**80**:565-574

[21] Nagashayana N et al. Association of L-DOPA with recovery following Ayurveda medication in Parkinson's disease. Journal of the Neurological Sciences. 2000;**176**:124-127

[22] González-Maldonado R. Tratamientos heterodoxos en la enfermedad de Parkinson. North Charleston: CreateSpace; 2013. ISBN: 9788461652815

[23] Misra L, Wagner H. Extraction of bioactive principles from mucuna pruriens seeds. Indian Journal of Biochemistry & Biophysics. 2007;**44**:56-60

[24] Vaidya AB et al. Treatment of Parkinson's disease with the cowhage plant-mucuna pruriens Bak. Neurology India. 1978;**26**:171-176

[25] Kempster PA et al. Motor effects of broad beans (Vicia faba) in Parkinson's disease: Single dose studies. Asia Pacific Journal of Clinical Nutrition. 1993;**2**:85-89

[26] Rabey JM et al. Broad bean (Vicia faba) consumption and Parkinson's disease. Advances in Neurology. 1993;**60**:681-684

[27] González-Maldonado R. El extraño caso del Dr. Parkinson. Grupo Editorial Universitario. Granada, 1997. ISBN: 978849223685x

[28] Parkinson's Disease Study Group, PDSG. An alternative medicine treatment for Parkinson's disease: Results of a multicenter clinical trial. HP-200 in PD study group. Journal of Alternative and Complementary Medicine. 1995;**1**:249-255

[29] Manyam BV, Dhanasekaran M, Hare TA. Neuroprotective effects of the antiparkinson drug Mucuna pruriens. Journal of Phytotherapy Research. 2004;**18**:706-712

[30] Suchowersky O et al. Practice parameter: Neuroprotective strategies and alternative therapies for Parkinson disease (an evidence-based review). Report of the quality standards Subcommittee of the American Academy of neurology. Neurology. 2006;**66**:976-972

[31] Ramya KB, Thaakur S. Herbs containing L- Dopa: An update. Ancient Science of Life. 2007;**27**:50-55

[32] Hussian G, Manyam BV. Mucuna pruriens proves more effective than L-DOPA in Parkinson's disease animal model. Phytotherapy Research. 1997;**11**:419-423

[33] Behari M et al. Experiences of Parkinson's disease in India. Lancet Neurology. 2002;**1**:258-262

[34] Cilia R, Laguna J, Cassani E, et al. Mucuna pruriens in Parkinson disease: A double-blind, randomized, controlled, crossover study. Neurology. 2017;**89**:432-438. Published Online before print July 5, 2017. DOI 10.1212/WNL.0000000000004175

[35] Lieu CA et al. The Antiparkinsonian and Antidyskinetic mechanisms of mucuna pruriens in the MPTP-treated nonhuman primate. Evidence-based Complementary and Alternative Medicine. 2012;**2012**:840247

[36] Lieu CA et al. A water extract of mucuna pruriens provides long-term amelioration of parkinsonism with reduced risk for dyskinesias. Parkinsonism & Related Disorders. 2010;**16**:458-465

[37] Pathan AA et al. Mucuna pruriens attenuates haloperidol-induced orofacial dyskinesia in rats. Natural Product Research. 2011;**25**:764-771

[38] Lampariello LR et al. The magic velvet bean of mucuna pruriens. Journal of Traditional and Complementary Medicine. 2012;**2**:331-339

[39] Kasture S et al. Assessment of symptomatic and neuroprotective efficacy of mucuna pruriens seed extract in rodent model of Parkinson's disease. Neurotoxicity Research. 2009; **15**:111-122

[40] Yadav SK et al. Comparison of the neuroprotective potential of mucuna pruriens seed extract with estrogen in 1-methyl-4-phenyl-1,2,3,6-tetrahydropyridine (MPTP)-induced PD mice model. Neurochemistry International. 2014;**65**:1-13

[41] Dhanasekaran M, Tharakan B, Manyam BV. Antiparkinson drug--mucuna pruriens shows antioxidant and metal chelating activity. Phytotherapy Research. 2008;**22**:6-11

[42] Tharakan B et al. Anti-Parkinson botanical mucuna pruriens prevents levodopa induced plasmid and genomic DNA damage. Phytotherapy Research. 2007;**21**:1124-1126

[43] Yadav SK et al. Mucuna pruriens seed extract reduces oxidative stress in nigrostriatal tissue and improves neurobehavioral activity in paraquat-induced Parkinsonian mouse model. Neurochemistry International. 2013;**62**:1039-1047

[44] Lees A, Olanow WC, Der Giessen RV, Wagner H. Mucuna pruriens and extracts thereof for the treatment of neurological diseases. Patent WO 2004039385-A2, May 13, 2004

[45] Mahajani SS et al. Bioavailability of L-DOPA from HP-200 : A formulation of seed powder of mucuna pruriens (Bak) : A pharmacokinetic and pharmacodynamic study. Phytotherapy Research. 1996;**10**:254-256

[46] Pruthi SC, Pruthy P. Ayurvedic composition for the treatment of disorders of the nervous system including Parkinson's disease. Patent US 6106839 (2003) A. https://www. google.com/patents/US6106839

[47] Manyam BV, Dhanasekaran M, Cassady JM. Anti-Parkinson's disease pharmaceutical and method of use. United States Patent 20050202111-A1. http://www.freepatentsonline. com/y2005/0202111.html

[48] González MR. Parkinson y estrés. North Charleston: CreateSpace; 2013. ISBN: 9781492254447

[49] González MR. Conjeturas de un neurólogo que escuchó a mil parkinsonianos. North Charleston: CreateSpace; 2014. ISBN: 9788461679997

[50] Munhoz RP, Teive HA. Darkening of white hair in Parkinson's disease during use of levodopa rich mucuna pruriens extract powder. Arquivos de Neuro-Psiquiatria. 2013;**71**:133

[51] Infante ME et al. Outbreak of acute toxic psychosis attributed to mucuna pruriens. Lancet. 1990;**336**:1129

[52] Soumyanath A, Denne T, Peterson A, Shinto L. Assessment of commercial formulations of mucuna pruriens seeds for levodopa content. P01.36. International research congress on integrative medicine and health, Portland, Oregon 2012. BMC Complementary and Alternative Medicine. 2012;**12**(Suppl 1):S36

[53] González-Maldonado R, González-Redondo R, Di Caudo C. Beneficio de la combinación de mucuna, té verde y levodopa/benseracida en la enfermedad de Parkinson. Revista de Neurologia. 2016;**62**:525-526

[54] González-Maldonado R, González-Redondo R, Di Caudo C. The clinical effects of mucuna and green tea in combination with levodopa-benserazide in advanced Parkinson's disease: Experience from a case report. International Parkinson and movement disorders society, berlin june 2016. Movement Disorders. 2016;**31**(Suppl 2):S639

[55] Bertoldi M, Gonsalvi M, Voltattorni CB. Green tea polyphenols: Novel irreversible inhibitors of dopa decarboxylase. Biochemical and Biophysical Research Communications. 2001 Jun;**284**(1, 1):90-93

[56] Kang KS, Wen Y, Yamabe N, Fukui M, Bishop SC, Zhu BT. Dual beneficial effects of (−)-epigallocatechin-3-gallate on levodopa methylation and hippocampal neurodegeneration: In vitro and in vivo studies. PLoS One. 2010 Aug 5;**5**(8):e11951

[57] Guo S, Yan J, Yang T, Yang X, Bezard E, Zhao B. Protective effects of green tea polyphenols in the 6-OHDA rat model of Parkinson's disease through inhibition of ROS-NO pathway. Biological Psychiatry. 2007 Dec 15;**62**(12):1353-1362 Epub 2007 Jul 12

[58] Cassani E, et al. Natural therapy: *Mucuna pruriens*. A possible alternative in developing countries. 18th Movement Disorders Society Meeting, Stockholm; June 2014

[59] Cassani E, et al. *Mucuna pruriens*: A new strategy for Parkinson's disease treatment in Africa. An update. 18th Movement Disorders Society Meeting, Stockholm; June 2014

4

Stem Cell Therapy for Parkinson's Disease

Fabin Han

Abstract

Parkinson's disease (PD) is the second most common neurodegenerative disorder of aging after Alzheimer's disease (AD). Pathologically, it is characterized by a degeneration of dopamine (DA) neurons in substantia nigra of middle brain, which causes the motor symptoms and nonmotor symptoms of PD. The dopamine replacement therapy using levodopa and surgical treatment of deep brain stimulation (DBS) can only improve the symptoms of PD, but cannot stop the disease progression. Because of the selective loss of DA neurons, cell transplantation provides an exciting potential for the treatment of Parkinson's disease. The available cell sources include mesenchymal stem cells (MSCs) from bone marrow, neural stem cells (NSCs) from fetal brain tissues, embryonic stem cells (ESCs) from blastocysts, and induced pluripotent stem cells (iPSCs) reprogrammed from somatic cells transfected with stem cell transcription factors of OCT4, SOX2, KLF4, and c-MYC. Here, we first review the research advance conducted in animal models and patients of PD with these cells, then moving forward to recent development of iPSCs as a future source for the treatment of PD, and highlight the current challenges to make good manufacturing practice (GMP) standard cells suitable for large-scale production to move the cell-based therapy from dish to clinic as soon as possible.

Keywords: cell-based therapy, dopamine neuron, embryonic stem cell, induced pluripotent stem cell, neural stem cell, Parkinson's disease

1. Introduction

Parkinson's disease (PD) is affecting 1–2% of the population over the age of 60 years old and 3–5% of the population above the age of 85. Clinically, PD patients are characterized with four cardinal symptoms of resting tremors, muscle rigidity, bradykinesia, and postural instability. These motor symptoms appear when 60–80% of dopamine (DA) neurons in the substantia nigra are degenerated and are used as diagnostic criteria. The nonmotor symptoms have recently been highlighted as some of these symptoms including depression, constipation, pain, genitourinary problems, and sleep disorders may precede the motor dysfunction and can be used as early diagnosis and treatment of PD [1].

Because of the decrease of dopamine release in brains of PD patients, either increasing dopamine levels using drugs such as levodopa or reducing the dopamine degradation by dopamine inhibitor carbidopa can play therapeutic effects on PD patients [2]. A surgical treatment called deep brain stimulation (DBS) using electrodes to stimulate to the nucleus subthalamicus is also effective. However, surgical DBS is only suitable for a small portion of the patients and has unclear long-term benefits, while the medications have been found to decline in effectiveness over time and moreover cause the side-effect of dyskinesias (involuntary muscle movements). Recently, great treatment potential has been provided through replacing lost DA neurons using embryonic stem cells (ESCs), induced pluripotent stem cells (iPSCs) reprogrammed from patients' somatic fibroblasts or blood cells, neural stem cells (NSCs), or fully differentiated DA neurons from fetal brain tissue and mesenchymal stem cells (MSCs) sourced from fetuses or adults [3]. A lot of efforts have been done to find suitable cells to improve treatments not just of PD, but of all neurodegenerative diseases.

2. Etiology and molecular genetics

The causes of PD can be divided into genetic susceptible genes and environmental toxic environmental substances such as the pesticide rotenone and manganese, which integrate to damage the DA neurons through oxidative stress and mitochondrial impairment to induce PD. The majority of PD cases are sporadic or idiopathic with unknown causes (80–90%); the remained cases (10–20%) are familial and can be associated with PD-related genes or linked to a particular monogenic mutation [4–6]. Genetic factors play a minor role in causing typical PD, particularly for the patients having PD after 50 years of age [7]. This suggested that genetic factors are an important factor when the disease begins at or before the age of 50.

Genetic linkage analysis has great power to identify the disease genes for inherited monogenic diseases. By now more than 200 genes or loci have been characterized for neurological diseases and more than 100 genes or loci were reported for neuromuscular diseases including PD. The public available database for the genes or loci can be found in online catalog of human inherited genes and disorders (http://www.ncbi.nlm.nih.gov/omim/). The first gene for PD is the α-synuclein gene that was identified in 1997 [8]. Afterward more genes or loci were found to be responsible for familial PD. The characterized mutated genes for the autosomal dominant form of PD are SNCA and LRRK2 whereas the early-onset autosomal recessive genes for PD are PARK2 (Parkin), PINK1, and PARK7, ATP13A2. Some susceptible genes were also reported to be associated with PD such as Tau, Nurr1, and β-glucocerebrosidase (GBA). SNCA, which codes for α-synuclein, has been particularly well-studied and different point mutations (A53T, A30P, and E46K) in SNCA were found in different families with PD. It seems that the missense mutations of the SNCA gene are rare and the genomic rearrangements including the duplication and triplications of SNCA are more common to induce the aggregation of α-synuclein in the dopamine neurons.

Leucine-rich repeat kinase 2 (LRRK2) is another disease gene for autosomal dominant form of PD. It contains more than 50 exons and codes an 832-amino acid protein, which plays GTPase and kinase functions. Mutations can occur in any exons of LRRK2 gene, but the most common missense mutations are R1441C, Y1699C, G2019A, and I2020T. The G2019S mutation in LRRK2 is worldly prevalent, constituting 4% of familial PD cases and 1% of sporadic PD cases. Identification of mutations in the enzymatic GTPase and kinase domains suggests change of these enzymatic activities leads to disease development. Studies have shown that R1441 and Y1699 mutations decrease GTPase activity of LRRK2 whereas G2019S and I2020T mutations increase kinase activity [9, 10].

The second locus for PD is PARK2 for parkin gene. Parkin mutations were first reported in the autosomal recessive families of PD. The total genomic size of parkin covered 1.4 Mb. It contains 12 exons, and the gene product is a protein with 462 amino acids. The parkin has 30% homology to ubiquitin in the amino terminal domain and has two RING-finger-like motifs in the carboxyl part of the protein. It was reported that the RING-like structures in parkin have some ubiquitin-ligase activity. By now, more than 100 different mutations of *parkin* were found in familial and sporadic cases of PD. Most of the Parkin mutations are exonic deletions but missense, nonsense mutations, and genomic rearrangements were also found in PD families.

In addition to the autosomal dominant or recessive genes, some other genes are also reported to be associated with PD. NURR1 is one of the important transcription factors to regulate the development and maturation of the dopamine neurons. We had ever screened 202 familial and sporadic patients with PD and identified one patient has missense mutation of the NURR1 gene. This mutation produced a truncated NURR1 protein that loses the important functional domain to bind the promoter region of the tyrosine hydroxylase (TH), the key kinase to control the synthesis of the dopamine neurotransmitter [11]. GBA is another susceptible gene involved with PD. This gene encodes the lysosomal hydrolase β-glucocerebrosidase in which mutations are associated with neurodegenerative diseases, such as PD and GD (Gaucher's disease). We have performed a case–control study in a Chinese Cohort with PD and a Chinese control cohort by sequencing all the 12 exons of the GBA gene and found that the PD patients have significantly higher frequency of mutations in the GBA gene. Totally, we found nine reported and three novel GBA mutations in 184 Chinese patients. These known GBA mutations are R163Q, F213I, E326K, S364S, F347L, V375L, L444P, RecNciI, and Q497R and the novel mutations are 5-bp deletion (c.334_338delCAGAA), L264I and L314V. Importantly, we identified the novel 5-bp deletion (CAGAA) that produces a nonfunctional GBA protein of 142 amino acids, which loses major enzymatic function domains of the full GBA protein [12].

3. Pathological mechanisms

The mainly pathological mechanism of PD is the degeneration and loss of dopamine (DA) neurons in the substantia nigra of the mesencephalon. These DA neurons project to the basal ganglia (the striatum), which is responsible for motor control and function. The loss of DA neurons is accompanied by Lewy neuritis and Lewy bodies, which cause motor dysfunctions accompanied by an intensification of the disease, including cognitive impairment which encompasses hallucinations, dementia, and speech difficulties. The Lewy neurites might hamper the survival and dendritic development of neurons and glial cells through forming insoluble aggregates of α-synuclein (coded by *SCNA*), ubiquitin, and other misfolded proteins [13].

To understand the molecular mechanism and replicate the phenotypic features of PD, different animal models have been studied to explore dopaminergic neurotoxicity mainly using transgenic models of the familial PD-causing genes such as SNCA and LRRK2. The transgenic mice expressing human SNCA showed pathological inclusions in some neurons and glial cells, motor behavior deficits, and loss of dopaminergic neuron terminals in the basal ganglia. Overexpression of SNCA in drosophila leads to age-dependent dopaminergic neuron degeneration. Furthermore, the slowness of movement in LRRK2-G2019S transgenic mouse models was shown to be associated with diminished dopamine release and axonal pathology. These results support a causal role for α-synuclein in the development of PD. Some studies also suggest that the cellular toxicity in dopamine neurons may be caused by the soluble cytoplasmic oligomeric α-synuclein protein, whereas the large insoluble protein aggregates may represent a cellular defense mechanism in which the cell eventually convert cytotoxic-soluble oligomeric proteins into insoluble inclusion bodies. The α-synuclein-containing fibrils in the degenerative dopamine neurons can disturb cell membrane, leading to increased membrane permeability and eventual cell death of affected neural cells [14, 15]. Some studies showed that genetic mutations in PD genes can affect protein trafficking and cellular degradation machinery and eventually lead to development of PD, but the precise role of these mutated genes in disease progression and interaction with need to be further explored. A recent study reported that accumulation of α-synuclein reduced lysosomal degradation capacity in human midbrain dopamine neurons. Continuous aggregation of α-synuclein in the neural cells disrupted the endoplasmic reticulum–Golgi localization of the key genes such as RAB1a for vesicular transport. Overexpression of RAB1a restored the protein trafficking in endoplasmic reticulum–Golgi pathway and reduced pathological accumulation of α-synuclein in neurons. This study proposes that enhancement of lysosomal trafficking probably play beneficial roles in synucleinopathies [16]. Another molecular mechanism of PD is lysosomal dysfunction and the accumulation of glucosylceramide induced by decreased activity of β-glucocerebrosidase (GBA). Glucosylceramide played roles in stabilizing toxic oligomeric forms of α-synuclein and blocking transport of newly synthesized β-glucocerebrosidase from the endoplasmic reticulum to endocytic compartments, increasing the pathological aggregation of α-synuclein in neuronal cells. A recent study revealed that mutation in GBA is a major risk factor for the development of PD and the molecular pathways of pathological accumulation of glucosylceramide, related lipids, and α-synuclein will need to be studied for the identification of new therapeutic drugs for PD [12, 17].

4. Current stem cell sources for cell-based therapy of PD

Stem cell sources for the treatment of PD have been studied in the past decades. These cells mainly include mesenchymal stem cells from bone marrow and placenta; neural stem cells

(NSCs) and dopamine neurons from fetal brain tissue; embryonic stem cells (ESCs) of the blastocysts from in vitro fertilization; and induced pluripotent stem cells (iPSCs) reprogrammed from autologous somatic cells by expressing transgenes of OCT4, SOX2, c-MYC, and KLF4.

4.1. Mesenchymal stem cells

Mesenchymal stem cells (MSCs) were first reported in 1966, and were described as plastic-adherent colony-forming-unit fibroblastic (CFU-F) cells. MSCs are multipotent with potential to differentiate into different cells of mesodermal lineage and transdifferentiate into epithelial, endothelial, and neuronal cells. MSCs can be isolated from various neonatal and adult tissues such as bone marrow, adipose tissue, umbilical cord, cord blood, amnion, placenta, peripheral blood, and dental pulp [18]. Bone marrow-derived MSCs (BM-MSCs) are a potentially promising source of cells for use in regenerative medicine because they are abundantly available, easy to isolate from the patient themselves, an autologous tissue, and there is no ethical dispute over their use. Several studies have shown that BM-MSCs have the potential to regenerate DA neurons for the treatment of PD. Human BM-MSCs also have a protective effect on the progressive loss of DA neurons induced by carbobenzoxy-L-leucyl-L-leucyl-L-leucinal (MG-132) in vitro and in PD rats [19]. After grafted into the striatum, BM-MSCs were shown to exert neuroprotective effects against nigrostriatal degeneration and to improve motor function in 6-OHDA lesioned rats [20]. BM-MSCs grown in neuronal differentiation medium have more pronounced effect and improve the motor defects in a 6-OHDA fully lesioned rat PD model. BM-MSCs were induced to have neural morphology and expressed markers of DA neurons, such as tyrosine hydroxylase (TH), and most of the cells survived in striatum, expressed TH and behavioral recovery was observed after the cells were transplanted to a 6-OHDA mouse model. A human MSCs-induced DA subpopulation combined with pharmacologically active microcarriers grafted in a rat PD model also led to protection and repair of the nigrostriatal pathway and behavioral recovery.

The role of genetically modified MSCs for the protection and repair of damaged DA neurons and their therapeutic effects have been studied after implanted into PD models. Park et al. investigated the potential of MSCs genetically engineered with glial derived neurotrophic factor (GDNF) by viral transduction to deliver this potent neurotrophic factor for DA neurons in the brain. They found that MPTP(1-Methyl-4-phenyl-1,2,3,6-tetrahydropyridine) mice that were intravenously injected with GDNF-modified BM-MSCs possessed more TH-IR neurons and fibers and showed more prominent behavioral recovery compared with control mice that were implanted naive BM-MSCs [21]. Barzilay et al. reprogrammed the BM-MSCs toward dopaminergic differentiation through delivery of LMX1a, which was reported to be a key transcriptional factor of dopaminergic differentiation in both embryonic stem cells and developmental animal models. They found that the LMX1a protein was concentrated in the cell nuclei, and the cells with forced expression of LMX1a expressed higher levels of tyrosine hydroxylase, secreted significantly higher level of dopamine comparison with nontransduced cells [22]. Wang et al. tested a cytotherapeutic strategy combining cell transplantation and NTN/Lmx1α gene therapy to ameliorate disease progression in hemiparkinsonian rhesus.

They found induced rh-BMSCs exhibited gene/protein expression phenotypes resembling nigral dopaminergic neurons, and these cells survived and retained dopaminergic function following stereotaxic injection into the MPTP-lesioned hemiparkinsonian rhesus [23].

4.2. Neural stem cells and dopamine neurons from fetal brain tissue

Neural stem cells (NSCs) were first described as granule cells with a high proliferative activity in the brain cortex and middle brains. These cells have self-renewal and neural differentiation potential and can differentiate into neurons, astrocytes, and oligodendrocytes. In the developing brain, the distribution of NSCs demonstrate regionalization. For instance, only NSCs isolated from the midbrain have been reported to differentiate into A9 mesencephalic DA neurons necessary for treatment of PD patients. Moreover, NSCs can also be isolated from the other regions of fetal brain or from the subventricular zone (SVZ) and hippocampus of the adult mammalian brain, the regions where neurogenesis continues throughout the mammalian's lifespan [24, 25]. Since initial discoveries of NSCs in 1965, research advances in the isolation, expansion, and differentiation of NSCs have been made [26]. After transplantation in the adult rat brain, undifferentiated NSCs show some promise in treatment of PD. Human NSCs transplanted into the rat brain migrate and differentiate to neurons in a site-specific manner. Moreover, in PD rats with depleted host DA levels, engrafted NSCs were sensitive to environmental factors, appearing to differentiate preferentially to DA neurons.

NSCs can also be modified to overexpress the neurotrophic factors, which can increase the survival of the transplanted cells. Cai et al. studied some homeodomain proteins selectively expressed in DA progenitor cells in the ventral midbrain, and found that Lmx1a and Msx1 function as key factors triggering generation of DA neurons. Overexpressing the transcription factor ASCL1 was reported to be able to regain neurogenesis from human neural progenitor cells and to produce larger neurons with more neurites [27]. Animal study showed that forcing expression of Nurr1 promoted the mouse NSCs to differentiate into DA neurons and survive in 6-OHDA-lesioned PD rats. After transplantation of rodent and human fetal brain dopamine neurons to the midbrain of the 6-OHDA-lesioned rats, the cells survived well in the host brains and the motor defects of the PD rats were improved [28, 29]. Based on the results of animal studies, Lindvall et al. started the first clinical trials by transplanting fetal dopaminergic neurons or tissue to PD patients. Since then the clinical assessment protocols have been modified and significant effects were found by detecting behavioral and histological improvement [30, 31]. Moreover, younger PD patients showed more significant improvements, implying that the treatment efficiency may be limited in certain subpopulations. Generally, long-term graft survival was poor and did not convincingly justify the use of three to five human embryos per procedure [32]. In general, variable functional outcome has been showed from the clinical trials, but solid improvements need to be determined by clinical and imaging evaluations in the future [33, 34]. Transplantation of NSCs in PD patients also showed some side-effects. Olanow et al. reported that 56% of patients transplanted with fetal midbrain tissue developed persistent dyskinesia after overnight withdrawal of dopaminergic medication [35], which was much more than Freed et al.'s result of 15% of patients showing dyskinesias [31]. Its exact prevalence may be argued, while the recurrence of dyskinesia following neural transplantation has been well-proved. Some evidence showed that grafts containing serotonin neurons were easier to have this detrimental effect, therefore dyskinesias symptom may be alleviated by ensuring a homogeneous cell population in transplanted tissue [36].

Long-term follow-up results were shown in three individual clinical studies. One study found transplanted fetal midbrain DA neurons survived up to 14 years without pathology [37], whereas others found that α-synuclein-positive Lewy bodies in eventual spread to the transplanted DA neurons in PD patients [38, 39]. These findings suggest that PD can be an ongoing process with pathological changes. The controversy may be the reason of the difference between environmentally and genetically caused PD—a case of PD caused by environmental factors might be cured by the infusion of healthy cells, whereas a case of PD, which has been caused by genetic mutations would be an ongoing process. In general, DA neuron engraftment cannot be stated as a universally permanent treatment for PD; follow-up implantations may be further required for optimal effectiveness. Like all other allogeneic treatments, there is also a risk of graft rejection which must be repressed in the study [40]. Overall, the clinical trials with NSCs of fetal brains showed the survival of the transplanted cells and some improvements of symptoms in PD patients, whereas some results are over in dispute because of the diversities or limited cases of the PD patients [34]. **Table 1** summarized some of the clinical trials with fetal brain-derived NSCs or dopamine neurons.

No. of patients transplanted with NSC	Observation time	Symptom improvement 0/0	Side effect of dyskinesia	References and publication year
1	12 months	1/1	No	[41]
6	10–72 months	4/6	No	[42]
5	18–24 months	2/5	No	[43]
20/40	3 years	17/20	No	[31]
23/34	24 months	6/23	Yes	[35]
2	8 years	2/2	Yes	[44]
5	9–14 years	Not available	Not available	[37]
1	14 years	1/1	Yes	[39]
2	11–16 years	Not available	Not available	[38]
33	2–4 years	45%	Not available	[45]
3	13–16 years	Yes	Not available	[46]
2	18 and 15 years	2/2	Not available	[47]

Note: 23/34 indicates that 23 of 34 cases are in the group transplanted with NSCs and the other cases are in the control group.

Table 1. The clinical trials in PD patients transplanted with fetal brain-derived neural stem cells.

To further address the clinical therapeutic effects of the transplanted NSCs, and to provide new guidelines for clinical trials of fetal brain-derived cell therapy for PD treatment, a new, multicenter and collaborative study of European Union (TRANSEURO) was formed in 2010. These need careful selection of patients: early in the course of their disease (disease duration 2–10 years); aged 30–68 at the time of inclusion, showing a good response to levodopa; systematically evaluation of cell preparation, and location of transplantation; immunosuppression after transplantation and follow-up time; numbers of patients and clinical assessment standards. The new clinical trial for more than 100 patients suffered with PD has completed in this study, and results are in the analysis [48, 49].

4.3. Human embryonic stem cells (hESCs)-derived neural stem cells and dopamine neurons

Embryonic stem cells (ESCs) are self-renewing, pluripotent, and isolated from the inner cell mass cells of the preimplantation blastocysts. ESC can be differentiated into any kind of tissue cells including neural stem cells (NSCs), neurons, and DA neurons under special microenvironment. The differentiated neural stem cells, or fully differentiated neurons and dopamine neurons from mouse embryonic stem cell have been proved to have effects for PD neuroprotection [50].

Originally, human embryonic stem cells (hESCs) were isolated through culturing inner cell mass cells using mouse embryonic fibroblasts (MEFs) as feeder cells [51]. Since then, many groups have developed methods to direct the hESC differentiation to the neural stem cells and neurons, in particular dopamine neurons for the treatment of PD. Cooper et al. employed sonic hedgehog (SHH) and FGF8a as patterning factors in DA neuron induction [52]. The differentiation of hESCs to mesencephalic dopamine neurons was promoted by the application of specific patterning molecules that regulate mesencephalon development [53] or by applying growth factors SHH and FGF8a in a specific sequence [54]. Early exposure of FGF8a and SHH instructs early precursors to adopt a region identity which promotes DA neuron differentiation from mesencephalic neuroepithelial cells. These hESC-derived dopamine neurons were able to improve the motor deficiency of PD rat models, suggesting that grafted hESC-derived dopamine neurons played a role in vivo. The efficiency of DA production from pluripotent stem cells was greatly improved by Chamber et al. using a developed protocol through inhibiting SMAD signaling using Noggin and SB431542, with enhancing survival of mesencephalic DA neurons from hESCs [55]. They found that addition of Noggin and SB431542 for inhibiting SMAD signaling is sufficient to induce complete neural conversion of more than 80% of hESCs under adherent culture conditions. Fasano et al. found complimentary results, showing that neurons in development did not form toward anterior regionalization, but may be shifted toward a midbrain-like identity after FGF8 or Wnt1 treatment [56]. The same group developed a floor-plate-based protocol for generating hESCs-derived DA neurons in differentiation medium containing activators of sonic hedgehog (SHH) and canonical WNT signaling in vitro, further improved complete conversion of hESCs to the dopamine neurons and decreased the teratoma formation in vivo. They found that these DA neurons efficiently grew for several months in vitro and restored the amphetamine-induced rotation behaviors and improvements in tests of akinesia and forelimb use after transplanted to Parkinsonian monkeys and 6-OHDA-lesioned rats [57]. Sanchez-Danes et al. reported that using lentiviral expression of LMX1A, the key DA neuron-regulating gene, in hESCs to obtain more than 60% ventral mesencephalic DA neurons of the A9 subtype of all neurons differentiated from LMX1A-modified hESC [58]. Grealish et al. studied the functional properties of hESC-derived DA neurons in vivo by implanting hESC-derived mesencephalic dopamine neurons and fetal brain DA neurons into the brains of PD rats. They found that grafted hESC-DA neurons survived, projected long neural branches and played functions to improve the locomotive deficits of PD rats as similar as fetal brain DA neurons by MRI and PET imaging analysis, which provided further preclinical basis of hESC-derived dopamine neurons for PD patients' treatment [59].

To dissolve the major concerns for clinical use with stromal cells as feeder cells for culturing hESCs, some groups developed the implementation of factors which substitute for feeder cells. For example, Schulz et al. used a serum-free suspension system for generating the neurons, which are clinically applicable use [60]. Vazin et al. succeeded in substituting growth factors SDF-1, PTN, IGF2, and EFNB1 for the PA6 stromal cells, resulting in the induction of differentiating hESCs directly to TH-positive DA neurons without requiring this initial induction step [61]. During differentiating hESCs to NSCs, Swistowski et al. reported that growth factors SHH and FGF8 substitute for PA6 stromal cells for generating DA cells after an initial induction step. They endeavored a culture protocol applicable to the clinic and following to the standards of good manufacturing protocol (GMP). In their culture process, serum is not involved, but they found cells could be stored at each of the intermediate stages in their four-step process (propagation of ESC→generation of neural stem cells (NSC)→induction of dopaminergic precursors→maturation of dopaminergic neurons) without loss of functional ability, which is an important discovery that allowing cells to be transplanted at an appropriate time point in neural development [62].

Though many studies demonstrated hESCs can be differentiated to DA neurons efficiently in vitro and showed solid functional results to restore the motor defects in PD animal models including mice, rats, and nonhuman primates, clinical trials have not been performed for treating the PD patients because of the immune-rejection and ethical issues.

4.4. Induced pluripotent stem cells (iPSCs)-derived neural stem cells or dopamine neurons

Previous studies showed an undifferentiated state of cells could be reprogrammed from differentiated somatic cells using the somatic cell nuclear transfer (SCNT). SCNT technology is available to make the cloned lambs and cows. However, no studies were described generating patient-specific cells using this SCNT technique [63, 64]. The successful induction of mouse iPSCs from mouse embryonic and adult fibroblasts were first demonstrated in Yamanaka lab in 2006 by introducing four transcription factors of Oct3/4, Sox2, c-Myc, and Klf4 [65]. Soon afterward, human iPSCs and patient-specific iPSCs with different diseases including PD were also generated from several labs by introducing the human orthologs of these four transcription factors (OCT4, SOX2, c-MYC, and KLF4) or OCT4, SOX2, NANOG, and LIN28 [66, 67]. The implication of Oct3/4 and Sox2 was shown to play an essential role in the propagation of undifferentiated ESCs in culture. The roles of Klf4 and c-Myc were equally undecided. Later studies described that the only genes indispensable in generating iPSCs were Oct3/4 and Sox2 but not Klf4 and c-Myc [68]. Similar to ESCs, iPSCs are self-renew indefinitely and pluripotent. However, iPSCs overcome the problems associated with BM-MSCs, fetal NSCs and hESCs, as they reprogram from the already-differentiated somatic cells of an organism back to their embryonic-like pluripotent state. iPSCs generated from patients will have wide applications for exploring the molecular mechanisms and cell-based therapy of neurodegenerative diseases such as PD [69, 70].

In clinical applications, one of the major advantages of iPSCs over BM-MSCs, fetal NSCs, and hESCs is that iPSCs can be generated from the cells of the individual being treated. As the cultured cells will be autologous, this key trait of iPSCs theoretically enhances their integration into the brain tissues of PD patients and minimizes the risk of rejection. Furthermore, the ethical problems of using aborted fetuses as a cell source are avoided. Once reprogrammed into iPSC state from the mature cells, the iPSCs can be systematically exposed to specific factors that promote their differentiation into a specific lineage (such as NSCs or DA neurons) [71]. Until now, a ton of work has been done to improve the generation, differentiation, and potential clinical applications of iPSCs, especially with great efforts made to bring these therapeutic cells to meet GMP (good manufacturing practice) standards, to translate them to the clinic for treatment of neurodegenerative diseases like PD. iPSCs have also been used in other fields such as diseases model to study the molecular mechanisms of the disease and as drug screening and discovery.

To determine the clinical potential of iPSCs-derived cells, the therapeutic effects of mouse iPSCs were analyzed after transplanting them into the rat brains. Wernig et al. reported that grafted iPSCs matured into midbrain-like dopamine neurons, resulting in behavioral improvements in rat PD models [72].

It was found that DA neurons from the iPSCs with LRRK2 mutation (G2019S) were sensitive to oxidative stress and had α-synuclein aggregation and more expression of key oxidative stress-response genes. The phenotypic neurodegeneration of the differentiated DA neurons could be rescued by correction of LRRK2 G2019S mutation in iPSCs, supporting LRRK2 mutation playing an important role in the pathogenesis of PD [73]. The virus-free PD-iPS cells-derived DA neurons were transplanted to the 6-OHDA-lesioned rats and it was found that these DA neurons survived and provided functional improvements in PD rats by alleviating motor defects induced by apomorphine [74]. Recently, our lab made efforts to generate of iPS cells by retrovirus-mediated expression of OCT4, SOX2, c-MYC, and KLF4 from skin fibroblasts of PD patients and control individuals, and studied the differentiation of iPSCs to NSCs and DA neurons, and then transplanted the iPSCs-derived NSCs into the striatums of the 6-OHDA-induced PD rats. iPSCs carrying the transgenes can also be differentiated to the NSCs and be fully differentiated to neurons and DA neurons in vitro and in vivo. The grafted iPS cells-derived NSCs significantly improved the rotational asymmetry of PD rats [4]. Further work are needed to improve the differentiation efficiency of neurons and DA neurons by incorporating growth factors and iPSCs together for transplantation, or elevating the dose of immune-suppressive agents to lower the immune-rejection against the human-derived cells, or renewing the cell culture protocols.

Much work has been done toward improving the efficiency of iPSCs generation in absence of c-Myc. Stadtfeld et al. reprogrammed mouse liver cells into iPSCs using nonintegrating, replication-incompetent adenoviruses carrying the classic four transcription factors [75]. Okita et al. developed an approach that repeated transfection of plasmids containing the appropriate genes (one containing the complementary DNAs of Oct3/4, SOx2, and Klf4; the other, c-Myc) into embryonic fibroblasts could generate iPSCs [76]. Yu et al. developed a further protocol to iPSC generation by using nonintegrating episomal vectors, which allows the derivation of iPSCs free of vector and transgene sequences completely [77]. The direct protein transduction system free of DNA vector was also proposed to generate iPSCs to remove potential risks in association with chromosomal integrations and mutations [78].

This claim is verified by the follow-up study through comparing the cellular properties of human iPSCs (hiPSC) generated by chromosome integrating with nonintegrating methods. They found consistent differences in cellular and differentiation properties between hiPSCs from nonintegrating and integrating reprogramming factors. According to their results, protein-based reprogramming of cells into hiPSCs resulted in cells showed no obvious exogenous reprogramming gene expression, therefore behaved most similar to hESCs [79].

Many efforts have been done to achieve clinical-grade DA neurons with a stable phenotype, the A9 subtype DA neurons. From both human ES/iPS cells, a strategy for efficient differentiation and sorting DA neurons has been developed by Isacson et al. From iPSC-differentiated neural cells, the NCAM (+)/CD29 (low)-enriched ventral mesencephalic DA neurons were sorted. The sorted neurons were positive for EN1/TH and FOXA2/TH and had elevated expression levels of GIRK2, FOXA2, PITX3, LMX1A, NURR1, TH, and EN1 which indicated that the sorted neural cells are DA neurons. These iPSC-derived DA neurons were able to restore behavior activity of PD rats after transplantation. The sorted cells transplanted to the PD rats were integrated into the brain tissue. Their results provided molecular basis for the safety and feasibility of iPSC-derived cell therapies [80].

The similarity and differences between iPSCs and ESC is another issue about iPSCs. Many studies succeeded in generating both human iPSCs and mouse iPSCs identical to ESCs developmentally and epigenetically by improving end points for the reprogramming process [81]. Other groups have also made modifications to reduce the mutagenic potential of the lentiviruses and retroviruses By using non-integrating methods or omitting the KLF4 or c-MYC. For instance, Muller et al. found that substituting Nanog and Lin28 for Klf4 and c-Myc [67] was one way to reduce this risk. The reactivation of the c-Myc retrovirus particularly promotes the risk of mutations, because of tumorigenicity [82]. However, the efficiency of iPSC formation was far lower after eliminations of c-Myc from the protocol. This suggests that the role of c-Myc is not being necessary in the establishing pluripotency itself but to accelerate proliferation or otherwise enhance the speed of events establishing pluripotency [83]. Although the generated iPSCs in morphology, growth properties, and differentiation into different germ layers were very similar to ESCs, differences between iPSCs and ESCs were detected, which may be the reason by using different iPSC lines [84]. Recently at the molecular levels, the similarity and difference between iPSCs and hESCs were studied. In one study, Koyanagi-Aoi et al found that only two hiPSC lines had different gene expression and DNA methylation through analyzing 49 hiPSC lines and 10 hESC lines. And they found that only seven hiPSC lines formed some undifferentiated cells by comparing neural differentiation in vitro between 40 hiPSC lines and 10 hESC lines. This study showed that hiPSCs are very similar to hESCs [85].

The important point is that such protocols need to meet a xeno-free, scalable system for the clinic. A suspension culture system was created for the neural differentiation of hESCs and hiPSCs [86]. Such systems allowed long-term cell culture while keeping appropriate marker expression, normal karyotype, and pluripotency. To decrease the effects of transgenes on iPSCs functions, several labs developed protocols to use two or three factors to generate iPSCs. Using single factor of OCT4 in combination of small molecules of VPA, TGF-β inhibitor (616452), CHIR 99021, iPSCs can be reprogrammed from mouse adult and embryonic fibroblasts [68]. Omitting the OCT4, the naive iPSCs derived from rhesus monkey fibroblasts can be obtained with only small molecules, which provided a valuable cell source for further use in disease modeling and preclinical study [87]. Though iPSCs bring great potentials to the cell-based PD therapy, much work is needed for the researchers to find other convenient method to obtain DA neurons as the complicated procedures for generation, characterization, and differentiation to the DA neurons. Directly reprograming the fibroblasts of PD patients to DA neurons is one of the other approaches. Using different combinations of transcription factors such as Nurr1 (Nr4a2), Mash1 (Ascl1), Sox2, Ngn2, Lmx1a, and Pitx3, DA neurons were directly reprogrammed from the fibroblasts [88, 89]. Since the lentiviral vectors were used to express the genes related in most direct reprogramming methods for development of DA neurons, this can cause the safety concerns for use of the directly reprogrammed DA neurons in PD patients. However, the research advance will overcome these issues and finally bring these cells to clinical trials for PD.

5. Future aspects and challenges for clinical application of iPSCs

The NSCs and DA neurons from fetal brain and hESCs are not suitable for wide clinical use because of their immune-rejections and ethical issues. The availability of iPSCs has great potential for autologous cell-based therapy of PD. The treatment of eye-disorders using iPSCs for clinical trial has been initiated in Japan. However, several aspects of iPSCs are further needed to be resolved for clinical use. These include genetic and epigenetic abnormalities, low yields of DA neurons, and the safety of iPSC-derived cells.

5.1. Low yield

Low yield of fully reprogrammed cells is by no means an inherent property of iPSC generation and there will continue to be yield improvements in the future. Low yield is a potential problem, addition of VPA and other chemicals increased the original yields of 0.05% [90]. iPSCs can theoretically be sourced from anywhere on the adult human, such as stomach cells, liver cells, and human hair cells, with varying yields across experiments [75]. In fact, Aasen et al. generated keratinocyte-derived iPSCs using cells from adult human hairs with a 100-fold increase in efficiency compared to human fibroblast reprogramming, and found these iPSCs were indistinguishable from ESCs [91]. In any case, with the goal of optimizing methods for maximum cell yield of iPS cells, avenues must include comparisons between method efficiencies in the future.

5.2. Genetic and epigenetic abnormalities

It is unclear whether iPSCs cells toward a cell fate related to their donor source or otherwise maintaining a reprogramming signature after differentiation [92]. For the generation of clinical applicable iPS cells, the lentivirus or retrovirus-mediated reprogramming methods should be replaced by nonintegrating vectors to express the reprogramming genes or combine with small molecules [93]. Some iPSCs from PD patients may also have gene mutations such as chromosomal structure variation, point mutation, gene deletions, and duplications [12, 94]. It is not suitable to use the cells derived from iPSCs with genetic mutations for direct transplantation as the functions of cells are affected by the genetic mutations. Many reports developed protocols to correct the mutation in PD patient-derived iPSCs. Reinhardt et al. showed that iPSCs with *LRRK2* G2019S mutation was corrected and the *LRRK2* correction produced phenotype rescue in differentiated neurons [73]. Soldner et al. reported that the iPSCs with *SNCA* mutation (A53T) was repaired using zinc-finger nuclease (ZFN)-mediated nuclease approach and genetic repair of the A53T mutation in the patient-derived iPSCs did not affect the differentiation ability to dopaminergic neurons. The correctly repaired patient-derived iPSC lines were confirmed through PCR genotyping and sequencing analysis [95].

5.3. Safety and purity

It is required that the residues of undifferentiated iPSCs should be less than 1% to avoid the teratoma formation after transplantation, in the aim to obtain iPSC-derived NSCs or DA neurons for transplantation. FACS or other noninvasive magnetic selections were used for developing the approaches to sort the iPSC-derived cells. Moreover, the cell culture in feeder-free conditions are needed to avoid the contamination of animal sources. Currently, murine-derived feeder cells are widely used to maintain hESCs and hiPSCs. In addition, these feeder cells are normally cultured in culture medium including fetal bovine serum (FBS). This would enhance the possibility to cause the allogenic cell contamination of the iPSC-derived cells. Nakagawa et al. developed a new feeder-free system to culture the hESCs and iPSCs in StemFit™ medium, which made a big step to make clinically applicable GMP-standard cells [96].

6. Conclusion: moving forward to the clinic

Cell-based therapy holds clinical potential for the treatment of many neurodegenerative disorders including PD. The use of BM-MSCs, fetal NSCs, and ESCs is facing with safety and ethical concerns. However, recently great advance is making in developing iPSC-derived cells for PD. Animal studies using injection iPSCs and their derivatives into animal models have shown promise in treatment of disorders such as PD. However in clinical trials for PD, iPSCs have not been used until their limitations are overcome. Therefore, a relevant therapeutic progenitor or mature cell type may be identified and grafted in such treatments; in the case of PD, the options are of course iPSC-derived DA neurons and iPSC-derived NSCs.

Acknowledgements

This work was supported by National Natural Science Foundation of China (NSFC 81571241) and Program of high-educated Foreign Scholars, Shandong Province, China (201309116SDWZ). The author also thanks Jing Duan and Qingfa Chen for their technical and editing the manuscript.

Author details

Fabin Han*

Address all correspondence to: fhan2013@126.com

The Institute for Tissue Engineering and Regenerative Medicine, Liaocheng University/The Liaocheng People's Hospital, Shandong, China

References

[1] Berg, D., R.B. Postuma, B. Bloem, P. Chan, B. Dubois, T. Gasser, C.G. Goetz, G.M. Halliday, J. Hardy, A.E. Lang, I. Litvan, K. Marek, J. Obeso, W. Oertel, C.W. Olanow, W. Poewe, M. Stern, and G. Deuschl. Time to redefine PD? Introductory statement of the MDS Task Force on the definition of Parkinson's disease. Mov Disord. 2014; 29(4): 454–62.

[2] Olanow, C.W., R.L. Watts, and W.C. Koller. An algorithm (decision tree) for the management of Parkinson's disease (2001): treatment guidelines. Neurology. 2001; 56(11 Suppl 5): S1–S88.

[3] Takahashi, K., K. Tanabe, M. Ohnuki, M. Narita, T. Ichisaka, K. Tomoda, and S. Yamanaka. Induction of pluripotent stem cells from adult human fibroblasts by defined factors. Cell. 2007; 131(5): 861–72.

[4] Han, F., W. Wang, B. Chen, C. Chen, S. Li, X. Lu, J. Duan, Y. Zhang, Y.A. Zhang, W. Guo, and G. Li. Human induced pluripotent stem cell–derived neurons improve motor asymmetry in a 6-hydroxydopamine–induced rat model of Parkinson's disease. Cytotherapy. 2015; 17(5): 665–79.

[5]   Lesage, S. and A. Brice. Parkinson's disease: from monogenic forms to genetic suscept-
       ibility factors. Hum Mol Genet. 2009; 18(R1): R48–59.

[6]   Chen, M.L., C.H. Lin, M.J. Lee, and R.M. Wu. BST1 rs11724635 interacts with environ-
       mental factors to increase the risk of Parkinson's disease in a Taiwanese population.
       Parkinsonism Relat Disord. 2014; 20(3): 280–3.

[7]   Tanner, C.M., R. Ottman, S.M. Goldman, J. Ellenberg, P. Chan, R. Mayeux, and J.W.
       Langston. Parkinson disease in twins: an etiologic study. JAMA. 1999; 281(4): 341–6.

[8]   Polymeropoulos, M.H., C. Lavedan, E. Leroy, S.E. Ide, A. Dehejia, A. Dutra, B. Pike, H.
       Root, J. Rubenstein, R. Boyer, E.S. Stenroos, S. Chandrasekharappa, A. Athanassia-
       dou, T. Papapetropoulos, W.G. Johnson, A.M. Lazzarini, R.C. Duvoisin, G. Di Iorio, L.I.
       Golbe, and R.L. Nussbaum. Mutation in the alpha-synuclein gene identified in families
       with Parkinson's disease. Science. 1997; 276(5321): 2045–7.

[9]   Grimes, D.A., L. Racacho, F. Han, M. Panisset, and D.E. Bulman. LRRK2 screening in
       a Canadian Parkinson's disease cohort. Can J Neurol Sci. 2007; 34(3): 336–8.

[10] Martin, I., J.W. Kim, V.L. Dawson, and T.M. Dawson. LRRK2 pathobiology in
       Parkinson's disease. J Neurochem. 2014; 131(5): 554–65.

[11] Grimes, D.A., F. Han, M. Panisset, L. Racacho, F. Xiao, R. Zou, K. Westaff, and D.E.
       Bulman. Translated mutation in the Nurr1 gene as a cause for Parkinson's disease. Mov
       Disord. 2006; 21(7): 906–9.

[12] Yu, Z., T. Wang, J. Xu, W. Wang, G. Wang, C. Chen, L. Zheng, L. Pan, D. Gong, X. Li,
       H. Qu, F. Li, B. Zhang, W. Le, and F. Han. Mutations in the glucocerebrosidase gene
       are responsible for Chinese patients with Parkinson's disease. J Hum Genet. 2015; 60(2):
       85–90.

[13] Dawson, T.M., H.S. Ko, and V.L. Dawson. Genetic animal models of Parkinson's
       disease. Neuron. 2010; 66(5): 646–61.

[14] Gonzalez-Horta, A. The Interaction of Alpha-synuclein with Membranes and its
       Implication in Parkinson's Disease: a literature review. Nat Prod Commun. 2015; 10(10):
       1775–8.

[15] Fares, M.B., N. Ait-Bouziad, I. Dikiy, M.K. Mbefo, A. Jovicic, A. Kiely, J.L. Holton, S.J.
       Lee, A.D. Gitler, D. Eliezer, and H.A. Lashuel. The novel Parkinson's disease linked
       mutation G51D attenuates in vitro aggregation and membrane binding of alpha-
       synuclein, and enhances its secretion and nuclear localization in cells. Hum Mol Genet.
       2014; 23(17): 4491–509.

[16] Mazzulli, J.R., F. Zunke, O. Isacson, L. Studer, and D. Krainc. alpha-Synuclein-in-
       duced lysosomal dysfunction occurs through disruptions in protein trafficking in
       human midbrain synucleinopathy models. Proc Natl Acad Sci U S A. 2016; 113(7): 1931–
       6.

[17] Blanz, J. and P. Saftig. Parkinson's disease: acid-glucocerebrosidase activity and alpha-synuclein clearance. J Neurochem. 2016.

[18] Hass, R., C. Kasper, S. Bohm, and R. Jacobs. Different populations and sources of human mesenchymal stem cells (MSC): a comparison of adult and neonatal tissue-derived MSC. Cell Commun Signal. 2011; 9: 12.

[19] Park, H.J., P.H. Lee, O.Y. Bang, G. Lee, and Y.H. Ahn. Mesenchymal stem cells therapy exerts neuroprotection in a progressive animal model of Parkinson's disease. J Neurochem. 2008; 107(1): 141–51.

[20] Blandini, F., L. Cova, M.T. Armentero, E. Zennaro, G. Levandis, P. Bossolasco, C. Calzarossa, M. Mellone, B. Giuseppe, G.L. Deliliers, E. Polli, G. Nappi, and V. Silani. Transplantation of undifferentiated human mesenchymal stem cells protects against 6-hydroxydopamine neurotoxicity in the rat. Cell Transplant. 2010; 19(2): 203–17.

[21] Park, K.W., M.A. Eglitis, and M.M. Mouradian. Protection of nigral neurons by GDNF-engineered marrow cell transplantation. Neurosci Res. 2001; 40(4): 315–23.

[22] Barzilay, R., T. Ben-Zur, S. Bulvik, E. Melamed, and D. Offen. Lentiviral delivery of LMX1a enhances dopaminergic phenotype in differentiated human bone marrow mesenchymal stem cells. Stem Cells Dev. 2009; 18(4): 591–601.

[23] Wang, W.P., Z.L. He, S.Y. Lu, M. Yan, Y. Zhou, T.H. Xie, N. Yin, W.J. Wang, D.H. Tang, H.J. Li, and M.S. Sun. Dopaminergic neuron-like cells derived from bone marrow mesenchymal stem cells by Lmx1alpha and neurturin overexpression for autologous cytotherapy in hemiparkinsonian rhesus monkeys. Curr Stem Cell Res Ther. 2015; 10(2): 109–20.

[24] Eriksson, P.S., E. Perfilieva, T. Bjork-Eriksson, A.M. Alborn, C. Nordborg, D.A. Peterson, and F.H. Gage. Neurogenesis in the adult human hippocampus. Nat Med. 1998; 4(11): 1313–7.

[25] Taupin, P. and F.H. Gage. Adult neurogenesis and neural stem cells of the central nervous system in mammals. J Neurosci Res. 2002; 69(6): 745–9.

[26] Kallur, T., V. Darsalia, O. Lindvall, and Z. Kokaia. Human fetal cortical and striatal neural stem cells generate region-specific neurons in vitro and differentiate extensively to neurons after intrastriatal transplantation in neonatal rats. J Neurosci Res. 2006; 84(8): 1630–44.

[27] Kim, H.J., E. McMillan, F. Han, and C.N. Svendsen. Regionally specified human neural progenitor cells derived from the mesencephalon and forebrain undergo increased neurogenesis following overexpression of ASCL1. Stem cells. 2009; 27(2): 390–8.

[28] Studer, L., V. Tabar, and R.D. McKay. Transplantation of expanded mesencephalic precursors leads to recovery in parkinsonian rats. Nat Neurosci. 1998; 1(4): 290–5.

[29] Monni, E., C. Cusulin, M. Cavallaro, O. Lindvall, and Z. Kokaia. Human fetal striatum-derived neural stem (NS) cells differentiate to mature neurons in vitro and in vivo. Curr Stem Cell Res Ther. 2014; 9(4): 338–46.

[30] Lindvall, O., G. Sawle, H. Widner, J.C. Rothwell, A. Bjorklund, D. Brooks, P. Brundin, R. Frackowiak, C.D. Marsden, P. Odin, et al. Evidence for long-term survival and function of dopaminergic grafts in progressive Parkinson's disease. Ann Neurol. 1994; 35(2): 172–80.

[31] Freed, C.R., P.E. Greene, R.E. Breeze, W.Y. Tsai, W. DuMouchel, R. Kao, S. Dillon, H. Winfield, S. Culver, J.Q. Trojanowski, D. Eidelberg, and S. Fahn. Transplantation of embryonic dopamine neurons for severe Parkinson's disease. N Engl J Med. 2001; 344(10): 710–9.

[32] Hagell, P. and P. Brundin. Cell survival and clinical outcome following intrastriatal transplantation in Parkinson disease. J Neuropathol Exp Neurol. 2001; 60(8): 741–52.

[33] Lindvall, O. and A. Bjorklund. Cell therapy in Parkinson's disease. NeuroRx. 2004; 1(4): 382–93.

[34] Barker, R.A., J. Barrett, S.L. Mason, and A. Bjorklund. Fetal dopaminergic transplantation trials and the future of neural grafting in Parkinson's disease. Lancet Neurol. 2013; 12(1): 84–91.

[35] Olanow, C.W., C.G. Goetz, J.H. Kordower, A.J. Stoessl, V. Sossi, M.F. Brin, K.M. Shannon, G.M. Nauert, D.P. Perl, J. Godbold, and T.B. Freeman. A double-blind controlled trial of bilateral fetal nigral transplantation in Parkinson's disease. Ann Neurol. 2003; 54(3): 403–14.

[36] Politis, M., K. Wu, C. Loane, N.P. Quinn, D.J. Brooks, S. Rehncrona, A. Bjorklund, O. Lindvall, and P. Piccini. Serotonergic neurons mediate dyskinesia side effects in Parkinson's patients with neural transplants. Sci Transl Med. 2010; 2(38): 38ra46.

[37] Mendez, I., A. Viñuela, A. Astradsson, K. Mukhida, P. Hallett, H. Robertson, T. Tierney, R. Holness, A. Dagher, and J.Q. Trojanowski. Dopamine neurons implanted into people with Parkinson's disease survive without pathology for 14 years. Nat Med. 2008; 14(5): 507.

[38] Li, J.Y., E. Englund, J.L. Holton, D. Soulet, P. Hagell, A.J. Lees, T. Lashley, N.P. Quinn, S. Rehncrona, A. Bjorklund, H. Widner, T. Revesz, O. Lindvall, and P. Brundin. Lewy bodies in grafted neurons in subjects with Parkinson's disease suggest host-to-graft disease propagation. Nat Med. 2008; 14(5): 501–3.

[39] Kordower, J.H., Y. Chu, R.A. Hauser, T.B. Freeman, and C.W. Olanow. Lewy body-like pathology in long-term embryonic nigral transplants in Parkinson's disease. Nat Med. 2008; 14(5): 504–6.

[40] Michel-Monigadon, D., V. Nerriere-Daguin, X. Leveque, M. Plat, E. Venturi, P. Brachet, P. Naveilhan, and I. Neveu. Minocycline promotes long-term survival of neuronal

transplant in the brain by inhibiting late microglial activation and T-cell recruitment. Transplantation. 2010; 89(7): 816–23.

[41] Lindvall, O., P. Brundin, H. Widner, S. Rehncrona, B. Gustavii, R. Frackowiak, K.L. Leenders, G. Sawle, J.C. Rothwell, C.D. Marsden, and et al. Grafts of fetal dopamine neurons survive and improve motor function in Parkinson's disease. Science. 1990; 247(4942): 574–7.

[42] Wenning, G.K., P. Odin, P. Morrish, S. Rehncrona, H. Widner, P. Brundin, J.C. Rothwell, R. Brown, B. Gustavii, P. Hagell, M. Jahanshahi, G. Sawle, A. Bjorklund, D.J. Brooks, C.D. Marsden, N.P. Quinn, and O. Lindvall. Short- and long-term survival and function of unilateral intrastriatal dopaminergic grafts in Parkinson's disease. Ann Neurol. 1997; 42(1): 95–107.

[43] Hagell, P., A. Schrag, P. Piccini, M. Jahanshahi, R. Brown, S. Rehncrona, H. Widner, P. Brundin, J.C. Rothwell, P. Odin, G.K. Wenning, P. Morrish, B. Gustavii, A. Bjorklund, D.J. Brooks, C.D. Marsden, N.P. Quinn, and O. Lindvall. Sequential bilateral transplantation in Parkinson's disease: effects of the second graft. Brain. 1999; 122 (Pt 6): 1121–32.

[44] Pogarell, O., W. Koch, F.J. Gildehaus, A. Kupsch, O. Lindvall, W.H. Oertel, and K. Tatsch. Long-term assessment of striatal dopamine transporters in Parkinsonian patients with intrastriatal embryonic mesencephalic grafts. Eur J Nucl Med Mol Imaging. 2006; 33(4): 407–11.

[45] Ma, Y., C. Tang, T. Chaly, P. Greene, R. Breeze, S. Fahn, C. Freed, V. Dhawan, and D. Eidelberg. Dopamine cell implantation in Parkinson's disease: long-term clinical and (18)F-FDOPA PET outcomes. J Nucl Med. 2010; 51(1): 7–15.

[46] Politis, M., K. Wu, C. Loane, N.P. Quinn, D.J. Brooks, W.H. Oertel, A. Bjorklund, O. Lindvall, and P. Piccini. Serotonin neuron loss and nonmotor symptoms continue in Parkinson's patients treated with dopamine grafts. Sci Transl Med. 2012; 4(128): 128ra41.

[47] Kefalopoulou, Z., M. Politis, P. Piccini, N. Mencacci, K. Bhatia, M. Jahanshahi, H. Widner, S. Rehncrona, P. Brundin, A. Bjorklund, O. Lindvall, P. Limousin, N. Quinn, and T. Foltynie. Long-term clinical outcome of fetal cell transplantation for Parkinson disease: two case reports. JAMA Neurol. 2014; 71(1): 83–7.

[48] Moore, S.F., N.V. Guzman, S.L. Mason, C.H. Williams-Gray, and R.A. Barker. Which patients with Parkinson's disease participate in clinical trials? One centre's experiences with a new cell based therapy trial (TRANSEURO). J Parkinsons Dis. 2014; 4(4): 671–6.

[49] Evans, J.R., S.L. Mason, and R.A. Barker. Current status of clinical trials of neural transplantation in Parkinson's disease. Prog Brain Res. 2012; 200: 169–98.

[50] Liu, T.W., Z.G. Ma, Y. Zhou, and J.X. Xie. Transplantation of mouse CGR8 embryonic stem cells producing GDNF and TH protects against 6-hydroxydopamine neurotoxicity in the rat. Int J Biochem Cell Biol. 2013; 45(7): 1265–73.

[51] Thomson, J.A., J. Itskovitz-Eldor, S.S. Shapiro, M.A. Waknitz, J.J. Swiergiel, V.S. Marshall, and J.M. Jones. Embryonic stem cell lines derived from human blastocysts. Science. 1998; 282(5391): 1145–1147.

[52] Cooper, O., G. Hargus, M. Deleidi, A. Blak, T. Osborn, E. Marlow, K. Lee, A. Levy, E. Perez-Torres, A. Yow, and O. Isacson. Differentiation of human ES and Parkinson's disease iPS cells into ventral midbrain dopaminergic neurons requires a high activity form of SHH, FGF8a and specific regionalization by retinoic acid. Mol Cell Neurosci. 2010; 45(3): 258–66.

[53] Zeng, X., J. Cai, J. Chen, Y. Luo, Z.B. You, E. Fotter, Y. Wang, B. Harvey, T. Miura, C. Backman, G.J. Chen, M.S. Rao, and W.J. Freed. Dopaminergic differentiation of human embryonic stem cells. Stem Cells. 2004; 22(6): 925–40.

[54] Yan, Y., D. Yang, E.D. Zarnowska, Z. Du, B. Werbel, C. Valliere, R.A. Pearce, J.A. Thomson, and S.C. Zhang. Directed differentiation of dopaminergic neuronal subtypes from human embryonic stem cells. Stem Cells. 2005; 23(6): 781–90.

[55] Chambers, S.M., C.A. Fasano, E.P. Papapetrou, M. Tomishima, M. Sadelain, and L. Studer. Highly efficient neural conversion of human ES and iPS cells by dual inhibition of SMAD signaling. Nat. Biotechnol. 2009; 27(3): 275–80.

[56] Fasano, C.A., S.M. Chambers, G. Lee, M.J. Tomishima, and L. Studer. Efficient derivation of functional floor plate tissue from human embryonic stem cells. Cell Stem Cell. 2010; 6(4): 336–47.

[57] Kriks, S., J.W. Shim, J. Piao, Y.M. Ganat, D.R. Wakeman, Z. Xie, L. Carrillo-Reid, G. Auyeung, C. Antonacci, A. Buch, L. Yang, M.F. Beal, D.J. Surmeier, J.H. Kordower, V. Tabar, and L. Studer. Dopamine neurons derived from human ES cells efficiently engraft in animal models of Parkinson's disease. Nature. 2011; 480(7378): 547–51.

[58] Sanchez-Danes, A., A. Consiglio, Y. Richaud, I. Rodriguez-Piza, B. Dehay, M. Edel, J. Bove, M. Memo, M. Vila, A. Raya, and J.C. Izpisua Belmonte. Efficient generation of A9 midbrain dopaminergic neurons by lentiviral delivery of LMX1A in human embryonic stem cells and induced pluripotent stem cells. Hum Gene Ther. 2012; 23(1): 56–69.

[59] Grealish, S., E. Diguet, A. Kirkeby, B. Mattsson, A. Heuer, Y. Bramoulle, N. Van Camp, A.L. Perrier, P. Hantraye, A. Bjorklund, and M. Parmar. Human ESC-derived dopamine neurons show similar preclinical efficacy and potency to fetal neurons when grafted in a rat model of Parkinson's disease. Cell Stem Cell. 2014; 15(5): 653–65.

[60] Schulz, T.C., S.A. Noggle, G.M. Palmarini, D.A. Weiler, I.G. Lyons, K.A. Pensa, A.C. Meedeniya, B.P. Davidson, N.A. Lambert, and B.G. Condie. Differentiation of human

embryonic stem cells to dopaminergic neurons in serum-free suspension culture. Stem Cells. 2004; 22(7): 1218–38.

[61] Vazin, T., K.G. Becker, J. Chen, C.E. Spivak, C.R. Lupica, Y. Zhang, L. Worden, and W.J. Freed. A novel combination of factors, termed SPIE, which promotes dopaminergic neuron differentiation from human embryonic stem cells. PLoS One. 2009; 4(8): e6606.

[62] Swistowski, A., J. Peng, Y. Han, A.M. Swistowska, M.S. Rao, and X. Zeng. Xeno-free defined conditions for culture of human embryonic stem cells, neural stem cells and dopaminergic neurons derived from them. PLoS One. 2009; 4(7): e6233.

[63] Wilmut, I., A.E. Schnieke, J. McWhir, A.J. Kind, and K.H. Campbell. Viable offspring derived from fetal and adult mammalian cells. Nature. 1997; 385(6619): 810–3.

[64] Jullien, J., V. Pasque, R.P. Halley-Stott, K. Miyamoto, and J.B. Gurdon. Mechanisms of nuclear reprogramming by eggs and oocytes: a deterministic process? Nat Rev Mol Cell Biol. 2011; 12(7): 453–9.

[65] Takahashi, K. and S. Yamanaka. Induction of pluripotent stem cells from mouse embryonic and adult fibroblast cultures by defined factors. Cell. 2006; 126(4): 663–76.

[66] Park, I.H., R. Zhao, J.A. West, A. Yabuuchi, H. Huo, T.A. Ince, P.H. Lerou, M.W. Lensch, and G.Q. Daley. Reprogramming of human somatic cells to pluripotency with defined factors. Nature. 2008; 451(7175): 141–6.

[67] Yu, J., M.A. Vodyanik, K. Smuga-Otto, J. Antosiewicz-Bourget, J.L. Frane, S. Tian, J. Nie, G.A. Jonsdottir, V. Ruotti, R. Stewart, Slukvin, II, and J.A. Thomson. Induced pluripotent stem cell lines derived from human somatic cells. Science. 2007; 318(5858): 1917–20.

[68] Li, Y., Q. Zhang, X. Yin, W. Yang, Y. Du, P. Hou, J. Ge, C. Liu, W. Zhang, X. Zhang, Y. Wu, H. Li, K. Liu, C. Wu, Z. Song, Y. Zhao, Y. Shi, and H. Deng. Generation of iPSCs from mouse fibroblasts with a single gene, Oct4, and small molecules. Cell Res. 2011; 21(1): 196–204.

[69] Isobe, K., Z. Cheng, N. Nishio, T. Suganya, Y. Tanaka, and S. Ito. Reprint of "iPSCs, aging and age-related diseases". N Biotechnol. 2015; 32(1): 169–79.

[70] Han, F. The Applications of the Induced Pluripotent Stem Cells in Studying the Neurodegenerative Diseases. Chin J Cell Biol. 2012; 34(5): 13.

[71] Kiskinis, E. and K. Eggan. Progress toward the clinical application of patient-specific pluripotent stem cells. J Clin Invest. 2010; 120(1): 51–9.

[72] Wernig, M., J.-P. Zhao, J. Pruszak, E. Hedlund, D. Fu, F. Soldner, V. Broccoli, M. Constantine-Paton, O. Isacson, and R. Jaenisch. Neurons derived from reprogrammed fibroblasts functionally integrate into the fetal brain and improve symptoms of rats with Parkinson's disease. Proc Natl Acad Sci. 2008; 105(15): 5856–61.

[73] Reinhardt, P., B. Schmid, L.F. Burbulla, D.C. Schondorf, L. Wagner, M. Glatza, S. Hoing, G. Hargus, S.A. Heck, A. Dhingra, G. Wu, S. Muller, K. Brockmann, T. Kluba, M. Maisel,

R. Kruger, D. Berg, Y. Tsytsyura, C.S. Thiel, O.E. Psathaki, J. Klingauf, T. Kuhlmann, M. Klewin, H. Muller, T. Gasser, H.R. Scholer, and J. Sterneckert. Genetic correction of a LRRK2 mutation in human iPSCs links parkinsonian neurodegeneration to ERK-dependent changes in gene expression. Cell Stem Cell. 2013; 12(3): 354–67.

[74] Hargus, G., O. Cooper, M. Deleidi, A. Levy, K. Lee, E. Marlow, A. Yow, F. Soldner, D. Hockemeyer, P.J. Hallett, T. Osborn, R. Jaenisch, and O. Isacson. Differentiated Parkinson patient-derived induced pluripotent stem cells grow in the adult rodent brain and reduce motor asymmetry in Parkinsonian rats. Proc Natl Acad Sci U S A. 2010; 107(36): 15921–6.

[75] Stadtfeld, M., M. Nagaya, J. Utikal, G. Weir, and K. Hochedlinger. Induced pluripotent stem cells generated without viral integration. Science. 2008; 322(5903): 945–9.

[76] Okita, K., M. Nakagawa, H. Hyenjong, T. Ichisaka, and S. Yamanaka. Generation of mouse induced pluripotent stem cells without viral vectors. Science. 2008; 322(5903): 949–53.

[77] Yu, J., K. Hu, K. Smuga-Otto, S. Tian, R. Stewart, Slukvin, II, and J.A. Thomson. Human induced pluripotent stem cells free of vector and transgene sequences. Science. 2009; 324(5928): 797–801.

[78] Kim, D., C.H. Kim, J.I. Moon, Y.G. Chung, M.Y. Chang, B.S. Han, S. Ko, E. Yang, K.Y. Cha, R. Lanza, and K.S. Kim. Generation of human induced pluripotent stem cells by direct delivery of reprogramming proteins. Cell Stem Cell. 2009; 4(6): 472–6.

[79] Rhee, Y.H., J.Y. Ko, M.Y. Chang, S.H. Yi, D. Kim, C.H. Kim, J.W. Shim, A.Y. Jo, B.W. Kim, H. Lee, S.H. Lee, W. Suh, C.H. Park, H.C. Koh, Y.S. Lee, R. Lanza, and K.S. Kim. Protein-based human iPS cells efficiently generate functional dopamine neurons and can treat a rat model of Parkinson disease. J Clin Invest. 2011; 121(6): 2326–35.

[80] Sundberg, M., H. Bogetofte, T. Lawson, J. Jansson, G. Smith, A. Astradsson, M. Moore, T. Osborn, O. Cooper, and R. Spealman. Improved cell therapy protocols for Parkinson's disease based on differentiation efficiency and safety of hESCcy ion -, and non-human primate iPSC-derived dopaminergic neurons. Stem Cells. 2013; 31(8): 1548–62.

[81] Maherali, N., R. Sridharan, W. Xie, J. Utikal, S. Eminli, K. Arnold, M. Stadtfeld, R. Yachechko, J. Tchieu, R. Jaenisch, K. Plath, and K. Hochedlinger. Directly reprogrammed fibroblasts show global epigenetic remodeling and widespread tissue contribution. Cell Stem Cell. 2007; 1(1): 55–70.

[82] Okita, K., T. Ichisaka, and S. Yamanaka. Generation of germline-competent induced pluripotent stem cells. Nature. 2007; 448(7151): 313–7.

[83] Muller, L.U., G.Q. Daley, and D.A. Williams. Upping the ante: recent advances in direct reprogramming. Mol Ther. 2009; 17(6): 947–53.

[84] Hu, B.Y., J.P. Weick, J. Yu, L.X. Ma, X.Q. Zhang, J.A. Thomson, and S.C. Zhang. Neural differentiation of human induced pluripotent stem cells follows developmental principles but with variable potency. Proc Natl Acad Sci U S A. 2010; 107(9): 4335–40.

[85] Koyanagi-Aoi, M., M. Ohnuki, K. Takahashi, K. Okita, H. Noma, Y. Sawamura, I. Teramoto, M. Narita, Y. Sato, T. Ichisaka, N. Amano, A. Watanabe, A. Morizane, Y. Yamada, T. Sato, J. Takahashi, and S. Yamanaka. Differentiation-defective phenotypes revealed by large-scale analyses of human pluripotent stem cells. Proc Natl Acad Sci U S A. 2013; 110(51): 20569–74.

[86] O'Brien, C. and A.L. Laslett. Suspended in culture--human pluripotent cells for scalable technologies. Stem Cell Res. 2012; 9(2): 167–70.

[87] Fang, R., K. Liu, Y. Zhao, H. Li, D. Zhu, Y. Du, C. Xiang, X. Li, H. Liu, Z. Miao, X. Zhang, Y. Shi, W. Yang, J. Xu, and H. Deng. Generation of naive induced pluripotent stem cells from rhesus monkey fibroblasts. Cell Stem Cell. 2014; 15(4): 488–96.

[88] Caiazzo, M., M.T. Dell'Anno, E. Dvoretskova, D. Lazarevic, S. Taverna, D. Leo, T.D. Sotnikova, A. Menegon, P. Roncaglia, G. Colciago, G. Russo, P. Carninci, G. Pezzoli, R.R. Gainetdinov, S. Gustincich, A. Dityatev, and V. Broccoli. Direct generation of functional dopaminergic neurons from mouse and human fibroblasts. Nature. 2011; 476(7359): 224–7.

[89] Kim, H.S., J. Kim, Y. Jo, D. Jeon, and Y.S. Cho. Direct lineage reprogramming of mouse fibroblasts to functional midbrain dopaminergic neuronal progenitors. Stem Cell Res. 2014; 12(1): 60–8.

[90] Wang, Q., X. Xu, J. Li, J. Liu, H. Gu, R. Zhang, J. Chen, Y. Kuang, J. Fei, C. Jiang, P. Wang, D. Pei, S. Ding, and X. Xie. Lithium, an anti-psychotic drug, greatly enhances the generation of induced pluripotent stem cells. Cell Res. 2011; 21(10): 1424–35.

[91] Aasen, T., A. Raya, M.J. Barrero, E. Garreta, A. Consiglio, F. Gonzalez, R. Vassena, J. Bilic, V. Pekarik, G. Tiscornia, M. Edel, S. Boue, and J.C. Izpisua Belmonte. Efficient and rapid generation of induced pluripotent stem cells from human keratinocytes. Nat Biotechnol. 2008; 26(11): 1276–84.

[92] Lister, R., M. Pelizzola, Y.S. Kida, R.D. Hawkins, J.R. Nery, G. Hon, J. Antosiewicz-Bourget, R. O'Malley, R. Castanon, S. Klugman, M. Downes, R. Yu, R. Stewart, B. Ren, J.A. Thomson, R.M. Evans, and J.R. Ecker. Hotspots of aberrant epigenomic reprogramming in human induced pluripotent stem cells. Nature. 2011; 471(7336): 68–73.

[93] Hou, P., Y. Li, X. Zhang, C. Liu, J. Guan, H. Li, T. Zhao, J. Ye, W. Yang, K. Liu, J. Ge, J. Xu, Q. Zhang, Y. Zhao, and H. Deng. Pluripotent stem cells induced from mouse somatic cells by small-molecule compounds. Science. 2013; 341(6146): 651–4.

[94] Laurent, L.C., I. Ulitsky, I. Slavin, H. Tran, A. Schork, R. Morey, C. Lynch, J.V. Harness, S. Lee, M.J. Barrero, S. Ku, M. Martynova, R. Semechkin, V. Galat, J. Gottesfeld, J.C. Izpisua Belmonte, C. Murry, H.S. Keirstead, H.S. Park, U. Schmidt, A.L. Laslett, F.J. Muller, C.M. Nievergelt, R. Shamir, and J.F. Loring. Dynamic changes in the copy

number of pluripotency and cell proliferation genes in human ESCs and iPSCs during reprogramming and time in culture. Cell Stem Cell. 2011; 8(1): 106–18.

[95] Soldner, F., J. Laganiere, A.W. Cheng, D. Hockemeyer, Q. Gao, R. Alagappan, V. Khurana, L.I. Golbe, R.H. Myers, S. Lindquist, L. Zhang, D. Guschin, L.K. Fong, B.J. Vu, X. Meng, F.D. Urnov, E.J. Rebar, P.D. Gregory, H.S. Zhang, and R. Jaenisch. Generation of isogenic pluripotent stem cells differing exclusively at two early onset Parkinson point mutations. Cell. 2011; 146(2): 318–31.

[96] Nakagawa, M., Y. Taniguchi, S. Senda, N. Takizawa, T. Ichisaka, K. Asano, A. Morizane, D. Doi, J. Takahashi, M. Nishizawa, Y. Yoshida, T. Toyoda, K. Osafune, K. Sekiguchi, and S. Yamanaka. A novel efficient feeder-free culture system for the derivation of human induced pluripotent stem cells. Sci Rep. 2014; 4: 3594.

5

Neuro-Ophthalmologic Evaluation as a Biomarker for Diagnosis and Progression in Parkinson Disease

María Satue, Vicente Polo, Sofía Otin,
Jose M. Larrosa, Javier Obis and Elena Garcia-Martin

Abstract

Objectives: The purpose of current neuro-ophthalmologic research is to evaluate visual dysfunction and its correlation with structural changes in the retina of patients with Parkinson's disease and to examine whether there is an association between retinal thinning and disease progression.

Methods: Patients with Parkinson's disease and controls were included in a series of observational cross-sectional studies and underwent visual function evaluation. Structural measurements of different layers of the retina were obtained using spectral domain optical coherence tomography (SD-OCT). Disease severity was assessed using the Schwab–England Activities of Daily Living scale, the Unified Parkinson Disease Rating Scale, and the Hoehn and Yahr (HY) scale. Comparison of obtained data and correlation analysis between functional and structural results and disease severity was performed. The diagnostic ability of SD-OCT for the detection of Parkinson disease was also tested by the development of two linear discriminant functions (LDFs).

Results: Patients with Parkinson's disease had altered visual function and presented retinal thinning in different sectors. Disease progression correlated with retinal parameters and measurements of retinal thickness was differentiated between healthy subjects and those with advanced Parkinson's disease.

Keywords: Parkinson's disease, optical coherence tomography, retinal nerve fiber layer, retinal ganglion cells, macular thickness

1. Introduction

Parkinson's disease (PD) is well known for its motor symptoms, such as bradykinesia, rigidity, resting tremor, and postural instability. However, the loss of dopaminergic neurons also leads to non-motor alterations, such as depression, dementia, and autonomic dysfunction [1].

Vision is one of the non-motor systems altered in PD. Patients suffering from Parkinson's are reported to have decreased visual acuity (VA), contrast sensitivity, and color vision [2–8]. Recent research demonstrated that retinal thinning in PD patients and axonal damage can be detected and quantified using ocular imaging technologies, such as optical coherence tomography (OCT). The retina is part of the central nervous system and is easily accessible to clinical examination. The retinal nerve fiber layer (RNFL) comprises mainly non-myelinated axons of retinal ganglion cells (RGCs), so RNFL thickness measurements provide a relatively direct assessment of the axons and axonal damage.

OCT provides cross-sectional images of the retina and optic disc based on interference patterns produced by low coherence light reflected from retinal tissues. This technology includes the development of parameters to provide quantitative, objective, and reproducible measurements of the different retinal layers. Recent research on segmentation and analysis of different retinal layers has shown that measures of specific layers, such as the RGC layer provide more accurate information about axonal loss in neurodegenerative diseases [9].

Dopamine in the human retina is released by a set of amacrine cells. These dopaminergic cells are located in the proximal inner nuclear layer of the retina and send long processes to other retinal layers. Dopamine in the mammalian retina modulates color vision and contrast sensitivity through dopaminergic receptors (D1 and D2), which are differentially located in the retinal layers. A complete lack of D1 and D2 receptor activation leads to signal dispersion and alterations in color vision and contrast sensitivity.

The diagnosis of idiopathic PD is based on medical history and neurologic examination, and it sometimes takes several years to obtain a definitive diagnosis. Thus, new technologies and accurate tests are needed to improve and accelerate the diagnostic procedure in early stages of PD.

Recent research using OCT technology has demonstrated that parameters provided by OCT are accurate to detect various inner retinal or optic nerve pathologies, such as multiple sclerosis, PD, or Alzheimer disease [10–15]. At present, no clear guidelines are available on whether one, several, or all of the retinal parameters provided by OCT can be used in the diagnosis of PD.

Current research in the field of neuro-ophthalmology focuses on the evaluation of visual dysfunction in PD and its correlation with retinal alterations in these patients. Recent studies in PD have evaluated the association between macular, ganglion cell layer, and RNFL defects and PD severity, as well as the possible diagnostic ability of OCT technology [9, 15, 16].

The main objective of this study was to provide a better understanding of the role of retinal layers in PD and a diagnostic tool for the early detection of this neurodegenerative pathology.

2. Neuro-ophthalmologic evaluation of PD patients

2.1. Visual dysfunction in PD

Vision comprises many simultaneous functions that are important for daily life activities, such as mobility, reading, driving, and facial recognition [17–20]. Thus, it is important to assess the functional capability of the visual pathways by measuring VA, color vision, visual fixation, objects visual tracking, and contrast sensitivity and to evaluate the impact of vision loss on a person's ability to perform everyday visual tasks.

PD patients are reported to have decreased contrast sensitivity and color vision [2–8]. Previous studies have indicated that PD patients lose foveal contrast sensitivity to patterns to which normal observers are most sensitive (that is, requiring the least contrast for detection of letters, shapes, and figures) [3, 4]. In the retina, ganglion cells adapt to visual contrast and pool the visual information of their receptive fields through a network of parallel bipolar cells with smaller receptive fields [21]. Additionally, contrast sensitivity and color vision are modulated through dopaminergic receptors, which are located in the inner retinal layers. A complete lack of activation of these receptors leads to signal dispersion and alterations in color vision and contrast sensitivity [22].

In our hospital, we evaluated a cohort of 37 patients with PD and analyzed possible alterations in their visual function. We assessed VA, contrast sensitivity vision (CSV), and color vision in these patients and compared the results with healthy controls.

The diagnosis of PD was based on standard clinical and neuroimaging criteria [23]. Patients with significant refractive errors (>5 diopters of spherical equivalent refraction or 3 diopters of astigmatism), intraocular pressure ≥21 mm Hg, media opacifications, concomitant ocular diseases including history of glaucoma or retinal pathology, and systemic conditions that could affect the visual system were excluded from the study. The healthy controls had no history and no evidence of ocular or neurologic disease of any nature, and their best-corrected visual acuity (BCVA) was >20/30 based on the Snellen scale, to ensure all of them could complete the visual function evaluation tests. All subjects underwent a complete neuro-ophthalmic evaluation that included pupillary, anterior segment, and funduscopic examination. All procedures adhered to the tenets of the Declaration of Helsinki, and all participants provided informed consent to participate in the study.

Visual function was assessed by evaluating different functional parameters: BCVA using an ETDRS chart; CSV using the CVS-1000E test and Pelli–Robson chart; and color vision using the Farnsworth D15 and L'Anthony D15 tests.

VA is a measure of the spatial resolution of the visual processing system and is dependent on optical and neural factors, that is, the sharpness of the retinal focus within the eye, the health and functioning of the retina, and the sensitivity of the interpretative faculty of the brain. Thus, the VA in a patient with PD and a healthy eye will depend solely on their neurologic condition. VA can be evaluated using different optotypes (with letters or numbers). For clinical research, the ETDRS chart is considered the gold standard and consists of a set of 10 letters from the Roman alphabet, each of them equally visible (**Figure 1**).

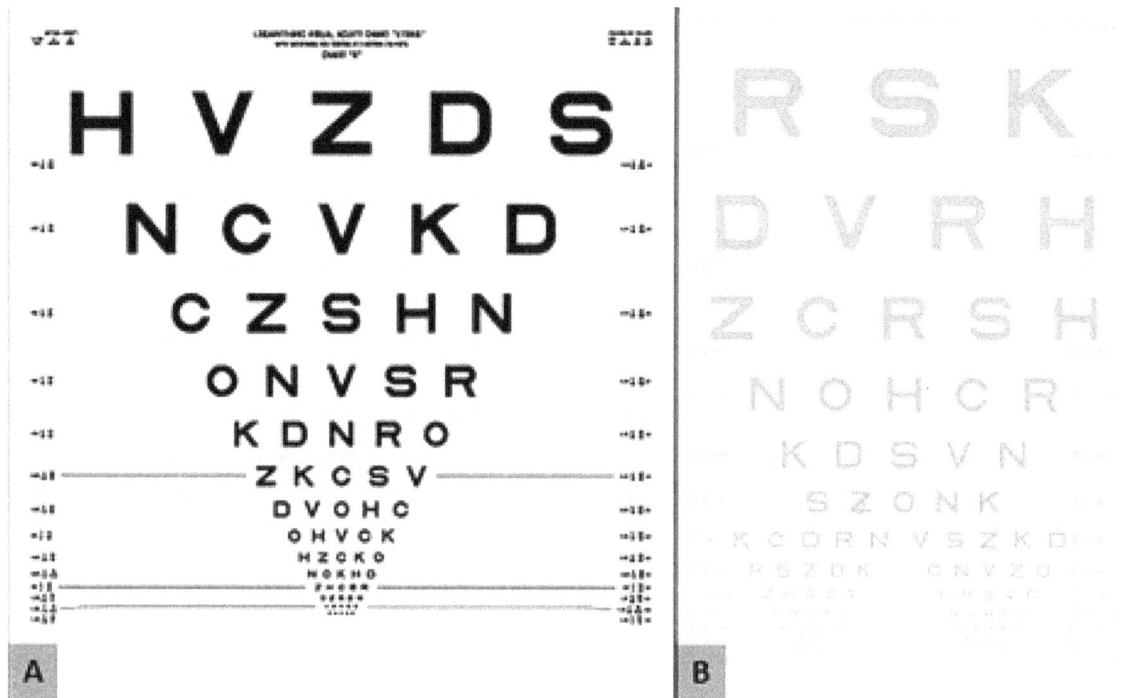

Figure 1. ETDRS charts for evaluation of high and low contrast visual acuity. (A): 100% contrast ETDRS chart. (B:) 2.50% contrast ETDRS chart.

The letters are arranged in 14 rows, with 5 letters each, and decrease in size progressively. Results can be expressed as 6/6, 10/10, decimal value or logarithmic scale (LogMar). In the expression 6/6, at 6 m, a human eye with a VA of 6/6 is able to separate contours that are approximately 1.75 mm apart; 6/12 means that a person with 6/6 vision would discern the same optotype from 12 m away (i.e., at twice the distance). The equivalent to 6/6 in decimal digits would be 1.0 and 0.0 in logarithmic scale (LogMar). In our patients, LogMAR VA was evaluated at three different contrast levels: 100, 2.50, and 1.25% (using Low-Contrast Sloan Letter Charts), the percentage indicating the level of contrast, that is, 100% representing black letters over white background and 1.25% light grey letters over white background (**Figure 1**).

CSV provides more complete information about visual function than VA tests. CSV was evaluated in our patients using the Pelli–Robson chart and the CSV-1000E test. The Pelli–Robson is a commonly used test for the evaluation of contrast sensitivity, assessing CSV at one spatial frequency (1 cycle/degree [cpd]). This chart comprises horizontal lines of capital letters organized into groups of three (triplets) with two triplets per line. Within each triplet, all letters have the same contrast. The contrast decreases from one triplet to the next, even within each line. All patients were evaluated at a distance of 1 m from the chart and under controlled fotopic conditions (85 cd/m^2). The score corresponding to the last triplet of letters seen by the patient was recorded. The CSV-1000E instrument is used worldwide for standardized CSV and glare testing and evaluates CSV at 4 different spatial frequencies (3, 6, 12, and 18 cpd). The chart comprises four rows with 17 circular patches each. The patches present a grating that decreases in contrast moving from left to right across the row (**Figure 2**). Each contrast value for each spatial frequency was transformed into a logarithmic scale according to standardized values.

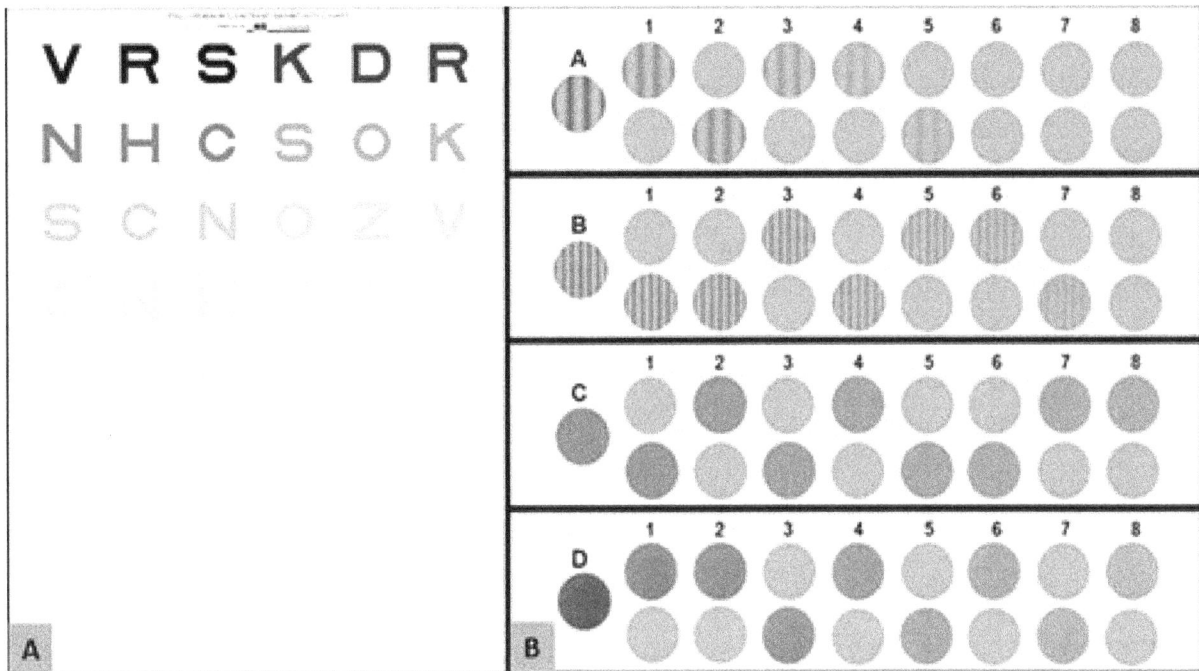

Figure 2. Contrast sensitivity vision tests. (A) Pelli–Robson chart explores contrast sensitivity in one spatial frequency (1 cycle per degree). (B) CSV 1000E test evaluates contrast sensitivity at four different spatial frequencies (3, 6, 12, and 18 cycles per degree).

Color vision was evaluated using the Color Vision Recorder (CVR) program. CVR software is designed for the Windows operating system and analyzes chromatic discrimination by classification of colors (color arrangement using colored caps). CVR includes several classic color tests. All patients in the study were evaluated using the Farnsworth D15 and L´Anthony D15 tests. These tests are often used to differentiate between subjects with severe loss of color vision and those with milder color defects or normal color vision. Different output parameters, such as the age-corrected color confusion index (AC CCI, which represents the ratio between the radius or distance between caps), the Confusion angle (Conf angle, which represents the axis of color deficiency), and the Scatter index (S-index, which represents the parallelism of confusion vectors to the personal confusion angle) were recorded [24, 25]. All these parameters evaluate the severity of dyschromatopsia. For example, an AC CCI score higher than 1, indicates altered color vision perception; the higher the score in the AC CCI and the S-index, the worse the color deficiency.

We found that our patients with PD had a lower BCVA at all three contrast levels of the ETDRS chart compared to the controls (0.18 ± 0.26 in patients vs. -0.065 ± 0.9 in controls at 100%, $p = 0.001$; 0.59 ± 0.21 vs. 0.44 ± 0.13 at 2.50%, $p = 0.01$; and 0.61 ± 0.23 vs. 0.58 ± 0.16 at 1.25%, $p = 0.009$). The Pelli– Robson results revealed a significant reduction in CSV in PD patients ($p = 0.02$). CSV was also affected in patients at all four spatial frequencies of the CSV 1000E chart (3, 6, 12, and 18 cpd; $p = 0.001$, <0.001, <0.001, and 0.004 respectively). Color vision was also affected in PD: In our patients, only the L´Anthony test results were significantly altered. L´Anthony test is less saturated than the Farnsworth color test; thus, it is designed to detect very subtle color deficiencies. Our patients performed worse than controls in both tests (higher C-index and S-index, reaching ranges similar to protanomalies), although only the differences in L'Anthony S-index were statistically significant, indicating that our patients had a (subtle) protanomaly (**Table 1**).

	Healthy controls		Parkinson's disease		P
	Mean	**SD**	**Mean**	**SD**	
VA ETDRS 100	−0.06	0.096	0.18	0.26	**0.001**
VA ETDRS 2.5	0.44	0.13	0.59	0.22	**0.010**
VA ETDRS 1.25	0.58	0.16	0.62	0.23	**0.009**
Pelli–Robson	1.89	0.11	1.71	0.17	**0.002**
CSV 1000 3 cpd	1.72	0.16	1.49	0.35	**0.001**
CSV 1000 6 cpd	1.94	0.13	1.62	0.34	**0.000**
CSV 1000 12 cpd	1.62	0.17	1.26	0.41	**0.000**
CSV 1000 18 cpd	1.11	0.22	0.73	0.34	**0.004**
Farnsworth AC CCI	1.11	0.22	0.73	0.34	0.851
Farnsworth Conf Angle	63.90	11.15	65.84	7.49	0.392
Farnsworth S-index	1.56	0.22	1.64	0.39	0.278
Farnsworth time	78.67	28.96	82.91	33.10	0.616
L'Anthony AC CCI	1.05	0.19	1.02	0.18	0.489
L' Anthony Conf Angle	62.31	14.74	71.91	9.25	**0.002**
L' Anthony S-index	1.69	0.43	1.95	0.48	**0.020**
L' Anthony time	77.14	25.99	84.09	39.31	0.431

Results in bold letters indicate statistical significance ($p < 0.05$).
AC CCI, age-corrected color confusion index; Conf Angle, confusion angle; cpd, cycles per degree; ETDRS, early treatment diabetic retinopathy study; PD, Parkinson disease; S-index, scatter index; VA, visual acuity.

Table 1. Mean and standard deviation (SD) of visual functional parameters in healthy controls and subjects with Parkinson's disease. Results in bold letters indicate statistical significance ($p < 0.05$).

Ganglion cells in the retina show adaptation to visual contrast. The parvo- and magnocellular ganglion cells are located in the RGC layer and take two different pathways for the identification of color and contrast at different frequencies [26]. RGC loss was recently identified as the cause of visual impairment in patients suffering from another neurodegenerative process (multiple sclerosis) [27]. Thus, a similar process could be the cause of the contrast and color deficiencies in PD.

The results found in this study highlight the importance of visual function tests in the evaluation of PD patients and may have important implications for clinical diagnosis of functional deficits in these patients.

2.2. Retinal changes in PD

Parkinson's disease has been associated with alterations in foveal vision. This visual alteration seems to be caused by a dysfunction of the intraretinal dopaminergic circuitry and final retinal output to the brain [2].

Thanks to the new digital imaging technologies applied in the field of ophthalmology, an objective assessment of the retinal layers is now possible. OCT provides a rapid, objective, non-invasive, and reproducible method for the assessment of eye structures thicknesses and volumes.

OCT is an established medical imaging technique that uses light to capture micrometer-resolution, three-dimensional images from within optical scattering media. OCT is based on low-coherence interferometry, usually employing near-infrared light. The use of relatively long wavelength light allows it to penetrate into the scattering medium. The interference of light (caused by the different tissues) occurs at a distance of micrometers. Light with broad bandwidths can be generated using superluminescent diodes or lasers with extremely short pulses.

The OCT device combines the reflected light from two arms (one arm containing the object of study, and a second arm containing usually a mirror) to rise an interference pattern. A reflectivity profile of the sample is obtained by scanning the mirror in the reference arm [28]. Parts of the sample that reflect a lot of light will create greater interference than areas that do not. These higher interference areas will be seen as bright patterns and will correlate with fibrosis or dense retinal layers, whereas low interference areas will be seen as dark patterns and will correlate with fluid. Any light that is outside the short coherence length will not interfere.

There are many studies on neurodegenerative diseases using OCT to detect changes in the RNFL thickness and macular morphology. Regarding PD and the alteration of macular thickness, recent studies have shown a significant thinning in the retinal inner layers of the macular area in patients with PD. Alterations of the retinal layers in PD patients were first demonstrated in 2004 [29]. Since then, various studies have reported different results [29–33].

For the past 5 years, the neuro-ophthalmology research team of Miguel Servet University Hospital has studied retinal structural alterations in PD patients using different OCT devices. Various software applications were used in the evaluation of these patients.

A first cohort of 153 subjects with PD underwent OCT examinations using the Cirrus high-definition (HD) OCT device and the Spectralis OCT device. Two different applications were used for Spectralis OCT, for the analysis of the optic nerve: the *Glaucoma* application (which scans the optic nerve head starting and finishing in the temporal quadrant), and the *Axonal Analytics* application for neurodegenerative diseases (which scans the optic nerve from and to the temporal quadrant) (**Figure 3.**).

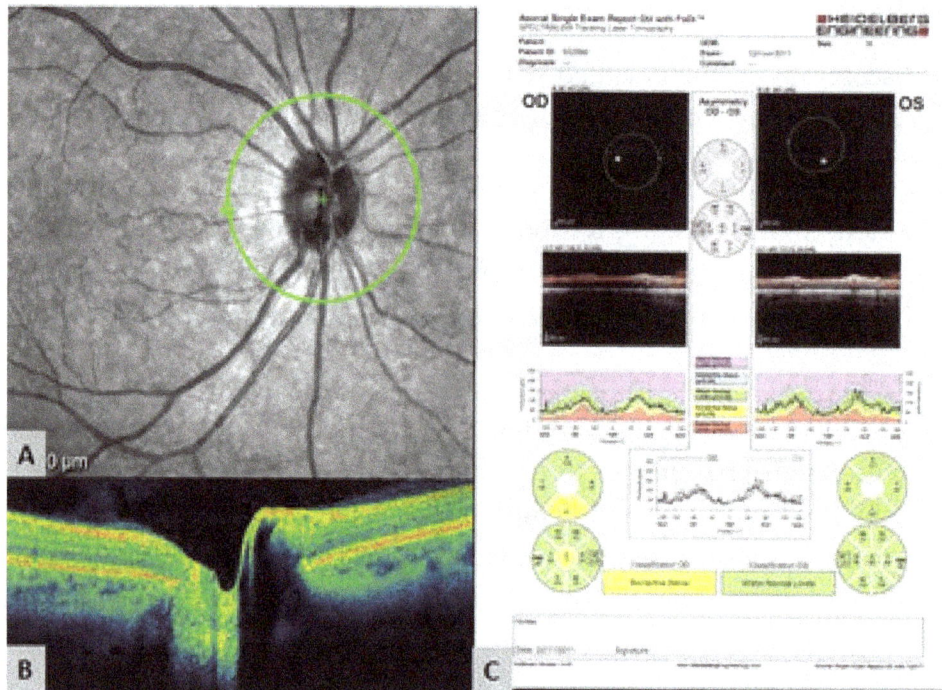

Figure 3 Evaluation of the retinal nerve fiber layer using Axonal Analytics application for Spectralis OCT. (A) Arrow marks the direction of the scan in the optic nerve head. (B) Cross-sectional image of the peripapillary retinal thickness. The retinal layers can be observed in different colors, depending on their interference pattern. (C) OCT report with measurements of the retinal nerve fiber layer in μm.

The difference between both applications resides in the sector with the most accurate measurements: With Glaucoma application, the most accurate sector is nasal, and with Axonal Analytics application is the temporal sector, which is precisely the sector with earlier affectation in neurodegenerative diseases. Macular and peripapillary RNFL thicknesses were evaluated and compared with thicknesses of a group of 242 healthy individuals [9].

The Spectralis OCT measurements revealed significant differences in most of the RNFL sectors using the traditional *Glaucoma* application, and in the mean thickness, the inferior quadrant, the inferonasal, and the inferotemporal RNFL sectors using the *Axonal* Analytics application. The Cirrus OCT measurements revealed significant RNFL differences in mean thickness, and thickness of superior, inferior, and temporal quadrants. Macular thickness was also reduced in patients with PD for all measurements of the inner and outer macular sectors using the Spectralis OCT device; and for the central sector (fovea thickness) and the nasal outer and inferior outer sectors with the Cirrus OCT. Results from this study were published in the *British journal of Ophthalmology* in 2014.

A different cohort of patients underwent retinal evaluation with a new prototype technique for retinal segmentation using the Spectralis OCT [16]. This new software is designed to identify each retinal layer and to measure its thickness. Segmentation of the retinal layers in single horizontal foveal scans was performed automatically by the segmentation application into 10 different layers [16] (**Figure 4.**).

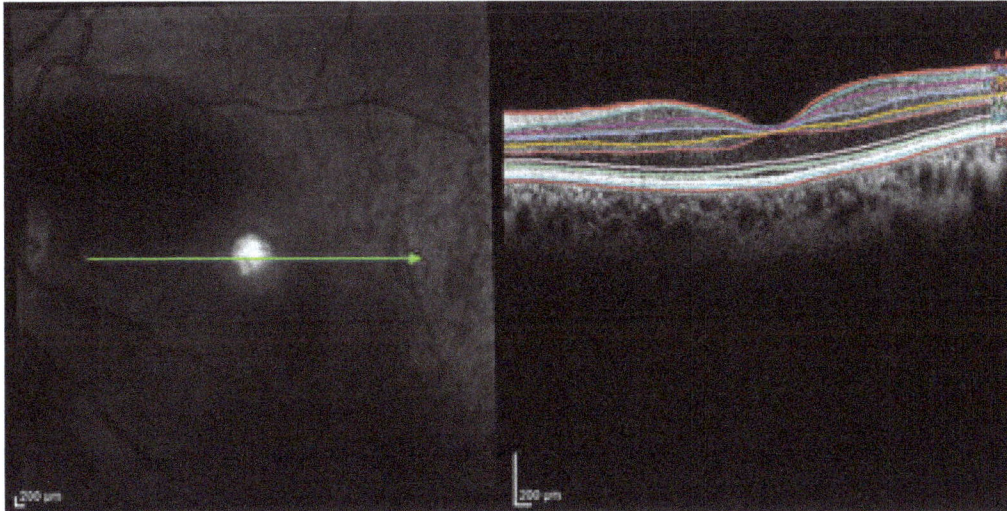

Figure 4 Macular cross-sectional image of a patient with Parkinson's disease, as provided by the segmentation application of Spectralis OCT. The different retinal layers can be observed marked in different colored lines.

All measurements of the macular and peripapillary thickness of the 10 layers were registered in a database for all eyes, and mean thickness of each retinal layer was calculated. A total of 129 eyes from 129 PD patients and 129 eyes of 129 healthy subjects were included in the study.

The segmentation application revealed a significant reduction of the RNFL, ganglion cell layer, the inner plexiform, and outer plexiform layer thickness in PD patients compared with controls. Surprisingly, the inner nuclear layer was significantly thicker in PD patients compared with healthy subjects (**Table 2**). These results were published in 2013 in the *American Journal of Ophthalmology*.

LAYER	Parkinson's disease (n = 129)	Healthy subjects (n = 129)	P*
Inner glial limiting membrane	5.69 ± 2.01	5.68 ± 1.72	0.563
Retinal nerve fiber layer	6.06 ± 1.90	6.26 ± 1.80	**0.036**
Ganglion cell layer	6.30 ± 1.89	6.49 ± 1.86	**0.011**
Inner plexiform layer	6.64 ± 1.95	6.77 ± 1.92	**0.016**
Inner nuclear layer	7.39 ± 1.94	7.14 ± 1.90	**0.033**
Outer plexiform layer	7.17 ± 1.93	7.31 ± 1.91	**0.028**
Outer nuclear layer	7.89 ± 1.91	7.95 ± 1.92	0.085
Outer glial limiting membrane	8.20 ± 1.90	8.25 ± 1.96	0.220
Photoreceptors	8.26 ± 1.98	8.29 ± 1.95	0.139
Retinal pigment epithelium	8.58 ± 1.88	8.63 ± 1.89	0.397

Table 2. Mean and standard deviation of retinal thickness in the 10 different retinal layers automatically provided by the segmentation application of the Spectralis optical coherence tomography and comparison between patients with Parkinson's disease and healthy subjects.

The correlation between retinal changes and visual dysfunction in patients suffering from PD was also investigated. A small cohort of 37 patients with PD (37 eyes) underwent visual function tests (see previous section *Visual dysfunction in Parkinson's disease*) and structural analysis of macular thickness, ganglion cell layer (GCL) and RNFL thickness, and linear correlations between functional and structural results were calculated using Pearson's correlation coefficient.

Results demonstrated that CSV was the functional parameter most frequently associated with structural measurements in PD. The Pelli– Robson CSV results correlated with GCL thickness in all sectors, although the association was not strong ($r < 0.5$, $p < 0.05$). The Pelli– Robson measurements also correlated with the thicknesses in different sectors of the peripapillary RNFL (average, superior, and inferior sectors). The CSV-1000E measurements at different spatial frequencies correlated significantly with most GCL measurements: The spatial frequency of 6 cpd correlated with the superonasal thickness ($r = 0.40$, $p = 0.013$), with the superotemporal thickness ($r = 0.44$, $p = 0.006$), with the average GCL + IPL thickness ($r = 0.40$, $p = 0.012$), and with the minimum GCL + IPL ($r = 0.40$, $p = 0.011$). The spatial frequency of 18 cpd correlated with the superotemporal thickness ($r = 0.41$, $p = 0.01$) and the minimum GCL + IPL thickness ($r = 0.43$, $p = 0.006$), showing here the strongest correlations with GCL thickness. Spatial frequencies of 6 and 18 cpd were strongly correlated with average macular thickness ($r = 0.79$, $p = 0.012$; $r = 0.77$, $p = 0.016$, respectively) and macular volume ($r = 0.78$, $p = 0.013$; $r = 0.78$, $p = 0.014$, respectively). Color vision was also associated with the structural parameters, but only those measurements (the C-index and CCI) assessed by the L'Anthony test were significantly correlated with all outer macular parameters and most of the GCL measurements. A significant association between color vision and the RNFL parameters was only found in isolated sectors.

The VA ETDRS results (high and low contrast) correlated strongly with average macular thickness and macular volume (**Table 3**). This was particularly interesting, since this is the first time such a strong correlation between macular thickness, macular volume, and functional parameters (VA and CSV) is reported ($r > 0.70$).

	Macular thickness (correlation coefficient)	P value	Macular volume (correlation coefficient)	P value
VA ETDRS 100	−0.765	**0.006**	−0.761	**0.007**
VA ETDRS 1.25	−0.718	**0.013**	−0.715	**0.013**
VA ETDRS 2.50	−0.738	**0.010**	−0.729	**0.011**

Correlation data in bold type are statistically significant (p value < 0.05).
ETDRS, early treatment diabetic retinopathy study; VA, visual acuity.

Table 3. Correlation between visual acuity measured with ETDRS chart at different levels of contrast (in %) and macular structural measurements (thickness and volume) in patients with Parkinson disease. Results in bold letters indicate statistical significance (p < 0.05).

The study on the association between structural and functional parameters is currently pending acceptance for its publication in a peer- reviewed journal.

2.3. Correlation between structural changes and disease severity

The stage and severity of PD were determined in all our patients based on three different rating scales: the Hoehn and Yahr (HY), the Schwab–England activities of daily living (ADL), and the Unified Parkinson's disease rating score (UPDRS). Patients were tested by a trained neurologist who was blind to the ophthalmology results. Disease duration was also recorded, setting the appearance of the first symptoms as the onset time of the disease.

A correlation analysis between disease severity and structural changes as measured by OCT was performed in the first cohort of patients (153 patients with PD). Correlations between structural data (measured with Cirrus OCT and Spectralis OCT) and the different rating scales were examined by Pearson's test. The results of this study were published in the *British Journal of Ophthalmology*, in 2014 [9].

The correlation analysis revealed an inverse correlation between most macular thickness measurements assessed by Spectralis OCT and the scores on the HY scale. This means that increased neurological effects and severity of PD progression are linked to thinning of macular tissue. There was a significant correlation between the Schwab–England ADL scores and the outer temporal macular thickness measured with the Cirrus OCT device (r = 0.284, p = 0.010); and between the Schwab–England ADL scores and the inner inferior macular thickness measured with the Spectralis OCT device (r = 0.217, p = 0.039). The UPDRS scores were significantly correlated with the inner inferior macular thickness and measured using the Cirrus OCT device (r = −0.331, p = 0.032). Disease duration was correlated with RNFL thickness measured by the Spectralis OCT device (nasal quadrant using glaucoma application, p = 0.036; nasal quadrant and mean thickness using axonal application, p = 0.016 and p = 0.038, respectively). No correlation between disease duration and Cirrus OCT values was found.

In the second cohort (129 patients and 129 healthy controls), PD patients were divided into two groups depending on disease duration: <10 years (67% of the patients) or at least 10 years (33%). The thickness of the different retinal layers was compared between both patient's groups using Student's t-test. Linear agreement between the mean thickness of each retinal layer and three neurologic parameters (duration of disease, HY, and UPDRS scores) was obtained using the Pearson correlation coefficient. A logistical regression analysis was performed to identify which retinal layer thicknesses predicted axonal damage in PD patients.

When analyzing the results, the inner retinal layer thicknesses (RNFL, ganglion cell, and inner plexiform layers) were more affected in PD patients with disease duration of at least 10 years (**Table 4**). GCL thickness correlated inversely with PD duration (r = −0.221, p = 0.046) and the HY scale (r = −0.311, p = 0.041), but not the UPDRS scale.

Layer	Parkinson's disease patients with disease duration < 10 years (n:86)	Parkinson's disease patients with disease duration ≥ 10 years (n:43)	P*
Inner glial limiting membrane	5.70 ± 1.95	5.68 ± 1.96	0.211
Retinal nerve fiber layer	6.06 ± 1.87	5.89 ± 1.91	**0.028**
Ganglion cell layer	6.40 ± 1.92	5.96 ± 1.85	**0.031**
Inner plexiform layer	6.47 ± 1.91	6.11 ± 1.89	**0.009**
Inner nuclear layer	7.37 ± 1.91	7.41 ± 1.75	0.111
Outer plexiform layer	7.19 ± 1.91	7.08 ± 1.99	0.136
Outer nuclear layer	7.89 ± 1.98	7.82 ± 1.93	0.356
Outer glial limiting membrane	8.21 ± 1.79	8.20 ± 1.95	0.457
Photoreceptors	8.27 ± 1.90	8.24 ± 1.89	0.665
Retinal pigment epithelium	8.60 ± 1.85	8.57 ± 1.93	0.763

Table 4. Mean and standard deviation of thicknesses in the 10 retinal layers automatically provided by the new segmentation application of the Spectralis optical coherence tomography and comparison between Parkinson disease patients with disease duration of <10 years or at least 10 years.

The regression analysis showed that only the GCL thickness could predict axonal atrophy in PD. Based on the OCT measurements, PD patients with thinner GCL thickness showed a greater decrease in average RNFL thickness. However, thickness of the other retinal layers was not predictive of axonal damage. These results were published in the *American Journal of Ophthalmology*, in 2013 [16].

Our data clearly revealed that disease duration has an impact on the thickness of the RNFL, the GCL, and the inner plexiform layer. The negative correlation between macular thickness, the thickness of the RNFL, and the Hoehn and Yahr score indicates that patients with greater axonal damage tend to have more severe PD symptoms. Our results also indicated that GCL thickness could predict axonal damage in PD patients. GCL atrophy is thought to be a component of RNFL loss, which is suggested to produce consecutive degeneration of the RGC layer and its axons as disease progresses [34, 35].

2.4. The role of OCT in the diagnosis of Parkinson's disease

Because of the difficulty in diagnosing PD, medical organizations have created diagnostic criteria to standardize and simplify the diagnostic process. Diffusion magnetic resonance imaging is a specific technique that may help discriminate between typical and atypical parkinsonism, but its exact diagnostic value is still under investigation.

A definitive diagnosis for PD may take years. Thus, new technologies and accurate tests are needed to improve and accelerate the diagnostic procedure in early stages of the disease. Currently, there are no clear guidelines available on which retinal or RNFL parameters provided by OCT can be used in the diagnosis of PD. Previous research demonstrated that overall RNFL mean thickness provided by OCT is a good parameter to detect various inner retinal or optic nerve pathologies, such as glaucoma [11], and neurodegenerative disease [10]. Optimal neurodegenerative disease detection, however, is liable to depend on a combination of several parameters. In 2013, our research team published a study in the journal *Retina* that evaluated whether a selective combination of RNFL and retinal OCT parameters could further optimize PD diagnosis. The purpose of this study was to evaluate the diagnostic ability of a linear discriminant function (LDF) for PD, based exclusively on ophthalmologic parameters.

Two independent samples of 100 consecutive healthy subjects and 60 idiopathic patients with PD were recruited from two clinics in the hospital area. The diagnosis of PD was based on the United Kingdom's BrainBank criteria and the United States National Institute of Neurological Disorders and Stroke criteria [36].

All subjects underwent OCT evaluation to obtain measurements of the peripapillary RNFL and retinal thickness using the Spectralis OCT device. Regression analysis was used, when the dependent variable (to have PD) was dichotomous (yes/no) and the independent variables (all OCT measurements) were of any kind. For logistic regression analysis, the probability that a subject has PD was set as the predicted-dependent variable. The relative importance of each independent variable was evaluated using the forward Wald method, which tests the unique contribution of each predictor in the context of the other predictors. The LDF was calculated by taking the weighted sum of the predictor variables. The significant OCT parameters were combined to generate a new variable (LDF) in such a way that the measurable differences between healthy eyes and eyes with PD were maximized. One hundred and eleven eyes from 60 patients with PD were evaluated. All RNFL scans and retinal measurements provided by the Spectralis OCT were analyzed to calculate three LDFs: the Retinal LDF using the 9 retinal measurements (macular area), the RNFL LDF with 768 RNFL measurements, and the definitive LDF (which combined all OCT measurements). The statistical analysis showed that the Retinal LDF was the best formula. Retinal LDF was defined as follows: 31.173 + temporal outer thickness × 0.026 − superior outer thickness × 0.267 + nasal outer thickness × 0.159 − inferior outer thickness × 0.197 − superior inner thickness × 0.060 + foveal thickness × 0.049 [36].

For the Retinal LDF, the area under the ROC curves was 0.900 (**Table 5**).

OCT parameters	AUC	95% CI	AUC P-value	Cut-off point	Sens (%)	Spec (%)
Retinal LDF	0.900	0.862–0.933	**<0.001**	>−58.4	89.5	80.5
Foveal thickness	0.467	0.409–0.525	0.345	>305	22.4	96.5
Temporal inner thickness	0.737	0.684–0.787	**<0.001**	≤327	66.3	75.5
Temporal outer thickness	0.680	0.624–0.733	**<0.001**	≤277	47.2	83.5
RNFL LDF	0.824	0.777–0.865	**<0.001**	>−0.84	85.6	63.5
RNFL average thickness	0.535	0.478–0.592	0.185	<86	17.1	96.5
RNFL temporal thickness	0.574	0.517–0.630	0.083	>77	32.4	86.5

OCT parameters	AUC	95% CI	AUC P-value	Cut-off point	Sens (%)	Spec (%)
RNFL PMB sector	0.567	0.510–0.623	0.037	>52	65.7	50.0
RNFL N/T index	0.586	0.529–0.641	0.016	≤1.16	65.7	52.5

AUC, area under the receiver operating characteristic curve; CI, confidence interval; LDF, linear discriminant function; OCT, optical coherence tomography; RNFL, retinal nerve fiber layer; Sens, Sensitivity; Spec, Specificity.

Table 5. In the validating set, areas under the receiver operating characteristic curves, best sensitivity-specificity balance, and likelihood ratios of retinal nerve fiber layer parameters of the Nsite Axonal Analytics software of Spectralis optical coherence tomography (OCT) to discriminate between normal subjects and patients with Parkinson's disease.

The largest areas under the ROC curves were those for the Temporal Inner and Outer retinal thickness [36].

3. Discussion

Parkinson's disease patients present decreased high and low contrast VA and CSV, and mild anomalies in color perception. Visual dysfunction in PD is frequently underdiagnosed, since tests designed to detect abnormalities in visual function are not routinely performed in eye examination, and symptoms often go unnoticed by patients.

Neurodegeneration caused by PD can be detected using OCT. Our studies, along with previous research, revealed a reduction in retinal thickness (specifically in the macular area), RNFL and RGC thicknesses in patients suffering from PD. The loss of RGCs has been linked to visual dysfunction and may also be responsible for visual function anomalies in PD patients.

The loss of RGCs leads to a corresponding decrease in retinal and RNFL thicknesses that can be detected using OCT [37, 38]. In PD patients, this loss could be due to primary neurodegeneration of the RGCs and their axons or to retrograde degeneration of the RGC layer plus its axons produced by PD lesions of the posterior visual pathways [39]. Retrograde RGC degeneration produced by retrogeniculate lesions was previously reported in patients with homonymous hemianopia [40], which suggests that OCT measurements reveal combined anterior and posterior visual pathway disease [40, 41].

Our results revealed macular thinning of all areas in patients with PD compared with controls, an inverse correlation with HY and UPDRS severity, and a positive correlation with the Schwab–England ADL scale. Therefore, increased neurologic alterations and severity of PD progression are linked to thinning of macular tissue. The degree of correlation, although significant, was low moderate. These results, however, are consistent with findings in other neurodegenerative diseases [42].

Our segmentation analysis revealed that the GCL thickness was inversely correlated with disease duration and PD severity and was predictive of axonal damage in PD patients. We believe that further research with segmentation application is needed to establish the extent to which each retinal layer can predict PD in particular circumstances (e.g., recognizing PD when in an early stage), or to evaluate the effectiveness of different treatments.

The retinal measurements provided by Fourier domain OCT technology are tools that can be used in combination with other parameters and clinical explorations. LDF calculated upon OCT parameters may be more sensitive and specific than the methods currently used for diagnosis. Our Retinal LDF yielded higher sensitivity (at a high specificity) than any single parameter determined using OCT. The high sensibility and specificity demonstrated by OCT may be better than some of the accepted neuroimaging criteria in the current PD diagnosis procedure.

The LDFs presented in our study, however, demonstrate better accuracy for PD diagnosis in patients with advanced disease. Clinical application of our findings may help diagnosis in patients who suffer from movement alterations, and PD is suspected. Our results indicate that retinal thinning may be useful for detecting patients with PD. However, larger studies using OCT technology are needed to evaluate the sensitivity, specificity, and the ability of retinal thickness measurements to detect PD. Longitudinal prospective studies should be carried out in the future, to assess disease progression and treatment effectiveness.

Author details

María Satue*, Vicente Polo, Sofía Otin, Jose M. Larrosa, Javier Obis and Elena Garcia-Martin

*Address all correspondence to: mariasatue@gmail.com

IIS Aragon, Ophthalmology Department, Institute for Health Sciencies of Aragon (IACS), Miguel Servet University Hospital, Zaragoza, Spain

References

[1] Park A, Stacy M. Non-motor symptoms in Parkinson's disease. J Neurol 2009; 256(Suppl 3): 293–298.

[2] Bodis-Wollner I. Retinopathy in Parkinson disease. J Neural Transm 2009;116:1493–501.

[3] Bodis-Wollner I. Visual acuity and contrast sensitivity in patients with cerebral lesions. Science 1972;178:769–71.

[4] Bodis-Wollner I, Diamond S. The measurement of spatial contrast sensitivity in cases of blurred vision associated with cerebral lesions. Brain 1976;99:695–710.

[5] Price MJ, Feldman RG, Adelberg D, Kayne H. Abnormalities in color vision and contrast sensitivity in Parkinson's disease. Neurology 1992;42:887–90.

[6]   Oh YS, Kim JS, Chung SW, Song IU, Kim YD, Kim YI, Lee KS. Color vision in Parkinson's disease and essential tremor. Eur J Neurol 2011;18: 577–83.

[7]   Hipp G, Diedericha NJ, Pieria V, Vaillant M. Primary vision and facial emotion recognition in early Parkinson's disease. J Neurol Sci 2014;338: 178–82.

[8]   Archibald NK, Clarke MP, Mosimann UP, Burn DJ. Retinal thickness in Parkinson's disease. Parkinsonism Relat Disord 2011; 17(6):431–6.

[9]   Satue M, Seral M, Otin S, Alarcia R, Herrero R, Bambo MP, Fuertes MI, Pablo LE, Garcia-Martin E. Retinal thinning and correlation with functional disability in patients with Parkinson's disease. Br J Ophthalmol 2014;98(3):350–5.

[10] Garcia-Martin E, Pueyo V, Ara JR, Almarcegui C, Martin J, Pablo L, Dolz I, Sancho E, Fernandez FJ. Effect of optic neuritis on progressive axonal damage in multiple sclerosis patients. Mult Scler 2011;17:830–837.

[11] Burgansky-Eliash Z, Wollstein G, Chu T, Glymour C, Noecker RJ, Ishikawa H, Schuman JS. Optical coherence tomography machine learning classifiers for glaucoma detection: a preliminary study. Investig Ophthalmol Vis Sci 2005;46:4147–4152.

[12] Garcia-Martin E, Pueyo V, Martin J, Almarcegui C, Ara JR, Dolz I, Honrubia FM, Fernandez FJ. Progressive changes in the retinal nerve fiber layer in patients with multiple sclerosis. Eur J Ophthalmol 2010;20:167–173.

[13] Garcia-Martin E, Pablo LE, Herrero R, Satue M, Polo V, Larrosa JM, Martin J, Fernandez J. Diagnostic ability of a linear discriminant function for Spectral domain optical coherence tomography in multiple sclerosis patients. Ophthalmology 2012;119(8): 1705–11.

[14] Larrosa JM, Garcia Martin E, Bambo MP, Pinilla J, Polo V, Otin S, Satue M, Herrero R, Pablo LE. Potential new diagnostic tool for Alzheimer's disease using a linear discriminant function for Fourier domain optical coherence tomography. Investig Ophthalmol Vis Sci 2014;55(5):3043–51.

[15] Garcia-Martin E, Satue M, Otin S, Fuertes I, Alarcia R, Larrosa JM, Polo V, Pablo LE. Retina measurements for diagnosis of Parkinson disease. Retina 2014;34(5):971–80.

[16] Garcia-Martin E, Larrosa JM, Polo V, Satue M, Marques ML, Alarcia R, Seral M, Fuertes I, Otin S, Pablo LE. Distribution of retinal layer atrophy in patients with Parkinson disease and association with disease severity and duration. Am J Ophthalmol 2014;157(2):470–478.

[17] Turano KA, Broman AT, Bandeen-Roche K, Munoz B, Rubin GS, West SK. Association of visual field loss and mobility performance in older adults: salisbury eye evaluation study. Optom Visi Sci 2004;81(5):298–307.

[18] Leat SJ, Woo GC. The validity of current clinical tests of contrast sensitivity and their ability to predict reading speed in low vision. Eye 1997;11(6):893–9.

[19] Wood JM. Age and visual impairment decrease driving performance as measured on a closed-road circuit. Hum Factors 2002;44(3):482–94.

[20] West SK, Rubin GS, Broman AT, Muñoz B, Bandeen-Roche K, Turano K. How does visual impairment affect performance on tasks of everyday life? The SEE project. Arch Ophthalmol 2002;120(6):774–80.

[21] Kim, KJ, Rieke, F. Temporal contrast adaptation in the input and output signals of salamander retinal ganglion cells. J. Neurosci 2001;21:287–99.

[22] Hajee ME, March WF, Lazzaro DR, Wolintz AH, Shrier EM, Glazman S, Bodis-Wollner IG. Inner retinal layer thinning in Parkinson's disease. Arch Ophthalmol 2009;127:737–41.

[23] Gelb DJ, Oliver E, Gilman S. Diagnostic criteria for Parkinson disease. Arch Neurol 1999;56:33–9.

[24] Vingrys AJ, King-Smith PE. A quantitative scoring technique for panel tests of color vision. Investig Ophthalmol Vis Sci 1988;29(1):50–63.

[25] Bowman AJ. A method for quantitive scoring of the Farnsworth panel D15. Acta Ophthalmol 1982;60:907–16.

[26] Laycock R, Crewther SG, Crewther DP. A role for the 'magnocellular advantage' in visual impairments in neurodevelopmental and psychiatric disorders. Neurosci Biobehav Rev 2007;31:363–76.

[27] Lampert EJ, Andorra M, Torres-Torres R, Ortiz-Pérez S, Llufriu S, Sepúlveda M, Sola N, Saiz A, Sánchez-Dalmau B, Villoslada P, Martínez-Lapiscina EH. Color vision impairment in multiple sclerosis points to retinal ganglion cell damage. J Neurol 2015;262(11):2491–7.

[28] Besharse J, Dana J, editors. Corneal Imaging: Clinical. Encyclopedia of the Eye, 1st ed. Academic Press Inc; Elsevier 2010. 9780123741981.

[29] Inzelberg R, Ramirez JA, Nisipeanu P, Ophir A. Retinal nerve fiber layer thinning in Parkinson's disease. Vis Res 2004;44:2793–7.

[30] Cubo E, Tedejo RP, Rodriguez Mendez V. Retina thickness in Parkinson's disease and essential tremor. Mov Disord 2010;25:2461–77.

[31] Satue M, Garcia-Martin E, Fuertes I, Otin S, Alarcia R, Herrero R, Bambo MP, Pablo LE, Fernandez FJ. Use of Fourier-domain OCT to detect retinal nerve fiber layer degeneration in Parkinson's disease patients. Eye (Lond) 2013;27:507–14.

[32] Garcia-Martin E, Satue M, Fuertes, Otin S, Alarcia R, Herrero R, Bambo MP, Fernandez J, Pablo LE. Ability and reproducibility of Fourier domain optical coherence tomography to detect retinal nerve fiber layer atrophy in Parkinson's disease. Ophthalmology 2012;119:2161–7.

[33] Altintaş O, Işeri P, Ozkan B, Cağlar Y. Correlation between retinal morphological and functional findings and clinical severity in Parkinson's disease. Doc Ophthalmol 2008;116:137–46.

[34] Almarcegui C, Dolz I, Pueyo V, Garcia E, Fernandez FJ, Martin J, Ara JR, Honrubia F. Correlation between functional and structural assessments of the optic nerve and retina in multiple sclerosis patients. Neurophysiol Clin 2010;40(3):129–135.

[35] Davies EC, Galetta KM, Sackel DJ, Talman LS, Frohman EM, Calabresi PA, Galetta SL, Balcer LJ. Retinal ganglion cell layer volumetric assessment by spectral-domain optical coherence tomography in multiple sclerosis: Application of a high precision manual estimation technique. J Neuroophthalmol 2011;31(3):260–264.

[36] Garcia-Martin E, Satue M, Otin S, Fuertes I, Alarcia R, Larrosa JM, Polo V, Pablo LE. Retina measurements for diagnosis of Parkinson disease. Retina 2014;34(5):971–80.

[37] Maresca A, la Morgia C, Caporali L, Valentino ML, Carelli V. The optic nerve: a "mito-window" on mitochondrial neurodegeneration. Mol Cell Neurosci 2013;55:62–76.

[38] La Morgia C, Barboni P, Rizzo G, Carbonelli M, Savini G, Scaglione C, Capellari S, Bonazza S, Giannoccaro MP, Calandra-Buonaura G, Liguori R, Cortelli P, Martinelli P, Baruzzi A, Carelli V. Loss of temporal retinal nerve fibers in Parkinson disease: a mitochondrial pattern? Eur J Neurol 2013;20:198–201.

[39] Albrecht P, Ringelstein M, Müller AK, Keser N, Dietlein T, Lappas A, Foerster A, Hartung HP, Aktas O, Methner A. Degeneration of retinal layers in multiple sclerosis subtypes quantified by optical coherence tomography. Mult Scler 2012;18(10):1422–1429.

[40] Jindahra P, Petrie A, Plant GT. Retrograde trans-synaptic retinal ganglion cell loss identified by optical coherence tomography. Brain 2009;132(Pt3):628–634

[41] Reich DS, Smith SA, Gordon-Lipkin EM, Ozturk A, Caffo BS, Balcer LJ, Calabresi PA. Damage to the optic radiation in multiple sclerosis is associated with retinal injury and visual disability. Arch Neurol 2009;66(8):998–1006.

[42] Garcia-Martin E, Rodriguez-Mena D, Herrero R, Almarcegui C, Dolz I, Martin J, Ara JR, Larrosa JM, Polo V, Fernández J, Pablo LE. Neuro-ophthalmologic evaluation, quality of life and functional disability in MS patients. Neurology 2013;81:1–8.

Understanding Pathophysiology of Sporadic Parkinson's Disease in *Drosophila* Model: Potential Opportunities and Notable Limitations

Priyanka Modi, Ayajuddin Mohamad,

Limamanen Phom, Zevelou Koza,

Abhik Das, Rahul Chaurasia, Saikat Samadder,

Bovito Achumi, Muralidhara,

Rajesh Singh Pukhrambam and

Sarat Chandra Yenisetti

Abstract

Parkinson's disease (PD) is the second most common neurodegenerative disorder affecting approximately 1% of the population over age 50. PD is widely accepted as a multifactorial disease with both genetic and environmental contributions. Despite extensive research conducted in the area the precise etiological factors responsible remain elusive. In about 95% Parkinsonism is considered to have a sporadic component. There are currently no established curative, preventative, or disease-modifying interventions, stemming from a poor understanding of the molecular mechanisms of pathogenesis. Here lies the importance of animal models. Pharmacological insults cause Parkinsonian like phenotypes in *Drosophila*, thereby modelling sporadic PD. The pesticides paraquat and rotenone induced oxidative damage causing cluster specific DA neuron loss together with motor deficits. Studies in fly PD model have deciphered that signaling pathways such as phosphatidylinositol 3-kinase (PI3K/Akt and target of rapamycin (TOR), c-Jun N-terminal kinase (JNK) have been defective. Further, these studies have demonstrated that fruit fly can be a potential model to screen chemical compounds for their neuroprotective efficacy.

This chapter overviews current knowledge on the pathophysiology of sporadic PD employing *Drosophila* model and discusses the future perspectives. Further we emphasize the importance of performing genome wide screens in fly model, which may lead to identification of novel pathways involved in PD, which may provide clues to develop therapeutic strategies that help to reduce the burden of PD.

Keywords: Parkinson's disease, *Drosophila*, dopaminergic neurons, neurotoxicants, genome-wide screens

1. Introduction

Parkinson's disease (PD) is the second most common neurodegenerative disorder after Alzheimer disease, affecting approximately 1% of the population over the age of 50. Frequency of PD increases with age, but an expected 4% of people with this disease are detected earlier the age of 50. It is assessed that 7–10 million people worldwide are suffering from PD. About one million Americans are surviving with PD, which is more than the collective number of sufferers diagnosed with muscular dystrophy, Lou Gehrig's disease, and multiple sclerosis. Further, about 60,000 Americans are diagnosed with PD each year and this number does not mirror thousands of unnoticed cases [1]. Studies illustrate that prevalence of PD in men is significantly higher (one and half times more) than in women. In poor and developing nations of Asia and Africa no systematic data are available about the number of sufferers. Painful truth is that in these regions, millions of elderly suffer in silence due to poverty and ignorance.

PD is widely accepted as a multifactorial disease with both genetic and environmental contributions. Clinical signs comprise bradykinesia, resting tremble, muscular rigidity, and postural unsteadiness. Supplementary symptoms are characteristic postural anomalies, dystonic spams, and dementia. PD is progressive and usually has a devious onset in mid to late adult life. Pathogenic characters of typical PD comprise loss of dopaminergic neurons in the *substantia nigra* (SN) and the manifestation of Lewy bodies, intracellular cytoplasmic inclusions, in enduring neurons in various areas of the brain, mainly the SN [2].

Despite intensive research conducted in the field of PD, the etiology of this neurodegenerative disease remains elusive. Although genetic elements and exposure to environmental toxins, such as pesticides, are thought to play a crucial role in disease onset, aging remains the predominant risk factor [3]. In about 95% patients, Parkinsonism is considered to have a sporadic component. Some findings suggest that environmental factors may be more important than genetic factors in familial aggregation of PD. In maximum PD cases the cause is environmental influence, probably toxic, overlaid on a background of slow, sustained neuronal loss due to progressing age [4]. Finding PD in 1-methyl-4-phenyl-1,2,3,6-tetrahydropyridine (MPTP) drug consumers rejuvenated curiosity in reassessing environmental influences [5]. Another theory of Parkinsonism suggests that genetic predisposition may be transmitted through mitochondrial inheritance.

Current therapeutic strategies for PD mitigate symptoms by the replacement of dopamine, with variable efficacy and considerable side effects. Levodopa (L-dopa), a dopamine precursor, the leading treatment of PD for over 40 years, improves motor impairment by increasing dopamine levels [6]. However, continued use of L-dopa leads to other motor dyskinesias that undermine the benefits of treatment. The development of effective treatment for PD is difficult because pathology is affected by several pathways that may act serially or in parallel. However, there are currently no established curative, preventative, or disease-modifying interventions, stemming from a poor understanding of the molecular mechanisms of pathogenesis.

This chapter primarily aims to present an overview of the sporadic PD, disease modeling in *Drosophila* and critically analyze the potential opportunities and the notable limitations associated with fly models. Further, we have also briefly discussed some of the current applications of the model to obtain insights into the underlying molecular mechanism/s related to PD.

2. Animal models of Parkinson's disease

Animal models have been invaluable tools for investigating the underlying mechanisms of the pathogenesis of PD. However, the usefulness of these models is dependent on how precisely they replicate the features of clinical PD. Nonmammalian models are a great cost-effective alternative to rodent and primate-based models, allowing rapid high-throughput screening of novel therapies and investigation of genetic and environmental risk factors. Thus far, the nonmammalian rotenone models have included worm (*Caenorhabditis elegans*), fly (*Drosophila*), zebrafish (*Danio rerio*), and pond snail (*Lymnea stagnalis*). A good model of PD should exhibit pathological and medical characteristics of PD including both dopaminergic and nondopaminergic systems, the central and peripheral nervous systems, also the motor and nonmotor symptoms associated with the disease. Furthermore, the age-reliant inception and progression of pathology should be reflected [7].

Contemporary knowledge on the potential pathogenic and pathophysiological mechanisms of PD derives from innumerable studies conducted, in the past four decades, on experimental models of PD. While animal models, in particular, have provided invaluable information, they also offer the opportunity of trying new therapeutic methods. These model systems have been traditionally grounded on the exposure of neurotoxins able to imitate *many* of the pathological and phenotypic characters of PD in mammals. Conversely in the previous decade, the dawn of the "genetic era" of PD has provided a significant growth in this field with a number of transgenic models for experimentation. It is well recognized that both these classes of animal PD models (genetic and neurotoxin) have their own specificities as well as limitations and employment of one model or the other depends on the specific questions that are being addressed.

Genetic models: Animal models are developed primarily based on identified target genes (i.e., by mutating or knocking out) associated with potential mechanisms known to cause PD in humans (**Table 1**) [8–21]. For example, the autosomal dominant transmission of LRRK2 mutations makes transgenic expression of pathogenic LRRK2 species suitable for modeling disease process in PD. The invertebrate transgenic models producing LRRK2 PD mutants phenotypes range from no change to apparent neuronal loss or deficits in DA systems and motor behavior [22] that were used to evaluate LRRK2 kinase inhibitors in neuroprotection, revealing the potential value of the invertebrate LRRK2 models in drug screening [23].

Symbol	Gene locus	Gene	*Drosophila* homolog	Inheritance	Disorder	Status and remarks
PARK1	4q21-22	SNCA [10]	No homolog	AD	Early-onset Parkinsonism	Confirmed
PARK2	6q25.2-q27	PARK2 encoding Parkin[11]	Parkin	AR	Early onset Parkinsonism	Confirmed
PARK3	2p13	Unknown	–	AD	Classical Parkinsonism	Unconfirmed
PARK4	4q21-q23	SNCA	No homolog	AD	Early-onset Parkinsonism	Erroneous locus (identical to PARK1)
PARK5	4p13	UCHL1	Uch	AD	Classical Parkinsonism	Unconfirmed
PARK6	1p35-p36	PINK1 [12]	Pink1	AR	Early onset Parkinsonism	Confirmed
PARK7	1p36	PARK7 encoding DJ-1[13]	Dj-1α and dj-1β	AR	Early onset Parkinsonism	Confirmed
PARK8	12q12	LRRK2 [14]	Lrrk	AD	Classical Parkinsonism	Confirmed
PARK9	1p36	ATP13A2 [15]	CG32000	AR	Kufor–Rakeb syndrome, a form of juvenile-onset atypical Parkinsonism with dementia, spasticity and supranuclear gaze palsy	Confirmed
PARK10	1p32	Unknown	–	Risk factor	Classical Parkinsonism	Confirmed susceptibility locus
PARK11	2q36-27	Unknown	–	AD	Late	Not

Sym bol	Gene locus	Gene	*Drosophila* homolog	Inheri tance	Disorder	Status and remarks
		(maybe GIGYF2)			onset Parkinsonism	independently confirmed
PARK12	Xq21-q25	Unknown	–	Risk factor	Classical Parkinsonism	Confirmed susceptibility locus
PARK13	2p12	HTRA2	HtrA2	AD or risk factor	Classical Parkinsonism	Unconfirmed
PARK14	22q13.1	PLA2G6 [16]	iPLA2-VIA	AR	Early-onset dystonia-Parkinsonism	Confirmed
PARK15	22q12-q13	FBXO7 [17]	No homolog	AR	Early-onset Parkinsonian-pyramidal syndrome	Confirmed
PARK16	1q32	Unknown (maybe RAB7L1)	–	Risk factor	Classical Parkinsonism	Confirmed susceptibility locus
PARK17	16q11.2	VPS35	Vps35	AD	Classical Parkinsonism	Unconfirmed
PARK18	6p21.3	EIF4G1	eIF4G	AD	Late onset Parkinsonism	Unconfirmed
PARK19	1p31.3	DNAJC6 [18]	Auxillin	AR	Juvenile-onset Parkinsonism	Confirmed
PARK20	21q22.11	SYNJ1 [19, 20]	Synj	AR	Early-onset Parkinsonism	Confirmed

AD, autosomal dominant; AR, autosomal recessive (adapted from Marras *et al.* [21]).

Table 1. Monogenetic forms of PD and its fly homolog(s).

Neurotoxic models: Several studies have been performed to model PD-associated neuron loss by neurotoxin intoxication in animals, the most common Parkinsonian neurotoxins being 6-hydroxydopamine (6-OHDA), 1-methyl-4-phenyl-1,2,3,6-tetrahydropyridine (MPTP), rotenone, and paraquat [24, 25], and the common neurotoxic models of PD include that produced by the toxin 6-hydroxydopamine (6-OHDA) commonly used in rats, mice and marmosets, and 1-methyl-4- phenyl-1,2,3,6 tetrahydropyridine (MPTP), used in mice and also in nonhuman primates. Administration of MPTP to animals, such as monkeys, mice, cats, rats, guinea pigs, dogs, sheep and even frogs and goldfish, has been shown to cause Parkinsonian-like motor disturbances [26, 27].

3. Pathophysiology of Parkinson's disease

3.1. Sporadic Parkinson's disease: an overview

A sporadic disease can be explained as a disease occurring randomly in a population with no known cause. In sporadic PD, the cause is considered to be environmental though the genetic influence is also present and hence the pathogenesis of PD is likely to be multifactorial which may involve gene–environment interactions. The discovery of MPTP (1-methyl-4-phenyl-1,2,3,6-tetrahydropyridine), which reproduces pathological features of idiopathic Parkinsonism by targeting the nigrostriatal system [28] and pesticides (such as rotenone and paraquat), has implicated environmental toxins in the induction of sporadic PD [29, 30]. Both epidemiological and experimental data suggest the potential involvement of specific agents such as neurotoxicants (e.g., pesticides) or neuroprotective compounds (e.g., tobacco products) in the pathogenesis of nigrostriatal degeneration, further supporting a relationship between the environment and PD [28]. Further, the identification of the mutated α-synuclein (SCNA) gene causing familial PD [10] as a risk factor for sporadic disease [31] provides a genetic context for the disease. The finding of α-synuclein as a key component of the Lewy body [32] further links this gene to potential molecular mechanisms of PD.

3.2. Environmental basis of sporadic PD

The study of environmental risk factors for PD is difficult because environmental exposures and gene–environment interactions may occur well before the onset of clinical symptoms since it remains undetected for many years. Moreover, the severe neurodegenerative changes that underlie the symptoms of PD may be the result of synergistic effects of multiple exposures and these effects could have been compounded by increased vulnerability of the aging nigrostriatal system to toxic injury over the years. Epidemiological and case–control studies suggest that rural residence, well water consumption, pesticide use, and certain occupations (farming, mining, and welding) are associated with an increased risk of PD [33–36].

Epidemiological studies have suggested an association with environmental toxins, mainly mitochondrial complex I inhibitors like rotenone [37, 38]. The results are consistent with a dose-dependent effect in agricultural workers and the risk increased with duration of pesticide use [39, 40]. Data also suggest that exposure to specific pesticide such as bipyridyl, organo-chlorine, and carbamate derivatives could have a causal role in PD [39, 41]. Further, chronic exposure to metals/pesticides is also associated with a younger age at onset of PD among patients with no family history of the disease and that duration of exposure is a factor in the magnitude of this effect [42]. For instance, a study in Taiwan, where the herbicide paraquat (PQ) is commonly spurted on rice fields, a robust relationship was testified between paraquat contact and PD menace and the danger was amplified by more than six times in individuals who had been exposed to PQ chronically [43].

3.3. Environment toxins and their mechanisms of action

The accidental discovery of MPTP leading to Parkinsonian syndrome stimulated the search for environmental factors as potential causes of PD. Several epidemiological studies have suggested that environmental toxins are one of the major causes of sporadic PD [44]. Sporadic PD's main cause is the accumulation of alpha-synuclein but by an uncertain causative agent and uneven occurrence point in age of patients. The mechanisms by which the neurotoxins induce PD-like symptoms are briefly described below.

MPTP: MPTP is a metabolite of the drug heroin. It is transported through the blood–brain barrier (BBB) by the plasma membrane dopamine transporter (DAT) and once it crosses the blood–brain barrier, MPTP is metabolically activated to the fully oxidized 1-methyl-4-phenylpyridinium species (MPP+) which is then taken up into dopaminergic neurons via DAT [45, 46]. After MPP+ gains access into dopaminergic neurons, it is accumulated into synaptic vesicles via the vesicular monoamine transporter (VMAT2) [47]. The modulation of MPTP/MPP+ toxicity by DAT and VMAT2, where DAT enhances and VMAT2 protecting against toxicant injury, provides a paradigm linking environmental exposures to nigrostriatal degeneration. The ratio of DAT to VMAT2 indicates the sensitivity of dopaminergic neurons to toxic injury [48].

6-Hydroxy dopamine (6-OHDA): 6-OHDA is the first catecholaminergic neurotoxin that was used to generate animal models of PD. Since this compound cannot cross BBB, it is needed to be injected and inserted systemically to aim dopamine pathways [49]. On injecting into *substantia nigra*, 6-OHDA causes severe loss of dopamine neurons within a day [50]. Inside neurons, 6-OHDA produces reactive oxygen species (ROS) and quinones that inactivate biological macromolecules. Till now, no Lewy body-like inclusion has been described in the 6-OHDA model. Owing to its inability to cross BBB, this model is less popular.

Rotenone (ROT): ROT is used as a broad-spectrum pesticide and belongs to the family of isoflavones naturally found in the roots and stems of several plants. Highly lipophilic, it easily crosses the BBB, and for cellular entry [51], it does not depend on the DAT. Within the cell rotenone mount up in mitochondria and inhibits complex I (where it impedes the transfer of electrons from iron–sulfur (Fe–S) centers to ubiquinone). It is opined that augmented ROS assembly is related with complex I inhibition, which may result in causing oxidative damage to DNA and proteins of neuronal cells. Further, nitric oxide may interact with ROS, particularly superoxide and hydroxyl radicals, resulting in peroxynitrite formation, eventually leading to cellular defects and impairment of dopaminergic neurons [52]. Further, ROT was shown to inhibit proteasome activity and dysfunction in proteasomes has been implicated in the pathogenesis of both genetic and sporadic forms of PD [53, 54].

Paraquat (PQ): PQ is one of the most widely used herbicides in the world. The structural similarity of PQ with 1-methyl-4-phenylpyridinium ion (MPP+) prompted the speculation that PQ might be dopaminergic neurotoxicant which may lead to PD. PQ is suspected to enter the brain by neutral amino acid transporters and subsequently the cells in a sodium-dependent fashion [55]. Once within cells of the CNS, PQ acts as a redox cycling compound at the cytosolic level, which potentially leads to indirect mitochondrial toxicity [56]. Recently, it has also been shown that PQ-induced apoptosis may involve Bak protein, a pro-apoptosis Bcl-2 family member [57].

Maneb (MB): MB, a commonly used fungicide, is an irritant to respiratory tracts and is capable of inducing sensitization by skin contact. Mechanistically, MB seems to cross the BBB. Although knowledge of the mechanisms of this toxin is very limited, MB preferentially inhibits mitochondrial complex III [58]. Further, MB was shown to induce apoptosis through Bak activation, whereas combination of PQ and MB inhibits the Bak-dependent pathway while potentiating apoptosis through Bak protein [59].

Metals: The potential role of metals due to prolonged exposure as risk factors for Parkinson's disease has been evaluated [60]. Chronic occupational exposure to high levels of manganese (Mn) in manganese miners causes accumulation of this metal in the basal ganglia, resulting in tremors, rigidity and psychosis that resemble PD [61]. The metal-induced Parkinsonian syndrome that results from Mn exposure differs significantly from idiopathic PD. The Parkinsonism caused by Mn does not respond to L-DOPA treatment and the primary target of Mn toxicity seems to be the globus pallidus rather than the nigrostriatal system [62]. The potential role of iron and other transition elements has also been studied. The level of ferritin (primary intracellular protein capable of keeping iron bound in a nonreactive status) in the nigral tissue of patients with PD was found to be decreased [63]. Thus, iron accumulation together with decreased binding capability may enhance the risk for iron-mediated toxic reactions in PD by generating the highly toxic hydroxyl radical in the presence of iron and hydrogen peroxide, thus leading to oxidative stress and ultimately neurodegeneration.

4. Molecular pathways in sporadic PD

Though Mendelian genes are responsible only for a small subset of PD patients, it is speculated that the same pathogenetic mechanisms could also play a relevant role in the development of more frequent sporadic PD [64]. With advancement in molecular biotechnological tools and techniques, a number of genes and proteins linked to PD have been identified, which reveal a complex network of molecular pathways involved in its etiology, suggesting that common mechanisms underlie both familial and sporadic forms of PD (**Table 2**) [65–79]. Three predominat pathways that can trigger the neurodegenerative process are as follows: (a) accumulation of aggregated and misfolded proteins, (b) impairment of the ubiquitin protein pathway (UPS) and the autophagy pathway, and (c) mitochondrial dysfunction [64]. Functional studies on the proteins encoded by PD-related genes supports these pathways and it is confirmed by both pathological and biochemical studies performed in patients with sporadic PD with no apparent genetic cause [80–82]. Further, critical cellular protective pathways, such as autophagy, UPS, and mitochondria dynamics, are shown to lose adeptness with increasing age and there is a progressive build-up of somatic mutations particularly in the mitochondrial DNA during aging process [64]. Recent studies have shown the role for chronic neuroinflammation and microglia activation in PD pathogenesis, suggesting that different molecular/cellular events may contribute to neurodegeneration by activating resident microglial populations in selected brain areas, with potential detrimental effects on vulnerable neuronal populations [83].

Compound treatment	Drosophila model	Modifies phenotype(s)	Pathway/ process	References
Sulforaphane and allyl Disulfide	parkin	DA neuron number	Oxidative stress	[65]
	α-synuclein	DA neuron number		[65]
S-Methyl-L-cysteine	α-synuclein	Locomotor activity		[66]
Polyphenols	α-synuclein	Lifespan, Locomotor activity		[67]
	Paraquat and Iron	Locomotor activity		[68]
α-Tocopherol	DJ-1β	Lifespan		[69]
	PINK1	Ommatidial degeneration		[70]
SOD	PINK1	Ommatidial degeneration		[70]
Melatonin	DJ-1β	Lifespan		[69]
	Paraquat	Locomotor activity		[71]
	Rotenone	Locomotor activity, Dopamine neuron number		[71]
Bacopa monieri leaf extract	Paraquat; Rotenone	Oxidative markers; Mitochondrial functions		[72, 73]
Minocycline	DJ-1α	DA neuron number, dopamine levels	Oxidative stress/ inflammatory process	[74]
Celestrol	DJ-1α	DA neuron number,		[74]

Compound treatment	*Drosophila* model	Modifies phenotype(s)	Pathway/ process	References
		dopamine levels, Locomotor activity and survival rate under oxidative stress conditions		
Rapamycin	Parkin/PINK1	Thoracic indentations, Locomotor activity, DA neuron number, and muscle integrity.	TOR signaling	[75]
Geldanamycin	α-synuclein	DA neuron number	Removal of excess or toxic protein forms	[76, 77]
Zinc Chloride	Parkin	Life span, Locomotor activity, and percentage of adulthood survivors.	Zinc homeostasis	[78]

Modified from Munoz-Soriano and Paricio [79].

Table 2. Therapeutic compounds shown to modify phenotype(s) in the *Drosophila* PD model.

4.1. Genetic basis of sporadic PD

The use of genetically tractable organisms to model gene–environment interactions has become an efficient means of identifying genetic risk factors [84, 85]. Functional characterization of the genes involved in familial PD has shown significant comprehensions into the molecular mechanism(s) responsible to the pathogenesis of PD. Abnormal protein and mitochondrial homeostasis are the crucial factors behind the development of PD, with oxidative stress playing a vital connection between the two events. Genome-wide association studies (GWAS) showed variations in α-synuclein and *LRRK2* (well-known familial PD genes), i.e., as important risk causes for the sporadic PD [86]. The elevation of dopamine synthesis in response to a variety of stressors [87] may subject DA neurons to an increased risk for oxidative stress-mediated impairment [88]. Nevertheless, connotation studies of polymorphisms within these genes have not proved the hypothesis [89, 90].

The recent application of high throughput whole genome and exome analysis technologies along with bioinformatics has provided valuable inputs in the identification of novel susceptibility loci involved in apparent sporadic PD. It is predicted that many more variants remained to be discovered despite the success of GWAS in discovering novel genetic variants in PD. In this regard, genome-wide complex trait analysis [91, 92] may prove useful for a more exhaustive screening for PD risk variants [93]. Groundbreaking efforts have begun to establish the relationship between single nucleotide polymorphisms (SNPs) identified by GWAS and gene expression levels to describe their functional meaning. This approach has provided significant insights into various potential novel mechanisms underlying the observed SNP associations with PD etiology.

4.2. Interaction between genetics and environment

The concept that gene–environment interactions affect PD susceptibility was proposed more than a decade ago [94]. Although many studies have described positive associations between genetic polymorphisms and increased risk for PD, only a few human association studies have examined gene–environment interactions. Occupational pesticide exposure as well as high exposure to PQ and MB in carriers of DAT genetic variants was shown to increase the PD risk [36, 95]. Further, SNP in *NOS1* (neuronal nitric oxide synthase 1) and *GSTP1* (glutathione S-transferase pi 1) have been linked to an increased risk for PD among pesticide-exposed individuals [96], although an association between *GSTP1* and pesticide exposure has not been supported by a large cohort study conducted subsequently [97]. However, European studies did not show noteworthy interaction between polymorphisms in 15 genes that impact metabolism of extraneous chemicals or dopamine and exposure to pesticides and metals [97].

Twin studies: Twin studies are particularly useful in distinguishing between the influence of genetics or the environment on the risks of a disease. If genetic factors predominate in etiology of a disease, it is expected that concordance in monozygotic (MZ) twins will be greater than dizygotic (DZ) twins. Using striatal ^{18}F[DOPA] positron emission tomography (PET) scan to detect dopaminergic dysfunction in asymptomatic cotwins of twin pairs with mostly sporadic and late onset PD, Piccini *et al.* [98] found a three-fold higher concordance rate of PD in MZ twins (55%) than in DZ twins (18%), suggesting a significant genetic contribution. Furthermore, when monitored over a period of 7 years, asymptomatic MZ cotwins all showed progressive loss of dopaminergic function and four developed clinical PD, while none of the DZ twin pairs became clinically concordant. Similarly, a recent longitudinal study carried out on Swedish twins with predominantly sporadic PD revealed concordance rates of 11% for MZ and 4% for same-sexed DZ twin pairs, with an overall heritability estimate of 34% [99].

Two-hit PD models: Present genetic PD models failed to reproduce nigrostriatal DA loss, hinting that a single genetic risk factor is not sufficient enough and an environmental factor may be required to initiate the process of neurodegeneration. To understand this paradigm and to decipher the interaction between genes and environment two hit animal models (animals with a genetic defect will be exposed to multiple environmental factors/toxicants to study if this synergy will lead to DA degeneration) will be of potential help.

5. Insights into sporadic PD pathophysiology through *Drosophila*

The fruit fly *Drosophila* has emerged as a suitable model for studying mechanisms of PD-related neurodegeneration in the past decade. Structural architecture and functional pathways involved in dopamine synthesis and degradation are well preserved between *Drosophila* and human. Transgenic flies (neuronal overexpression of *wt* or mutant (A53T or A50P) human alpha-synuclein) showed age-dependent and selective loss of dopaminergic neurons, formation of fibrillary inclusions containing alpha-synuclein, as well as a progressive loss of climbing activity, which could be alleviated by L-DOPA or DA agonists [100]. Mutational analyses of alpha-synuclein in *Drosophila* have permitted an extended evaluation of the protein domains involved and/or required for toxicity showing, for example, that truncated forms of alpha-synuclein have a central hydrophobic region, between residues 71 and 82, essential for the formation of oligomeric and fibrillary forms of the protein and toxicity. Importance of post-translational modification of alpha-synuclein (phosphorylation on serine 129 and tyrosine 125, on alpha-synuclein oligomerization and toxicity) was demonstrated using the *Drosophila* model. Using fly model it was also shown that early, soluble forms of aggregates of alpha-synuclein are more toxic.

Mutations that induce loss of function or inactivation of the fly homologs of mutations of fly homologs of PINK1, parkin, DJ-1, or LRKK2 lead to selective DA degeneration leading to mobility defects that can be characterized through behavioral assays. *Drosophila* parkin null mutants exhibit decreased life span, mitochondrial abnormalities, and flight muscle deterioration leading to mobility defects and diminished proteasome 26S activity. Overexpression of mutant but not with wild parkin (human gene) in *Drosophila* leads to dopaminergic deterioration and motor defects, signifying a dominant negative effect of the mutated protein in PD pathology. Further, PINK1 mutant flies also share PD characteristics with parkin mutants.

Drosophila models have been important to identify the role of both parkin and PINK1 in the regulation of mitochondrial physiology [101]. Unlike mammals, *Drosophila* expresses two DJ-1 homologs, viz., DJ-1 alpha, restricted to male germline, and DJ-1 beta that, similarly to mammals, is ubiquitously expressed. Different mutations of both genes have been induced. DJ-1beta KO flies showed enhanced susceptibility to cytotoxins, such as paraquat, H_2O_2, and rotenone, further supporting the protective redox function of DJ-1. Similarly, DJ-1beta mutations that cause loss of protein function lead to accumulation of ROS in fly's brain.

5.1. Induction of PD in *Drosophila*

Drosophila were first used to model PD, when Feany and Bender [100] produced transgenic flies that either expressed normal human α-synuclein or one of the mutant forms, A30P and A53T α-synuclein, which have both been linked to familial PD. This discovery revealed the potential of *Drosophila* system for modeling gain and loss-of-function genetic mutations that are associated with PD, thereby allowing the elucidation of the genes molecular functions and the pathways involved.

5.2. Toxin models of *Drosophila* for PD

Several environmental chemicals (neurotoxins) have been employed to recapitulate PD-like symptoms and pathology in *Drosophila* system [102]. *Drosophila* performs motor functions such as walking, climbing, and flying and has a well-developed nervous system which makes *Drosophila* a suitable model for understanding PD. These kinds of complex behavior phenotypes are similar from strain to strain and hence characterizing a toxin induced PD model for this organism becomes easy [100]. Extensively used chemical models with their salient features are briefly described below.

Rotenone (ROT) induced PD model in Drosophila: Inhibition of the mitochondrial respiratory chain by ROT has been widely used to study the role of the mitochondrial respiratory chain in apoptosis [103, 104]. The mitochondrial respiratory chain is the major site of ATP production in eukaryotes and it is well recognized that this organelle not only generates ATP, but also plays an important role in apoptosis [105–107]. It is now clear that upon apoptotic stimulation mitochondria can release several proapoptotic regulators, including cytochrome c [108], Smac/Diablo [109, 110], endonuclease G [111], and apoptosis-inducing factor [112] to the cytosol. These proapoptotic regulators will then activate cellular apoptotic programs downstream [105–107]. The release of proapoptotic regulators is further regulated by the translocation of Bcl-2 family proteins [113, 114]. Some of the salient pathophysiological features of the ROT fly model are: (a) being lipophilic, it can easily cross the blood–brain barrier but the final concentration of rotenone in the brain may probably be much lower than the initial because of these barriers and the powerful excretion system of flies. They have a tendency to stay at the bottom of vials and did not appear to coordinate their legs normally [37]. (b) Since neuronal dopaminergic clusters are normally present in each *Drosophila* adult brain hemisphere [115–117], abnormalities are characterized by the disappearance of part or the totality of dopaminergic cell clusters but this effect varies in intensity from one fly to another [37].

Paraquat (PQ) model of PD in Drosophila: Long-term exposure to environmental oxidative stressors, such as the herbicide PQ, has been linked to the development of PD. In view of this, PQ is frequently used in the *Drosophila system* and other animal models to study PD and the degeneration of dopaminergic neurons (DNs). Recently, it has been shown that expression of D_1 like dopaminergic receptor (DAMB receptor) was directly proportional to PQ induced toxicity in CNS of flies [118]. It is notable that a long-term neuronal DA synthesis decreases the DAMB expression and resists the PQ toxicity. Age-related decrement in PQ resistance is also observed with a significant increase in DAMB receptor. This evidence proves that there are more areas to be researched regarding DA related neurodegeneration in *Drosophila*. Some of the salient pathophysiological features of PQ fly model are: (a) flies exhibit rapid onset of movement disorders, including resting tremors, bradykinesis, rotational behaviors and postural instability which resemble Parkinsonian symptoms. Furthermore, the flies frequently freeze while attempting to climb vial walls and would often fall to the bottom of the vial. Males exhibit symptoms 12 hours earlier than females, but both males and females are strongly affected [71]; (b) PQ-dependent dopaminergic neuron loss is totally selective in a time-dependent loss of exposure where after 6 hours of exposure PPL1 and by 12 hours PPM2, PPM3 cluster will be affected whereas PPM1 and PPL2 clusters only get affected after 20–24 hour of exposure [71], and (c) changes in the neuronal cell are also a trait where cell bodies aggregate in a round shape, and fragment and then disappear [71].

6. Application of *Drosophila* model: screening platform for assessment of neuroprotective potential

Drosophila models are a great cost-effective alternative to rodent and primate-based models, allowing rapid high throughput screening of novel therapies. Studies done with *Drosophila* model coexposed to rotenone and melatonin (an antioxidant and free radical scavenger) showed that melatonin improved the movement behavior of rotenone-treated flies, even more evidently than L-dopa [119]. Quantification of the number of dopaminergic cells after 1 week of rotenone feeding revealed that the presence of melatonin significantly rescued the loss of neurons in all of the clusters [37]. Subsequently, the rotenone model of *Drosophila* has been extensively employed as a screening platform to assess the neuroprotective potential of various molecules and phytoconstituents. Over the last five years, numerous workers have employed the fly rotenone model (both wild type and genetically modified strains) to test potential neuroprotective treatments [72–73, 120, 121]. The majority of these studies used compounds that have multiple therapeutic properties such as antioxidant, anti-inflammatory, and anti-apoptotic properties, which largely yielded positive results such as reductions in ROS and inflammatory mediators, attenuation of TH-positive neuron loss and striatal dopamine loss as well as reversal of motor deficits [122].

6.1. Plant-derived neuroprotective agents in PD

The *Drosophila* model is extensively used due to the flies' rapid generation time, low cost, and amenability for genetic manipulation, and thus serves as an ideal model for identifying promising neuroprotective candidates that can then undergo further validation in mammalian models (**Table 2**) [65–79, 123]. Growing evidence indicate that the herbs used in traditional medicines contain neuroprotective compounds such as resveratol, curcumin or ginsenoside, green tea polyphenols or catechins, triptolide, etc. [124–128]. These compounds may help enhancing antioxidant activity, decrease loss of dopamine, inhibit activation of microglia, reduce the release of pro-inflammatory factors, prevent α-synuclein aggregation and fibrillation. These herbs also protect the dopaminergic neurons against neurotoxins like MTTP, 6-OHDA. Some of the major plant derived molecules suggested as therapeutic agents for PD are as follows.

Resveratol: This is a polyphenolic compound naturally found in grapes. This is able to cross the blood–brain barrier and is water soluble [129]. The numerous pharmacological functions include anti-inflammation, antiapoptosis, antioxidation, anticancer, etc.

Curcumin: In recent years curcumin has shown therapeutic potential for neurodegenerative diseases such as PD. It is a natural polyphenol found in the spice turmeric and is known for several biological and medicinal effects such as anti-inflammatory, antioxidant, anti-proliferative activities, etc. It is demonstrated to help in preventing the aggregation and fibrillation of α-synuclein [130]. Curcumin glucoside, a modified form, prevents the aggregation and enhances the solubility of α-synuclein [131]. Studies have shown that curcumin reduces the LRRK2 kinase activity and decreases the levels of oxidized proteins. Thus curcumin also acts as an inhibitor for LRRK2 kinase activity. Our laboratory has shown stage-specific neuroprotective efficacy of curcumin in *Drosophila* model of idiopathic PD [132].

Ginsenoside: There are two major categories of ginsenosides—protopanaxadiols and protopanaxatriols. In vitro and in vivo studies have shown ginsenosides to exert pharmacological effects against neuroinflammation, cerebral oxidative stress, radical formation, and apoptosis. It plays a neuroprotective role in regulation of synaptic plasticity, neurotransmitter release, and neuroinflammatory responses [126].

Blueberry extracts: Blueberry contains a large amount of polyphenols and has a greater antioxidant property than most fruits and vegetables. Consumption of blueberry has been reported to slow down the age-related functional and physiological deficits [133–135]. Peng *et al.* [136] were the first to show the anti-aging property of blueberry using *Drosophila* fly model. The study also showed that supplemented blueberry extracts increased the mRNA levels of SOD1, SOD2, and CAT in *Drosophila*. Blueberry extracts can partially reverse the chronic Paraquat exposure. Blueberry extracts in diet of flies could increase the mean life span, decrease Paraquat induced mortality, and partially reverse the locomotor deficiency.

7. Notable limitations

Animal models are absolutely necessary for reproducing physiologic and neurosystems aspects of neurodegenerative disorders. However, animal models are complicated by the differing expression levels and patterns of expression of target genes, with different promoters among other issues for genetic models, and complexities of drug administration, drug distribution, and metabolism for toxin models [79]. Rodent models have faced limitations due to lack of strong construct (i.e., genotype or intervention) and face validity (i.e., phenotype), as well as species and strain limitations. In general, toxin-induced PD models do not recapitulate the process of progressive neuron loss and the protein aggregation in LBs, due to the acute nature of the neurotoxin treatment [137, 138], but they have been useful to support the concept that alterations in mitochondrial biology are essential for the development of PD [139]. However, animal models allow studying a cellular process in the context of a whole organism and are thus more reliable.

Research on PD using cell cultures has many advantages in which they allow rapid screening for disease pathogenesis and drug candidates. Cellular models can be easily used for molecular, biochemical, and pharmacological approaches, but they can lead to misinterpretation and artifacts. *Vice versa* limitations include that the survival of neurons is dependent upon the culture conditions and the cells do not develop their natural neuronal networks. In most cases, neurons are deprived of the physiological afferent and efferent connections [140].

While there are many advantages of the fly PD model, the most common disadvantage is that the important pathogenetic factors which are vertebrate-specific may be ignored in invertebrate models. The differences between mammals and invertebrates represent potential drawbacks in modeling brain diseases such as PD [141].

8. Potential opportunities

Drosophila melanogaster was the first major complex organism to have its genome sequenced [142] and after the human genome was sequenced the homology between the two genomes greatly strengthened to understand human biology and the disease processes as a model [143]. More importantly, 75% of human disease-related loci have a *Drosophila* orthologue [144]. Fly model are less costly and time consuming to use when compared to mammals due to their rapid reproduction time and short lifespan [143, 145, 146]. In addition, flies are capable of performing complex motor behaviors such as walking, climbing, and flying and their brain is complex enough to make these behaviors relevant to humans [101, 147, 148].

Some of the unique features of the *Drosophila* model which have been identified are: (a) *Drosophila* models are instrumental in exploring the mechanisms of neurodegeneration, with several PD-related mutations eliciting related phenotypes including sensitivity to energy supply and vesicular deformities. These are leading to the identification of plausible cellular mechanisms, which may be specific to (dopaminergic) neurons and synapses rather than general cellular phenotypes. (b) Fly models show noncell autonomous signaling within the nervous system, offering the opportunity to develop our understanding of the way pathogenic signaling propagates, resembling Braak's scheme of spreading pathology in PD, (c) fly models link physiological deficits to changes in synaptic structure, and (d) the strong neuronal phenotypes observed in the fly models permit relevant *in vivo* drug testing [149]. Another key feature making *Drosophila* an attractive model is the range of genetic tools available to manipulate them and the ease of introducing human genes into the fly enables it to recapitulate the symptoms and progression of human disease in flies [150]. Two approaches employed are: the *reverse genetic approach* wherein a gene is tested for its potential functional role by using the GAL4/*UAS*-system and the *forward genetic approach* (function of a gene) for identification of genes based on phenotype, which is useful to understand diseases whose genetic basis is yet to determined [141]. The genomics era has played a crucial role in directing both the functional biology and the *in vitro/in vivo* modeling of neurodegenerative diseases in fly model.

9. Future perspectives

Drosophila has been used to model several aspects of neurodegenerative diseases, including aggregation toxicity of misfolding disease related proteins [151–156]. Ninety-five percent of the Parkinson's disease patients suffer from sporadic form. In those sporadic cases, no indication allows a decided inference about the underlying causes as well as the pathogenic mechanism involved [101]. The limitations of human genetics make it necessary to use model system to analyze affected genes and pathways knowledge of which is essential to develop therapeutic targets. During last three decades, genetically pliable fruit fly *Drosophila* has been a great model system to study human neurodegenerative disorders including PD human genetic screens, and pathological studies have been able to provide limited mechanistic insights into the molecular processes that determine disease susceptibility or age at onset of disease [157]. Genetic analysis has identified causative mutations for autosomal-dominant and recessive forms of familial PD. Functional studies of these genes have provided great insights into potential pathogenic mechanisms of inherited forms of PD; however it is unclear how these may relate to the more common sporadic forms of PD.

Identification of PD risk locus SREBF1 through GWAS (genome-wide association studies) analysis and substantiating its biological function as a regulator of mitophagy [158] remarkably emphasize the importance and potential to decipher the risk loci for idiopathic PD through genome-wide screens in animal models. However, no systematic genome-wide functional screens are performed in sporadic PD models. Here lies the importance and necessity to perform genome-wide screen to identify the risk locus for idiopathic PD. Comprehensive efforts in this direction will provide novel insights into the molecular mechanisms behind the dopaminergic neurodegeneration and also figure out genetic basis for sporadic PD. Here lies the potential relevance and advantage of fly genetics and available technologies such as UAS-Gal4, fly deletion lines, and RNAi lines, which can be of great help to figure out novel players, pathways, and mechanistic interactions among neurodegenerative disorders. Hence, it is worth placing future endeavors in this direction.

10. Conclusion

In this chapter, we have provided an overview of current knowledge on the pathophysiology of sporadic PD employing *Drosophila* system. We also presented the future perspectives on the subject matter and emphasize the utmost importance for the need to generate comprehensive data employing genome-wide association studies in this model that may lead to identification of newer pathways. We also discussed the importance and necessity to reexamine the strategies/methods of screens to assess the potential of neuroprotective compounds/molecules employing *late life stages* that may provide us better answers on successful utilization of therapeutic compounds in late onset neurodegenerative disorders such as PD.

Acknowledgements

This work is partly supported by the Department of Biotechnology (DBT), Ministry of Science and Technology, India (R&D grant nos. BT/249/NE/TBP/2011, 25-4-2012, and BT/405/NE/U-Excel/2013, 11-12-2014), to the corresponding author. Dr Muralidhara is a recipient of DBT (Department of Biotechnology, India) Visiting Research Professorship under the North–East scheme.

Author details

Priyanka Modi[1,2], Ayajuddin Mohamad[1,2], Limamanen Phom[1,2], Zevelou Koza[1,2], Abhik Das, Rahul Chaurasia[1,2], Saikat Samadder[1,2], Bovito Achumi[1,2], Muralidhara[1,2], Rajesh Singh Pukhrambam[1,2] and Sarat Chandra Yenisetti[1,2*]

*Address all correspondence to: yschandrays@rediffmail.com, sarat@nagalanduniversity.ac.in

1 These authors contributed equally to this work

2 Drosophila Neurobiology Laboratory, Department of Zoology, Nagaland University (Central), Lumami, Nagaland, India

References

[1] http://www.pdf.org/en/parkinson_statistics (Accessed 2016:04:09)

[2] Polymeropoulos MH, Higgins JJ, Golbe LI, Johnson WG, et al: Mapping of a gene for Parkinson's disease to chromosome 4q21-q23. Science. 1996;274:1197–1199

[3] Reeve A, Simcox E, Turnbull D: Ageing and Parkinson's disease: why is advancing age the biggest risk factor? Ageing Res Rev. 2014; 14:19–30

[4] Calne DB, Langston JW: Aetiology of Parkinson's disease. Lancet. 1983;2(8365–8366): 1457–1459

[5] Langston JW, Ballard P, Tetrud JW, Irwin I: Chronic Parkinsonism in humans due to a product of melperidine-analog, synthesis. Science. 1983;219:979–980

[6] Poewe W, Antonini A, Zijlmans JCM, Burkhard PR: Levodopa in the treatment of Parkinson's disease: an old drug still going strong. Clin Interv Aging. 2010;5:229–238

[7] Tieu K: A guide to neurotoxic animal models of Parkinson's disease. Cold Spring Harb Perspect Med. 2011;1(1):a009316

[8] Meredith GE, Sonsalla PK, Chesselet M-F: Animal models of Parkinson's disease progression. Acta Neuropathol. 2008;115(4):385–398

[9] Bezard E, Przedborski S: A tale on animal models of Parkinson's disease. Mov Disord. 2011;26(6):993–1002. DOI:10.1002/mds.23696

[10] Polymeropoulos MH, Lavedan C, Leroy E, Ide SE, et al: Mutation in the alpha-synuclein gene identified in families with Parkinson's disease. Science. 1997;276:2045–2047

[11] Kitada T, Asakawa S, Hattori N, Matsumine H, Yamamura Y, et al: Mutations in the parkin gene cause autosomal recessive juvenile Parkinsonism. Nature. 1998;392:605–608

[12] Valente EM, Abou-Sleiman PM, Caputo V, Muqit MMK, et al: Hereditary early-onset Parkinson's disease caused by mutations in PINK1. Science. 2004;304:1158–1160

[13] Bonifati V, Rizzu P, van Baren MJ, Schaap O, Breedveld GJ et al: Mutations in the DJ-1 gene associated with autosomal recessive early-onset Parkinsonism. Science. 2003;299:256–259

[14] Paisán-Ruíz C, Jain S, Evans EW, Gilks WP, et al: Cloning of the gene containing mutations that cause PARK8-linked Parkinson's disease. Neuron. 2004;44:595–600

[15] Ramirez A, Heimbach A, Grundemann J, Stiller B, Hampshire D, et al: Hereditary Parkinsonism with dementia is caused by mutations in ATP13A2, encoding a lysosomal type 5 P-type ATPase. Nat Genet. 2006;38:1184–1191

[16] Paisan-Ruiz C, Bhatia KP, Li A, Hernandez D, Davis M, et al: Characterization of PLA2G6 as a locus for dystoniaparkinsonism. Ann Neurol. 2009;65:19–23

[17] Shojaee S, Sina F, Banihosseini SS, Kazemi MH, Kalhor R, et al: Genome-wide linkage analysis of a Parkinsonian-pyramidal syndrome pedigree by 500 K SNP arrays. Am J Hum Genet. 2008;82:1375–1384

[18] Edvardson S, Cinnamon Y, Ta-Shma A, Shaag A, et al: A deleterious mutation in DNAJC6 encoding the neuronal-specific clathrin-uncoating co-chaperone auxilin, is associated with juvenile Parkinsonism. PLoS One. 2012;7:e36458. DOI:10.1371/journal.pone.0036458

[19] Krebs CE, Karkheiran S, Powell JC, Cao M, Makarov V, et al: The Sac1 domain of SYNJ1 identified mutated in a family with early-onset progressive Parkinsonism with generalized seizures. Hum Mutat. 2013;34:1200–1207

[20] Quadri M, Fang M, Picillo M, Olgiati S, Breedveld GJ, et al: Mutation in the SYNJ1 gene associated with autosomal recessive, early-onset Parkinsonism. Hum Mutat. 2013;34:1208–1215

[21] Marras C, Lohmann K, Lang A, Klein C: Fixing the broken system of genetic locus symbols: Parkinson disease and dystonia as examples. Neurology. 2012;78:1016–1024

[22] Yue Z: LRRK2 in Parkinson's disease: in vivo models and approaches for understanding pathogenic roles. FEBS J. 2009;276(22):6445–6454

[23] Liu Z, Hamamichi S, Lee BD, et al: Inhibitors of LRRK2 kinase attenuate neurodegeneration and Parkinson-like phenotypes in Caenorhabditis elegans and Drosophila Parkinson's disease models. Hum Mol Genet. 2011;20(20):3933–3942

[24] Bove J, Prou D, Perier C, Przedborski S: Toxin induced models of Parkinson's disease. NeuroRx. 2005;2:484–494

[25] Betarbet R, Sherer TB, DiMonte DA, Greenamyre JT: Mechanistic approaches to Parkinson's disease pathogenesis. Brain Pathol. 2002;12:499–510

[26] Gerlach M, Desser H, Youdim MBH, Riederer P: New horizons in molecular mechanisms underlying Parkinson's disease and in our understanding of the neuroprotective effects of selegiline. J Neural Transm. 1996;48:7–21

[27] Zigmond MJ, Stricker EM: Animal models of Parkinsonism using selective neurotoxins: clinical and basic implications. Int Rev Neurobiol. 1989;31:1–79

[28] Di Monte DA, Mitra Lavasani, Manning-Bog AB: Environmental factors in Parkinson's disease. NeuroToxicology. 2002;23:487–502

[29] McCormack AL, Thiruchelvam M, Manning-Bog AB, Thiffault C, et al: Environmental risk factors and Parkinson's disease: selective degeneration of nigral dopaminergic neurons caused by the herbicide paraquat. Neurobiol Dis. 2002;10:119 –127

[30] Uversky VN: Neurotoxicant-induced animal models of Parkinson's disease: understanding the role of rotenone, Maneb and paraquat in neurodegeneration. Cell Tissue Res. 2004;318:225–241

[31] Simon-Sanchez J, Schulte C, Bras JM, Sharma M, et al: Genome-wide association study reveals genetic risk underlying Parkinson's disease. Nat Genet. 2009;41(12):1308–1312

[32] Spillantini MG, Schmidt ML, Lee VM, Trojanowski JQ, et al: Alpha-synuclein in Lewy bodies. Nature. 1997;388:839–840

[33] Dhillon AS, Tarbutton GL, Levin JL, Plotkin GM, et al: Pesticide/environmental exposures and Parkinson's disease in East Texas. J Agromedicine. 2008;13:37–48

[34] Elbaz A, Clavel J, Rathouz PJ, Moisan F, et al: Professional exposure to pesticides and Parkinson disease. Ann Neurol. 2009;66:494–504

[35] Kamel F, Tanner C, Umbach D, Hoppin J, et al: Pesticide exposure and self-reported Parkinson's disease in the agricultural health study. Am J Epidemiol. 2007;165:364–374

[36] Ritz BR, Manthripragada AD, Costello S, Lincoln SJ, et al: Dopamine transporter genetic variants and pesticides in Parkinson's disease. Environ Health Perspect. 2009;117:964–969

[37] Coulom H, Birman S: Chronic exposure to rotenone models sporadic Parkinson's disease in Drosophila melanogaster. J Neurosci. 2004;24(48):10993–10998

[38] Ascherio A, Chen H, Weisskopf MG, O'Reilly E, et al: Pesticide exposure and risk for Parkinson's disease. Ann Neurol. 2006;60:197–203

[39] Liou HH, Tsai MC, Chen CJ, et al: Environmental risk factors and Parkinson's disease: a case-control study in Taiwan. Neurology. 1997;48:1583–1588

[40] Petrovitch H, Ross GW, Abbott RD, Sanderson WT, et al: Plantation work and risk of Parkinson's disease in a population-based longitudinal study. Arch Neurol. 2002;59:1787–1792

[41] Seidler A, Hellenbrand W, Robra BP, Veiregge P, et al: Possible environmental, occupational, and other etiologic factors for Parkinson's disease: a case-control study in Germany. Neurology. 1996;46:1275–1284

[42] Ratner MH, David HF, Josef O, Robert GF, Raymon D: Younger age at onset of sporadic Parkinson's disease among subjects occupationally exposed to metals and pesticides. Interdiscip Toxicol. 2014;7(3):123–133

[43] Di Monte DA: The environment and Parkinson's disease: is the nigrostriatal system preferentially targeted by neurotoxins? Lancet Neurol. 2003;2(9):531–538

[44] Uversky VN, Li J, Bower K, Fink AL: Synergistic effects of pesticides and metals on the fibrillation of alpha-synuclein: implications for Parkinson's disease. Neurotoxicology. 2002;23(4–5):527–536

[45] Chiba K, Trevor AJ, Castagnoli Jr. N :Active uptake of MPP+, a metabolite of MPTP, by brain synaptosomes. Biochem Biophys. Res Commun. 1985;128:1228–1232

[46] Javitch JA, D'Amato RJ, Strittmatter SM, Snyder SH: Parkinsonism inducing neurotoxin, N-methyl-4-phenyl-1,2,3,6-tetrahydropyridine: uptake of the metabolite N-methyl-4-phenylpyridine by dopamine neurons explains selective toxicity. Proc Natl Acad Sci USA. 1985;82:2173–2177

[47] Daniels AJ, Reinhard Jr. JF: Energy-driven uptake of the neurotoxin 1-methyl-4-phenylpyridinium into chromaffin granules via the catecholamine transporter. J Biol Chem. 1988;263:5034–5036

[48] Miller GW, Gainetdinov RR, Levey AI, Caron MG: dopamine transporters and neuronal injury. Trends Pharmacol Sci. 1999;20:424–429

[49] Javoy F, Sotelo C, Herbet A, Agid Y: Specificity of dopaminergic neuronal degeneration induced by intracerebral injection of 6-hydroxydopamine in the nigrostriatal dopamine system. Brain Res. 1976;102:201–215

[50] Jeon BS, Jackson-Lewis V, Burke RE: 6-Hydroxydopamine lesion of the rat substantia nigra: time course and morphology of cell death. Neurodegeneration. 1995;4:131–137

[51] Dauer W, Przedborski S: Parkinson's disease: mechanisms and models. Neuron. 2003;39:889–909

[52] Cicchetti F, Drouin-Ouellet L, Gross RE: Environmental toxins and Parkinson's disease: what we have learned from pesticides-induced animal models? Trends Pharmacol Sci. 2009;30(9):475–483

[53] Wang XF, Li S, Chou AP, Bronstein JM: Inhibitory effects of pesticides on proteasome activity: implication in Parkinson's disease. Neurobiol Dis. 2006;23:198–205

[54] Olanow CW: The pathogenesis of cell death in Parkinson's disease. Mov Disord. 2007;22(17):335–342

[55] Shimizu K, Ohtaki K, Matsubara K, Aoyama K, et al: Carrier-mediated processes in blood–brain barrier penetration and neural uptake of paraquat. Brain Res. 2001;906:135–142

[56] Miller GW: Paraquat: the red herring of Parkinson's disease research. Toxicol Sci. 2007;100:1–2

[57] Fei Q, McCormack AL, Di Monte DA, Ethell DW: Paraquat neurotoxicity is mediated by a Bak dependent mechanism. J Biol Chem. 2008;283:3357–3364

[58] Zhang J, Fitsanakis VA, Gu G, Jing D, et al: Manganese ethylene-bis-dithiocarbamate and selective dopaminergic neurodegeneration in rat: a link through mitochondrial dysfunction. J Neurochem. 2003;84:336–346

[59] Fei Q, Ethell DW: Maneb potentiates paraquat neurotoxicity by inducing key Bcl-2 family members. J Neurochem. 2008;105:2091–2097

[60] Gorell JM, Johnson CC, Rybicki BA, Peterson EL, et al: Occupational exposures to metals as risk factors for Parkinson's disease. Neurology. 1997;48:650–658

[61] Mergler D, Baldwin M: Early manifestations of manganese neurotoxicity in humans: an update. Environ Res. 1997;73:92–100

[62] Pal PK, Samii A, Calne DB: Manganese neurotoxicity: a review of clinical features. Neurotoxicology. 1999;20:227–238

[63] Dexter DT, Carayon A, Vidailhet M, Ruberg M, et al: Decreased ferritin levels in brain in Parkinson's disease. J Neurochem. 1990;55:16–20

[64] Valentea EM, Arenaa G, Torosantuccia L, Gelmettia V: Molecular pathways in sporadic PD. Parkinsonism Related Disorders. 2012;18(1):71–73

[65] Trinh K, Moore K, Wes PD, et al: Induction of the phase II detoxification pathway suppresses neuron loss in Drosophila models of Parkinson's disease, J Neurosci. 2008;28(2):465–472

[66] Wassef R, Haenold R, Hansel A, Brot N: Methionine sulfoxide reductase A and a dietary supplement S-methyl-L-cysteine prevent Parkinson's-like symptoms, J Neurosci. 2007;27(47):12808–12816

[67] Long JH, Gao L, Sun L, Liu J, Zhao-Wilson X: Grape extract protects mitochondria from oxidative damage and improves locomotor dysfunction and extends lifespan in a Drosophila Parkinson's disease model. Rejuvenation Res. 2009;12(5):321–331

[68] Jimenez-Del-Rio M, C Guzman-Martinez, C Velez-Pardo: The effects of polyphenols on survival and locomotor activity in Drosophila melanogaster exposed to iron and paraquat. Neurochem Res. 2010;35:227–238

[69] Lavara-Culebras E, Mu͂noz-Soriano V, G'omez-Pastor R, Matallana E, and Paricio N: Effects of pharmacological agents on the lifespan phenotype of Drosophila DJ-1β mutants. Gene. 2010;462(1–2):26–33

[70] Wang D, Qian L, Xiong H, et al: Antioxidants protect PINK1-dependent dopaminergic neurons in Drosophila. Proc Natl Acad Sci USA. 2006a;103(36):13520–13525

[71] Chaudhuri A, Bowling K, Funderburk C, Lawal H, et al: Interaction of genetic and environmental factors in a Drosophila Parkinsonism model. J Neurosci. 2007;27(10): 2457–2467

[72] Hosamani, R., Muralidhara: Neuroprotective efficacy of Bacopa monnieri against rotenone induced oxidative stress and neurotoxicity in Drosophila melanogaster. Neurotoxicology. 2009;30:977–985

[73] Hosamani R, Ramesh SR, Muralidhara: Attenuation of rotenone-induced mitochondrial oxidative damage and neurotoxicity in Drosophila melanogaster supplemented with creatine. Neurochem Res. 2010;35(9):1402–1412

[74] Faust K, Gehrke S, Yang Y, Yang L, et al: Neuroprotective effects of compounds with antioxidant and anti-inflammatory properties in a Drosophila model of Parkinson's disease. BMC Neurosci. 2009;10:109

[75] Tain LS, Chowdhury RB, Tao RN, et al: Drosophila HtrA2 is dispensable for apoptosis but acts downstream of PINK1 independently from Parkin. Cell Death Differentiation. 2009;16(8):1118–1125

[76] Auluck PK, Chan HY, Trojanowski JQ, Lee VM, Bonini NM: Chaperone suppression of alpha-synuclein toxicity in a Drosophila model for Parkinson's disease. Science. 2002;295:865–868.

[77] Auluck PK, Meulener MC, Bonini NM: Mechanisms of suppression of α-synuclein neurotoxicity by geldanamycin in Drosophila. J Biol Chem. 2005;280:2873–2878.

[78] Saini N, Schaffner W: Zinc supplement greatly improves the condition of parkin mutant Drosophila. BiolChem. 2010;391(5):513–518

[79] Munoz-Soriano V, Paricio N: Drosophila models of Parkinson's disease: discovering relevant pathways and novel therapeutic strategies. Parkinson's Disease. 2011;1–14. DOI:10.4061/2011/520640

[80] Burbulla LF, Kruger R: Converging environmental and genetic pathways in the pathogenesis of Parkinson's disease. J Neurol Sci. 2011;306:1–8

[81] Martin I, Dawson VL, Dawson TM: Recent advances in the genetics of Parkinson's disease. Annu Rev Genom Human Genet. 2011;12:301–325

[82] Cookson MR, Bandmann O: Parkinson's disease: insights from pathways. Hum Mol Genet. 2010;19:R1–R27

[83] Tansey MG, Goldberg MS: Neuroinflammation in Parkinson's disease: its role in neuronal death and implications for therapeutic intervention. Neurobiol Dis. 2010;37:510–518

[84] Bilen J, Bonini NM: Drosophila as a model for human neurodegenerative disease. Annu Rev Genet. 2005;39:153–171

[85] Cooper AA, Gitler AD, Cashikar A, Haynes CM, et al: α-Synuclein blocks ER-Golgi traffic and Rab1 rescues neuron loss in Parkinson's models. Science. 2006;313:324–328

[86] Chai C, Lim KL: Genetic insights into sporadic Parkinson's disease pathogenesis. Curr Genomics. 2013;14:486–501.

[87] De Bellis MD, Baum AS, Birmaher B, Keshavan MS, et al: Developmental traumatology, Part I: Biological stress systems. Biol Psychiatry. 1999;45:1259–1270

[88] Kim ST, Choi JH, Chang JW, Kim SW, Hwang O: Immobilization stress causes increase in tetrahydrobiopterin, dopamine, and neuromelanin and oxidative damage in the nigrostriatal system. J Neurochem. 2005;95:89–98

[89] Tan EK, Khajavi M, Thronby JI, Nagamitsu S, et al: Variability and validity of polymorphism association studies in Parkinson's disease. Neurology. 2000;5:533–538

[90] Warner TT, Schapira AHV: Genetic and environmental factors in the cause of Parkinson's disease. Ann Neurol. 2003;53(3):16–25

[91] Yang J, Benyamin B, McEvoy BP, Gordon S, Henders AK, et al: Common SNPs explain a large proportion of the heritability for human height. Nat Genet. 2010;42(7):565–569

[92] Yang J, Lee SH, Goddard ME, Visscher PM: GCTA: a tool for genome-wide complex trait. Am J Hum Genet. 2011;88(1):76–82

[93] Keller MF, Saad M, Bras J, Bettella F, et al: Using genomewide complex trait analysis to quantify 'missing heritability' in Parkinson's disease. Hum Mol Genet. 2012;21(22): 4996–5009

[94] Ross CA, Smith WW: Gene-environment interactions in Parkinson's disease. Parkinsonism Relat Disord. 2007;13(3):309–315.

[95] Kelada SN, Checkoway H, Kardia SL, Carlson CS, et al: 5′ and 3′ region variability in the dopamine transporter gene (SLC6A3), pesticide exposure and Parkinson's disease risk: a hypothesis generating study. Hum Mol Genet. 2006;15:3055 3062

[96] Hancock DB, Martin ER, Vance JM, Scott WK: Nitric oxide synthase genes and their interactions with environmental factors in Parkinson's disease. Neurogenetics. 2008;9:249–262

[97] Dick FD, De Palma G, Ahmadi A, Osborne A, et al: Gene environment interactions in Parkinsonism and Parkinson's disease: the Geoparkinson study. Occup Environ Med. 2007;64:673–680

[98] Piccini P, Burn DJ, Ceravolo R, Maraganore D, Brooks DJ: The role of inheritance in sporadic Parkinson's disease: evidence from a longitudinal study of dopaminergic function in twins. Ann Neurol. 1999;45(5):577–582

[99] Wirdefeldt K, Gatz M, Reynolds CA, Prescott CA, Pedersen NL: Heritability of Parkinson disease in Swedish twins: a longitudinal study. Neurobiol Aging. 2011;32(10):1921–1928

[100] Feany MB, Bender WW: A Drosophila model of Parkinson's disease. Nature. 2000;404:394–398

[101] Hirth F: Drosophila melanogaster in the study of human neurodegeneration. CNS Neurological Disorders. 2010;9:504–523

[102] Bonini NM, Fortini ME: Human neurodegenerative disease modeling using Drosophila. Annu Rev Neurosc. 2003;26:627–656

[103] Barrientos A, Moraes CT: Titrating the effects of mitochondrial complex I impairment in the cell physiology. J Biol Chem. 1999;274:16188–1619

[104] Chauvin C, De Oliveira F, Ronot X, Mousseau M, et al: Ubiquinone analogs: a mitochondrial permeability transition pore-dependent pathway to selective cell Death J Biol Chem. 2001;276,41394–41398

[105] Green DR, Reed JC: Mitochondria and apoptosis. Science. 1998;281:1309–1312

[106] Kroemer G, Reed JC: Mitochondrial control of cell death. Nat Med. 2000;6:513–519

[107] Wang X: The expanding role of mitochondria in apoptosis. Genes Dev. 2001;15:2922–2933

[108] Liu X, Kim CN, Yang J, Jemmerson R, Wang X: Induction of apoptotic program in cell-free extracts: requirement for dATP and cytochrome c. Cell. 1996;86:147–157

[109] Du C, Fang M, Li Y, Li L, Wang X: Smac, a mitochondrial protein that promotes cytochrome c-dependent caspase activation by eliminating IAP inhibition. Cell. 2000;102:33–42

[110] Verhagen AM, Ekert PG, Pakusch M, Silke J, Connolly LM, et al: Identification of DIABLO, a mammalian protein that promotes apoptosis by binding to and antagonizing IAP proteins. Cell. 2000;102:43–53

[111] Li LY, Luo X, Wang X: Endonuclease G is an apoptotic DNase when released from mitochondria. Nature. 2001;412:95–99

[112] Susin SA, Lorenzo HK, Zamzami N, Marzo I, et al: Molecular characterization of mitochondrial apoptosis-inducing factor. Nature. 1999;397:441–446

[113] Reed JC: Bcl-2 and the regulation of programmed cell death. J Cell Biol. 1994;124:1–6

[114] Reed JC: Double identity for proteins of the Bcl-2 family. Nature. 1997;387:773–776

[115] Budnik V, White K: Catecholamine containing neurons in Drosophila melanogaster: distribution and development. J Comp Neurol. 1988;268:400–413

[116] Nassel DR, Elekes K: Aminergic neurons in the brain of blowflies and Drosophila: dopamine- and tyrosine hydroxylase-immunoreactive neurons and their relationship with putative histaminergic neurons. Cell Tissue Res. 1992;267:147–167

[117] Friggi-Grelin F, Coulom H, Meller M, Gomez D, et al: Targeted gene expression in Drosophila dopaminergic cells using regulatory sequences from tyrosine hydroxylase. J Neurobiol. 2003;54:618–627

[118] Cassar M, Issa AR, Riemensperger T, Petitgas C, et al: A dopamine receptor contributes to paraquat-induced neurotoxicity in Drosophila. Hum Mol Genet. 2015;24(1):197–212

[119] Reiter LT, Potocki L, Chien S, Gribskov M, et al: A systematic analysis of human disease-associated gene sequences in Drosophila melanogaster. Genome Res. 2001;11:1114–1125

[120] Girish C, Muralidhara: Propensity of Selaginella delicatula aqueous extract to offset rotenone-induced oxidative dysfunctions and neurotoxicity in Drosophila melanogaster: implications. NeuroToxicology. 2012;33:444–456

[121] Manjunath MJ, Muralidhara: Standardized extract of Withania somnifera (Aswagandha) markedly offsets Rotenone-Induced locomotor deficits, oxidative impairments and neurotoxicity in Drosophila melanogaster. J Food Sci Technol. 2015;52:1971–1981

[122] Johnson ME, Bobrovskaya L: An update on the rotenone models of Parkinson's disease: their ability to reproduce the features of clinical disease and model gene–environment interactions. NeuroToxicology. 2015;46:101–116

[123] Marsh JL, Thompson LM: Drosophila in the study of neurodegenerative disease. Neuron. 2006;52:169–178

[124] Virmani A, Pinto L, Binienda Z, Ali S: Food nutrigenomics and neurodegeneration-neuroprotection by what you eat! Mol Neurobiol. 2013;48:353–362

[125] Lee WH, Lee CY, Bebaway M, Luk F, et al: Curcumin and its derivatives:their application in neuropharmacology and neuroscience in the 21st century. Curr Neuropharmacol. 2013;11:338–378

[126] Kim HJ, Kim P, Shin CY: A comprehensive review of the therapeutic and pharmacological effects of ginseng and ginsenosides in central nervous system. J Ginseng Res. 2013;37:8–29

[127] Sun AY, Wang Q, Simonyi A, Sun GY: Resveratol as a therapeutic agent for neurodegenerative diseases. Mol Neurobiol. 2010;41:375–383

[128] Chen LW, Wang YQ, Wei LC, Shi M, Chan YS: Chinese herbs and herbal extracts for neuroprotection of dopaminergic neurons and potential therapeutic treatment of Parkinson's disease. CNS Neurol Disord Drug Targets. 2007;6:273–281

[129] Chao J, Yu MS, Ho YS, Wang M, Chang RC: Dietary oxyresveratrol prevents Parkinsonian mimetic 6-hydroxydopamine neurotoxicity. Free Radic Biol Med. 2008;45:1019–1026

[130] Ji HF, Shen L: The multiple pharmaceutical potential of curcumin in Parkinson's disease. CNS Neurol Disord Drug Targets. 2014;13:369–373

[131] Gadad BS, Subramanya PK, Pullabhatla S, Shantharam IS, Rao KS: Curcumin-glucoside, a novel synthetic derivative of curcumin, inhibits alpha-synuclein oligomer formation: relevance to Parkinson's disease. Curr Pharm Des. 2012;18:76–84

[132] Phom L, Achumi B, Alone DP, Muralidhara, Yenisetti SC: Curcumin's neuroprotective efficacy in Drosophila model of idiopathic Parkinson's disease is phase specific: implication of its therapeutic effectiveness. Rejuvenation Res. 2014;17(6):481–489

[133] Prior RI, Cao G, Martin A, Sofic A, et al: Antioxidant capacity as influenced by total phenolic and anthocyanine content maturity and variety of vaccinium species. J Agri Food Chem. 1998;46:2586–2593

[134] Joseph JA, Hale-Shukitt B, Casadesus G: Reversing the deleterious effect of aging on neuronal communications and behavior: beneficial properties of fruit polyphenol compounds. Am J Clin Nutr. 2005;81:313S–316S

[135] Krikorian K, Slider MD, Nash TA, Kalt W, et al: Blueberry supplementation improves memory in older patients. J Agri Food Chem. 2010;58:3996–4000

[136] Peng C, Yuanyun Z, KinMing K, Yintong L, et al: Blueberry extract prolongs lifespan of Drosophila melanogaster. Exper Gerontol. 2012;47:170–178

[137] Lim LM, Ng CH: Genetic models of Parkinson disease. Biochimica Biophysica Acta. 2009;1792(7):604–615

[138] Dawson TM, Ko HS, Dawson VL: Genetic animal models of Parkinson's disease. Neuron. 2010;66(5):646–661

[139] Dagda RK, Zhu J, Chu CT: Mitochondrial kinases in Parkinson's disease: converging insights from neurotoxin and genetic models. Mitochondrion. 2009;9:289–298

[140] Falkenburger BH, Schulz JB: Limitations of cellular models in Parkinson's disease research. J Neural Transm. 2006;70:261–268

[141] Jeibmann A, Paulus W: Drosophila melanogaster as a model organism of brain diseases. Int J Mol Sci. 2009;10:407–440

[142] Adams MD, Celniker SE, Holt RA, Evans CA, et al: The genome sequence of Drosophila melanogaster. Science. 2000;287:2185–2219

[143] Pandey UB, Nichols CD: Human disease models in Drosophila melanogaster and the role of the fly in therapeutic drug discovery. Pharmacol Rev. 2011;63:411–436

[144] Cauchi RJ, vanden Heuvel M: The fly as a model for neurodegenerative diseases: is it worth the jump? Neurodegener Dis. 2006;3:338–356

[145] Chan HY, Bonini NM: Drosophila models of human neurodegenerative disease. Cell Death Differ. 2000;7:1075–1080

[146] Kohler RE: Drosophila: a life in the laboratory. J Hist Biol. 1993;26:281–310

[147] Lu B, Vogel H: Drosophila models of neurodegenerative diseases. Annu Rev Pathol. 2009;4:315–342

[148] Ambegaokar SS, Roy B, Jackson GR: Neurodegenerative models in Drosophila: polyglutamine disorders, Parkinson disease, and amyotrophic lateral sclerosis. Neurobiol Disease. 2010;40:29–39

[149] West RJH, Furmston R, Williams CAC, Elliott CJH: Neurophysiology of Drosophila models of Parkinson's disease. Parkinson's Disease. 2015;ID381281:11. DOI: 10.1155/2015/381281

[150] Stephenson R, Metcalfe NH: Drosophila melanogaster: a fly through its history and current use. J R Coll Physicians Edinb. 2013;43:70–75

[151] Fernandez-Funez P, Nino-Rosales ML, de Gouyon B, She WC, et al: Identification of genes that modify ataxin-1-induced neurodegeneration. Nature. 2000;408:101–106

[152] Ghosh S, Feany MB: Comparison of pathways controlling toxicity in the eye and brain in Drosophila model of human neurodegenerative diseases. Hum Mol Genet. 2004;13:2011–2018

[153] Hamamichi S, Rivas RN, Knight AL, Cao S, et al: Hypothesis based RNAi screening identifies neuroprotective genes in a Parkinson's disease model. Proc Natl Acad Sci USA. 2008;105:728–733

[154] Kazemi-Esfarjani P, Benzer S: Genetic suppression of polyglutamine toxicity in Drosophila. Science. 2000;287:1837–1840

[155] Menzies FM, Yenisetti YS, Min KT: Roles of Drosophila DJ-1 in survival of dopaminergic neurons and oxidative stress. Curr Biol. 2005;15(17):1578–1582

[156] Merzetti EM, Staveley BE: Spargel, the PGC-1 alpha homologue, in models of Parkinson disease in Drosophila melanogaster. BMC Neuroscience. 2015; 16(70): 1–8. DOI:10.1186/s12868-015-0210-2.

[157] Van Ham TJ, Breitling R, Morris A Swertz MA, Nollen EAA: Neurodegenerative diseases: lessons from genome-wide screens in small model organisms. EMBO Mol Med. 2009;1(8–9):360–370. DOI:10.1002/emmm.200900051

[158] Ivatt RM, Sanchez-Martinez A, Godena VK, Brown S, et al: Genome wide RNAi screen identifies the Parkinson disease GWAS risk locus SREBF1 as a regulator of mitophagy. Proc Nat Acad Sci USA. 2014;111(23):8494–8499

7

Cognitive Impairment in Parkinson's Disease: Historical Review, Past, and Present

Ivan Galtier, Antonieta Nieto and Jose Barroso

Abstract

Parkinson's disease (PD) is a neurodegenerative disorder of unknown etiology, not only characterized by motor signs but also by non-motor symptoms, including neuropsychiatric and cognitive dysfunction. The results obtained in the last decades show that the cognitive changes in PD are heterogeneous; impairment in different cognitive domains such as attention, executive, language, memory, and visuospatial functions can be present even in the early stages of the disease. Mild cognitive impairment is frequent in non-demented PD patients and is considered as a risk factor for the development of dementia. As a response to the heterogeneity of cognitive impairment associated with PD, the Movement Disorders Society has recently developed formal diagnostic criteria for mild cognitive impairment and dementia associated with PD. In the present chapter, the authors have conducted a revision of cognitive impairment in PD, describing the results obtained in numerous investigations, from the first studies in the1970s to the advances of the last few years.

Keywords: Parkinson's disease, review, mild cognitive impairment, dementia, predictors variables

1. Introduction

Parkinson's disease (PD) is a neurodegenerative disorder of unknown etiology, characterized by tremor, rigidity, bradykinesia, and impairment of balance that are usually of an asymmetric course. The neuropathology of PD affects several structures that are implicated in movement control. The main neuropathologic feature of PD is the loss of dopaminergic neurons in the substantia nigra pars compacta, leading to a dysfunction of the frontostriatal system.

Ever since James Parkinson published his best known medical study, entitled "an essay on the shaking palsy" in 1817, this pathology has awakened scientific interest. Initially, most research effort focused on the understanding of motor symptoms and the search for effective treatment options. Levodopa, a precursor of dopamine, was discovered in the 1960s, and years later would be used as an effective treatment for the motor symptoms of PD. Coinciding with this historic landmark, a significant increase in interest in the non-motor symptoms associated with PD began to be observed, with special attention being paid to the cognitive symptoms, because of their impact on the quality of life of patients.

This chapter focuses on cognitive impairment in PD, from the first studies that paid attention to cognitive deficits to the present day concept of dementia associated to PD (PDD). There is a description of the neuropsychological profile classically associated with PD, going into the concept of mild cognitive impairment in PD (PD-MCI) in greater depth, which has given rise to numerous investigations in recent years. There is also a summary of the most relevant clinical and demographic variables associated with cognitive impairment in PD.

2. Cognitive impairment in PD: a historical review

2.1. First studies

PD is a neurodegenerative disorder described for the first time in 1817 by James Parkinson [1]. In the monographic entitled "an essay on the shaking palsy," the author described the clinical characteristics of a limited series of PD patients (Paralysis agitans). He defined the pathology as *"Involuntary tremulous motion, with lessened muscular power, in parts not in action and even when supported; with a propensity to bend the trunk forwards, and to pass from a walking to a running pace"* and affirmed that *"the senses and intellects being uninjured"*. However, subsequent studies showed that the last statement is not correct.

Charcot [2], is among the first authors to describe changes in mental functioning in PD. The author stated that in PD patients *"...the mind becomes clouded and the memory is lost"*. However, it was not until the 1960s and 1970s, coinciding with the first levodopa treatments, that scientific interest of the cognitive disorders associated with this pathology increased significantly. Over the following years, and even during 1980s, investigations were carried out without excessive control over the clinical variables (cause of Parkinsonism, stage of disease, duration of illness, etc.). An example is the study of Reitan and Boll [3]. These authors selected a group of 25 PD patients and twenty five controls matched on sex, age, and education, which were evaluated with a battery of psychological tests. The results showed that PD patients suffered deterioration in general cognition, memory, problem-solving, abstract reasoning, and organizing abilities. This was a pioneer study in the use of a wide assessment of cognitive functions. However, information about the clinical features of the patients was not provided (disease stage, duration, motor symptoms, etc.).

The study of cognitive deficits associated with PD and other neurological diseases characterized by basal ganglia pathology, such as Huntington's disease and progressive supranuclear palsy, gave rise to the concept of subcortical dementia, as opposed to predominantly cortical dementia characteristic of Alzheimer's disease [4, 5]. In this period, the concept of subcortical dementia is frequently associated in the literature with descriptions of cognitive impairment in PD. However, different authors consider that this label is often inaccurate and misleading because its application is not always suitable when referring to the cognitive impairment in PD; patients with PD may have cognitive deficits, without significantly affecting their daily lives [6, 7].

The discussions generated by the association between PD and the concept of subcortical dementia led to the development of numerous investigations with an increase in the interest in the control of clinical variables (disease stage, duration, motor symptoms, depression, etc.) and with more exhaustive neuropsychological evaluations [8–11]. The investigation conducted by Lees and Smith [12] is among the first studies to consider these characteristics. The authors conducted a careful sample selection according to the different variables related to the disease; they selected a sample of PD patients, in early-mid-stage of the disease (Hoehn and Yahr stage I–II), under 65 years of old, without depression and without antiparkinsonian drugs. The instruments administered included measures of general intelligence, executive functions, and memory. The PD patients only showed deficits in executive functions. Various investigations, such as the study of Lees and Smith [12], were performed in the 1980s and 1990s, and they led to the establishment of the neuropsychological profile classically associated with PD.

2.2. Neuropsychological profile of PD

Cognitive deficits in PD have traditionally been seen as an executive dysfunction secondary to frontostriatal system impairment. In this schema, this executive dysfunction is responsible for other cognitive disturbances that can appear in this pathology. However, the recently obtained results, in the last few decades, show that the cognitive changes in PD are more heterogeneous than initially thought. PD patients can have deficits in multiple cognitive domains including the executive functions but also in processing speed, attention, visuospatial functions, memory, and language. As will be seen below, the heterogeneity of cognitive impairment associated with PD cannot be explained exclusively as a consequence of dysexecutive syndrome.

PD is associated with cognitive slowing (bradyphrenia). Numerous studies have used reaction time tasks to evaluate processing speed and found that PD patients have deficits in simple and choice reaction time tests [13–18]. However, other investigations show that PD patients only present an altered execution in the choice reaction time task [19, 20]. The results of a meta-analysis conducted by Gauntlett-Gilbert and Brown [21] showed that patients exhibit an altered performance in simple and choice reaction time tasks, but the magnitude of the deficits was associated with the test complexity. This result has been explained in terms of a limitation of resources in tasks with more cognitive demands. Processing speed was also measured by Symbol Digit test and similar instruments; PD patients showed an altered execution with this type of test [22].

As regards attention and working memory, PD patients tend to perform normally in verbal tasks, such as digit span [22, 23], while their execution in visuospatial tasks is altered (visual span) [23, 24]. Siegert et al. [25] conducted a meta-analysis including 56 studies. They differentiated the working memory tests according to the stimuli characteristic (verbal, visual) and difficulty level (direct, inverse). The results showed that PD patients performed poorly in all the working memory tasks. However, in the verbal tests, the difficulty was more significant in the more complex tasks (inverse), while patients showed significant difference in simple and complex tasks in visual tests. Other authors studied working memory based on the n-back paradigm and found that patients had deficits, compared to controls, unrelated to the level of demand or the nature of the stimuli [26].

Visuospatial functions tend to be altered in PD, even in the early stage of the disease. Different authors reported an altered performance in judgment of line orientation [23, 27], facial recognition test [28, 29], and visuospatial reasoning such as Raven's test [8, 10]. Block design [27–30] and the copy of Rey Complex figure test [27, 29] were other instruments in which PD patients showed poor execution. It should be noted that the motor component involving this type of tasks was not controlled in most of these investigations.

Executive functions include a complex set of processes that has been defined as wide and diverse. Lezak [31] define the executive functions as those skills to respond adaptively to novel situations: "*The executive functions can be conceptualized as having four components: (1) volition; (2) planning; (3) purposive action; and (4) effective performance. Each involves a distinctive set of activity-related behaviors. All are necessary for appropriate, socially responsible, and effectively self-serving adult conduct*" *(page 650)*.

The Wisconsin Cart Shorting Test (WCST) is one of the most widely used instruments for the assessment of executive functions; it measures the ability to form abstract concepts, develop strategies and use feedback to maintain or change the mental set on the objective. Numerous authors found that PD patients show an altered performance in this test, including less categories and a greater number of errors (e.g., see [32, 33]). Verbal fluency (VF) tests were also used to evaluate executive functions, as they are considered measures of cognitive flexibility and search strategy. Henry and Crawford [34] propose that phonetic fluency has more validity and specificity as a frontal impairment measure, compared with the WCST. The results obtained in PD with measures of VF are highly heterogeneous, both with phonetic and semantic fluency tests; different studies found an altered execution in PD patients [35–37], whereas other authors do not report the same results [38–40]. Henry and Crawford [41] studied the VF in PD by a meta-analysis that included 68 investigations and a total of 4644 participants. They found that PD is associated with a deficit in VF, with a greater involvement of semantic fluency in comparison with the phonetic fluency test. The difficulties are greater when versions of these tasks in which alternate consigns are used. According to the authors, the performance in VF in PD patients is not exclusively attributable to a deficit of executive functions (according to scores on the WCST); the relationship between the deficit of denomination task and VF performance suggests that PD is associated with a deficit in the recovery of information from semantic memory. Furthermore, the action fluency test has been considered an alternative VF measure of executive functions, since verb generation is strongly associated with the prefrontal cortex. PD patients show a poor performance with this task compared to controls [42].

Other instruments used to evaluate the executive functions in PD are the Trail Making Test (part B) and the Stroop test. As for the Trail Making Test, PD patients often have an altered performance [13, 19, 27]. However, with respect to the Stroop test, the results are heterogeneous: some authors report an altered performance in PD patients [15, 37, 43], whereas other research studies do not describe the same results [20, 22].

Regarding memory deficits in PD, classical descriptions consider that the alterations are confined to new information acquisition and spontaneous retrieval; the patients would show a normal performance in cued recall and recognition tasks. However, the results obtained in different investigations confirm that the affectation of memory functions in PD is more complex. PD patients often show an altered performance in different memory tests (Verbal Paired Associates, Logical Memory) [6, 44, 45], with a normal execution in recognition [44]. However, patients can perform poorly, compared to controls, even in recognition memory tasks [6]. Using tasks that allowed a more precise examination of different memory components (e.g., the Auditory Verbal Learning Test and the California Verbal Learning Test), some authors reported deficits in learning and spontaneous recall, without alteration in recognition [27, 37, 46]. However, this impairment pattern was not confirmed by other authors who found alterations in cued recall and recognition [47–50]. Whittington et al. [51] conducted a meta-analysis and concluded that PD patients have recognition deficits. Therefore, alteration of the verbal memory in PD is not exclusively limited to a deficit of information retrieval.

In regard to visual memory, there are fewer studies than those which are focused on verbal memory. The results obtained are diverse, probably as a consequence of the wide range of instruments used (Visual Retention Test, Visual Paired Associates, Face Memory Test, Complex Figure Test, etc.) [27, 45, 46, 52]. Visuospatial learning has been evaluated by Pillon et al. [53, 54] who found that PD patients present an altered execution. This result was confirmed in a more recent research study [23].

The first research studies into language functions in PD considered that the linguistic deficits observed in patients were a consequence of motor symptoms. Speech disorders were associated to alterations of phonation, facial musculature, reflections, articulation, and prosody [55–57]. However, in addition to the deficits described above, other alterations related to language production and comprehension are common in PD patients. The results of different studies show alterations in speech related to a lower proportion of sentences which are grammatically less complex [58–60]. On the other hand, the results obtained with the Boston naming test are not conclusive: some authors show an altered execution [8, 61], whereas other studies do not observe the same results [6, 44, 62]. Other investigations have been focused on the differentiation between the naming of actions and objects, based on the association of action generation with the frontal cortex. PD patients showed an altered performance in both naming tasks (naming and action), but the execution in the action naming was poorer than the naming of objects [63–65].

As for language comprehension in PD, it is worth mentioning the research line developed by the Grossman group. They reported the following results in a series of publications: patients had a normal performance in simple sentences and a deficient execution in complex sentences, with greater difficulty in those with subordinate clauses; patients show more difficulty when analyzing sentences with subordinate clauses, when the semantic information does not allow their understanding; patients make more mistakes in tasks requiring the matching of a sentence with a picture and patients show deficits when identifying phonetic errors in grammatical morphemes, such as pronouns. Taking all the results together, the authors concluded that PD patients show deficit in language comprehension, related to the limitation of cognitive resources including, attention, cognitive slowing and working memory [66–70]. However, other results do not confirm the conclusions of Grossman [66]. Skeel et al. [62] showed that the alterations of comprehension can be present even in simple sentences and that this deficit was not associated with the status of working memory. Other authors have recently described similar results to Skeel et al. [62]; Galtier et al. [47] reported deficits in language comprehension that cannot be exclusively explained by a limitation of cognitive resources.

In summary, the results obtained in a large number of research studies over the last 40 years confirm that the cognitive deficits associated with PD are heterogeneous, including alterations in different cognitive domains such as attention, memory, executive functions, language, and visuospatial functioning. In addition, these data also confirm that the cognitive alterations in PD patients cannot be exclusively reduced to an executive dysfunction, as has traditionally been thought.

3. Mild cognitive impairment in PD

3.1. Concept of PD-MCI

Reisberg et al. [71] published the Global Deterioration Scale (GDS) in 1982 describing seven stages from normal to severe dementia associated with Alzheimer's disease. The GDS differentiates between stage 2 in which persons complain of memory deficits (without objective evidence in clinical interview, in employment or social situations) and stage 3 which was initially termed "mild cognitive decline". Clinical deficits appear in stage 3 although the objective evidence of memory deficit is only obtained by means of an intensive interview conducted by a clinician. In addition, decreased performance becomes manifest in demanding employment and social situations. Stage 3 is different to a GDS 4 stage which is considered as the earliest stage of dementia. Deficits are manifest in many areas in stage 4 and patients can no longer perform complex tasks accurately and efficiently. A cross-sectional study in 1988 used the terminology "mild cognitive impairment" (MCI) for the first time to refer the GDS stage 3 [72]. The results showed that MCI patients performed poorly in different cognitive measures, compared to GDS stage 2 subjects group (subjective deficits only). In addition, the group with mild dementia (GDS stage 4) performed significantly more poorly than the MCI group in the Mini-Mental State Examination and other cognitive measurements.

The concept of MCI was developed and popularized years later by Petersen et al. [73] who proposed the following diagnostic criteria: (1) memory complaint, preferably corroborated by an informant; (2) objective memory impairment; (3) normal general cognitive function; (4) intact activities of daily living; (5) not demented. The International Working group on Mild

Cognitive Impairment statement in 2004 recommended the criteria which are currently accepted [74] (**Table 1**).

Inclusion criteria

• Not normal, not demented [does not meet criteria (DSM IV, ICD 10) for a dementia syndrome]

• Cognitive decline:

  -Self and/or informant report and impairment on objective cognitive tasks

  And/or

  -Evidence of decline over time on objective cognitive tasks

• Preserved basic activities of daily living and minimal impairment in complex instrumental functions

---

Adapted with permission from Winblad et al. [74]. © 2004 Blackwell Publishing Ltd.

Table 1. General criteria for MCI.

The construct of MCI in PD (PD-MCI) is a more recent concept, as a result of the gradual increase of interest in non-motor symptoms, the heterogeneity of cognitive deficits, and their impact on the quality of life of PD patients. The investigation of Janvin et al. [75] was the first study that focused on PD-MCI; it included 76 PD patients who were evaluated with a limited selection of neuropsychological tests (Benton Visual Retention Test, Judgment of Line Orientation test, Stroop Word Test). Forty-two patients had PD-MCI (55%), defined as scoring −2 standard deviations below the mean of the control group in at least one of the tests. In the PD-MCI group, 57% of the patients had an altered performance in one neuropsychological test, 33% in two tests while the remaining 10% had an altered execution in all the three tests.

In a recent review conducted by Litvan et al. [76], the authors reported that between 18.9% and 38.2% of PD patients met MCI criteria. However, the study of Janvin et al. [75], described above, and other investigations have reported results with higher percentages (51–55%) [77, 78]. These discrepancies can be explained by differences in the PD-MCI diagnostic criteria, number of cognitive domains explored or selection and number of neuropsychological tests used. Several studies used a less restrictive level (−1 standard deviation) to determine cognitive impairment, while other authors opted for a −1.5 standard deviation or −2 standard deviation cut-off. For example, Foltynie et al. [79] evaluated a group of 159 PD patients with different cognitive tests, including a pattern recognition memory, spatial recognition memory and the Tower of London task from the CANTAB battery. The results showed that 36% of PD patients were considered cognitively impaired, defined as scoring ≥1 standard deviation below the normative mean of at least one of the tests. Janvin et al. [80] conducted a study of cognitive function in a sample of 145 PD patients. Subjects with Mini-Mental State Examination score <25 were considered demented and excluded. Of the total sample, 72 PD patients without dementia were studied and compared to 38 normal controls. Of the nondemented PD patients, 52.8% were diagnosed with MCI, defined as impaired performance [−1.5 standard deviation or more below the mean of the control group) in one, two, or all three of the given neuropsychological tests (Benton Visual Retention Test, Judgment of Line Orientation test, Stroop Word Test). In the study of Muslimovic et al. [81], the authors opted for a −2 standard deviation cut-off. They assessed a sample of 115 nondemented newly diagnosed PD patients with neuropsychological tests which examined the following six cognitive domains: psychomotor speed, attention, language, memory, executive functions, and visuospatial. Cognitive dysfunction was considered to be present whether performance in three or more neuropsychological tests was impaired. The results showed that 27 PD patients (23.5%) had cognitive dysfunction.

As one can see, there has been no consensus on the number of tests that need to be considered as altered to establish a diagnosis of MCI; alteration in one or more tests was taken as a criterion for the diagnosis of MCI [80], while other authors consider that impairment should be present in at least three tests (either within a single cognitive domain or across different cognitive domains) [81]. Moreover, most of the studies used brief batteries or a set of neuropsychological tests that do not allow the evaluation of all cognitive domains with a sufficient level of accuracy. Some authors described cognitive impairment as defined by poor performance in a selection of tests from the CANTAB battery (pattern recognition memory, spatial recognition memory and the Tower of London task) [82]. Other research only evaluated four cognitive domains, including memory, executive, attention, and visuospatial. Only one test was used for the case of memory and attention. Moreover, visuospatial function was examined by one item of the Montreal Cognitive Assessment test, which is a screening instrument [83]. Muslimovic et al. [81] selected a wide range of neuropsychological tests to examine cognitive functions in the following six domains: psychomotor speed, attention, language, memory, executive functions, and visuospatial/constructive skills. However, not all the domains were studied in the same degree of detail; although the memory and executive domains were investigated in depth by up to six tests, only the Boston Naming Test was used for the language examination.

3.2. Diagnostic criteria for PD-MCI

As a response to the heterogeneity mentioned above, the Movement Disorder Society (MDS) commissioned a task force to develop formal diagnostic criteria for PD-MCI which were published in 2012 [84]. The criteria proposed by the MDS are intended to overcome most of the previously described limitations. The MDS task force proposes a uniform method to characterize and diagnose PD-MCI, providing a framework to advance the understanding of this pathology. The proposal of the task force sets out new objectives for the following years (**Table 2**).

I. Inclusion criteria

- Diagnosis of Parkinson's disease as based on the UK PD Brain Bank Criteria [124]

- Gradual decline, in the context of established PD, in cognitive ability reported by either the patient or informant, or observed by the clinician

- Cognitive deficits on either formal neuropsychological testing or a scale of global cognitive abilities

- Cognitive deficits are not sufficient to interfere significantly with functional independence, although subtle difficulties on complex functional tasks

II. Exclusion criteria

- Diagnosis of PD dementia based on MDS Task Force proposed criteria [123]

- Other primary explanations for cognitive impairment (e.g., delirium, stroke, major depression, metabolic abnormalities, adverse effects of medication, or head trauma)

- Other PD associated comorbid conditions (e.g., motor impairment or severe anxiety, depression, excessive daytime sleepiness, or psychosis) that, in the opinion of the clinician, significantly influence cognitive testing

Adapted with permission from Litvan et al. [84]. © 2012 Movement Disorder Society.

Table 2. MDS Criteria for the Diagnosis of PD-MCI.

The MDS criteria included a two-level operational schema that differs in the comprehensiveness of the neuropsychological testing. Level 1 criteria provide less diagnostic certainty than level 2: (A) Impairment on a scale of global cognitive abilities or impairment on a limited battery of neuropsychological tests. When a limited battery of tests is performed, impairment must be present in at least two tests for a diagnosis of PD-MCI (level 1); (B) Comprehensive neuropsychological testing that includes two tests in each of the five cognitive domains (attention and working memory, executive, language, memory, and visuospatial). Impairment should be present in at least two tests, either within a single cognitive domain or across different cognitive domains (level 2). In addition, impairment in neuropsychological tests may be demonstrated by performance approximately 1–2 standard deviations below age, education, gender, and culturally appropriate norms; or a significant decline demonstrated in serial cognitive testing; or a significant decline from estimated premorbid levels.

As proposed by the MDS task force, classification of PD-MCI subtypes is important for research purposes and for exploring whether impairments in different cognitive domains have a different neurobiological substrate and course. Comprehensive neuropsychological testing is required (level 2) for the PD-MCI sub-types classification. The use of two tests in each cognitive domain for the level 2 category examines all cognitive domains equally, can increase sensitivity and allow full subtyping of PD-MCI. The presence of two altered tests within a single cognitive domain, with the other domains unimpaired, represents a single domain subtype. Whether at least one test in two or more cognitive domains is impaired, then PD-MCI should be subtyped as multiple domain. The proposed MDS criteria recommend not using amnestic or nonamnestic terminology. Instead, specification of the affected domains is preferable so that potential differences among subtypes may be better analyzed in futures studies.

Up to now, only a few studies have provided data with the MDS PD-MCI criteria. Broeders et al. [85] examined a group of 123 newly diagnosed PD patients and found that PD-MCI was present in 35% of cases, when level 2 was applied (comprehensive assessment). In a more recent investigation, Stefanova et al. [86], applying level 2 of the MDS criteria, examined 111 early

PD patients and 105 healthy matched control subjects; PD-MCI was present in 24% of the patients. The differences in percentages compared to the study of Broeders et al. [85] can be explained by the clinical characteristics of PD patients; Stefanova et al. [86] included patients in stage 1 (Hoehn and Yahr] while the patient sample of the Broeders et al. [85] study were in stages 1 and 2. Pedersen et al. [87] examined a sample of 182 PD patients (Hoehn and Yahr stage 1–2), applying level 1 (brief assessment) of the MDS criteria and found that 20.3% of patients met MCI criteria. Other authors evaluated patients who had a mean PD duration of 5.2 and 14.1 years and found that PD-MCI was present in 33–42.6% of the patients respectively, when level 2 was used [88, 89]. Recently, Galtier et al. [90] showed that 60.5% of the patients were diagnosed with PD-MCI according to level 2 MDS criteria. The percentage of PD-MCI in this study was slightly higher than that obtained in previous studies. These differences could be explained by the tests used to assess the linguistic domain. The authors included an assessment of language comprehension, unlike the methodology used in previous investigations. Most of the studies that applied the MDS task force criteria used −1.5 SD cut-off [85, 87, 89, 90]. Goldman et al. [91], using a cut-off of 2 SD below norms, reported that 61.8% of patients (mean PD duration of 9.3 years) were classified as PD-MCI with level 2 of the MDS criteria. The subtype categorization showed the high predominance of the multiple-domain PD-MCI with percentages of between 84 and 96% [90, 92, 93].

4. Relationship between cognitive impairment in PD and clinical variables

There are many research studies which have studied the relationship between cognitive impairment and potential predictor variables. Cognitive performance has been related to the neurological impairment, duration of illness, age at onset of PD, depressive symptoms and educational level, among others. As we shall see, the results are diverse which could once again be interpreted as a reflection of the heterogeneity of cognitive impairment in PD.

Regarding neurological impairment, different investigations have opted for correlation analysis and found that the degree of neurological impairment was associated with poor performance in visuospatial functions [28, 94], processing speed [95], working memory [24], procedural learning [37] and executive functions [96, 97]. However, other authors have not confirmed these results finding no relationship between the neurological impairment and different cognitive functions, such as processing speed [98], visuospatial functions [99], or procedural learning [100, 101]. Neither has an association with declarative memory [53, 100, 102] or linguistic functions (comprehension sentences, verbs generation) [67, 103–105] been found.

Other investigations compared PD patients with different levels of neurological impairment according to the Hoehn and Yahr scale. Although these studies are less frequent, patients with mid-late PD (according to Hoehn and Yahr stage) often present more affectation in different cognitive domains. The investigation conducted by Huber et al. [8] was one of the first studies that examined cognitive performance by comparing patients with different stages of PD. Moderate-to-late stage patients performed poorly in visuospatial functions, memory, executive functions, and naming. The results of Huber et al. [8] are clear evidence that the deterioration in the PD is not homogeneous, but that it is linked to the severity of the disease. Other authors also found differences in cognitive functions related to neurological impairment. For example, late disease stage patients showed poor performance in immediate memory (verbal and visual) [106], and executive functions (alternating series) [20].

Quite a few investigations pay attention to the relationship between illness duration and cognitive impairment. Research studies using correlation analysis showed that disease duration was not associated to processing speed [95, 98], working memory [10, 102], procedural learning [37], visuospatial functions [107], executive functions [10, 96], or sentence comprehension [67, 108, 109]. The results are more heterogeneous for other cognitive functions such as memory; some authors showed that disease duration was related to poor performance in diverse memory tests [10], while others did not find similar results [53, 110].

Other authors have demonstrated that cognitive dysfunction occurs even at the time of PD diagnosis. Foltynie et al. [79] showed that 36% of newly diagnosed PD patients had signs of cognitive impairment based on their performance in a pattern recognition memory task and in the Tower of London task. Similarly, Muslimovic et al. [81] examined a sample of newly diagnosed PD patients and found poor performance in different cognitive tasks; the differences when compared to normative data could mainly be explained by measures of immediate memory and executive function.

The age at onset of the disease has been associated with an increased risk of cognitive impairment, in other words the older the age at onset, the greater risk of cognitive decline, as measured with the Mini-Mental State Examination [111]. The study of relationship between age at onset of the disease and different cognitive functions revealed that the older the patient was at onset, the more likely the patient was to perform poorly in declarative memory (verbal and visual), executive, visuospatial and language functions (naming) [10, 15, 112, 113].

Depression is among the most common neuropsychiatric disturbances in PD. Different studies have concluded that between 36 and 60% of patients show depressive symptoms [114–116]. Numerous investigations have focused on the association between cognitive impairment and depression in PD. Depression has been associated with poor performance in global cognition, as measured by instruments such as the Mini-Mental State Examination or the Dementia Rating Scale [116–118]. Some authors who have studied the relationship between depressive symptoms and specific cognitive functions showed that depression was related to poor performance in different measures of executive functions [11] and in the comprehension of complex sentences [62]. However, other authors did not find any connection between depression and different cognitive functions, including processing speed [95], visuospatial functions [99], declarative memory [48], procedural learning [101], or sentence comprehension [67].

Certain authors have compared PD patients with and without depression by means of a comprehensive neuropsychological assessment. The results showed that patients with depressive symptoms presented an altered performance in declarative memory and semantic fluency, without showing differences in verbal span, phonetic fluency, concept formation, or naming. However, when both groups of patients (with and without depression) were equated according to the Dementia Rating Scale no differences were found between the groups [119]. Ng et al. [120] recently looked into the influence of depression in cognitive functions using a longitudinal study. They examined eighty one PD patients who were classified into two groups; with and without depression, according to the score in the Geriatric Depression Scale (score ≥5 was required for depression diagnosis). The results showed that PD patients with depression had a slightly lower performance in global cognition, as measured by the Mini-Mental State Examination and the Montreal Cognitive Assessment test, although these differences did not reach statistical significance. On the other hand, no differences were found between patients with and without depression in a set of neuropsychological tests that included measures of attention, memory, executive, visuospatial, and language functions. An 18 month longitudinal study was conducted, and similar results to the baseline were found; both groups of patients did not differ in global cognition and cognitive measures. Therefore, although the depression in PD appears to have some effect on global cognition and some specific cognitive functions, the available results suggest that both depression and cognitive impairment evolve independently in this pathology.

As regards the study of clinical variables associated with PD-MCI, according to the new MDS task force criteria, the available data are still limited. The study of Pedersen et al. [87] found that patients with PD-MCI were older, had less education, longer disease duration and higher Hoehn and Yahr stage than patients without PD-MCI. Hobson and Meara [93] showed that PD-MCI was associated to increasing age and worsening motor function. Galtier et al. [90] reported that PD-MCI was associated with lower education and higher neurological impairment, as measured by the Hoehn and Yahr scale, although they did not find age of onset or duration to be important factors.

5. Dementia in PD

As we have seen in first section of the present chapter, the interest in dementia associated to PD patients dates back to the 1960s and over the last 30 years there have a large number of studies into the epidemiology of PDD. Aarsland et al. [121] conducted a review of 4336 patients in 27 studies and showed that the mean prevalence of PDD was 40%. The prevalence of dementia increased from 28% after 5 years of follow-up, to 48% at 15 years, and up to 83% after 20 years. Moreover, PDD has been associated with increased mortality; after 20 years of follow-up of newly diagnosed PD patients 100 of 136 (74%) have died [122].

The Movement Disorder Society (MDS) recruited a Task Force to define the clinical diagnostic criteria for PDD which were published in 2007 [123]. The defining feature of PDD is that dementia develops in the context of established PD. Hence, diagnosis of idiopathic PD (based on the UK PD Brain Bank Criteria) [124] before the development of dementia symptoms is the essential first step in the diagnosis. Diagnosis of dementia must be based on the presence of deficits in at least two of the four core cognitive domains (attention, memory, executive, and visuospatial functions) as shown in clinical and cognitive examination, and be severe enough to affect normal functioning. Neuropsychiatric and behavioral symptoms are frequent, but are not invariable (**Table 3**). Clinical diagnostic criteria for probable and possible PDD are proposed by the MDS (**Table 4**).

I. Core features

1.   Diagnosis of Parkinson's disease according to Queen Square Brain Bank criteria

2.   A dementia syndrome with insidious onset and slow progression, developing within the context of established Parkinson's disease and diagnosed by history, clinical, and mental examination, defined as:

- Impairment in more than one cognitive domain

- Representing a decline from premorbid level

- Deficits severe enough to impair daily life (social, occupational, or personal care), independent of the impairment ascribable to motor or autonomic symptoms

II. Associated clinical features

1.   Cognitive features:

- Attention: Impaired. Impairment in spontaneous and focused attention, poor performance in attentional tasks; performance may fluctuate during the day and from day to day

- Executive functions: Impaired. Impairment in tasks requiring initiation, planning, concept formation, rule finding, set shifting or set maintenance; impaired mental speed (bradyphrenia).

- Visuospatial functions: Impaired. Impairment in tasks requiring visual-spatial orientation, perception, or construction

- Memory: Impaired. Impairment in free recall of recent events or in tasks requiring learning new material, memory usually improves with cueing, recognition is usually better than free recall

- Language: Core functions largely preserved. Word finding difficulties and impaired comprehension of complex sentences may be present

2.   Behavioral features:

- Apathy: decreased spontaneity; loss of motivation, interest, and effortful behavior

- Changes in personality and mood including depressive features and anxiety

- Hallucinations: mostly visual, usually complex, formed visions of people, animals or objects

- Delusions: usually paranoid, such as infidelity, or phantom boarder (unwelcome guests living in the home) delusions

- Excessive daytime sleepiness

III. Features which do not exclude PD-D, but make the diagnosis uncertain

- Co-existence of any other abnormality which may by itself cause cognitive impairment, but judged not to be the cause of dementia, e.g. presence of relevant vascular disease in imaging

- Time interval between the development of motor and cognitive symptoms not known

IV. Features suggesting other conditions or diseases as cause of mental impairment, which, when present make it impossible to reliably diagnose PDD

- The cognitive and behavioral symptoms appearing solely in the context of other conditions such as:

    Acute confusion due to

    a. Systemic diseases or abnormalities

    b. Drug intoxication

    Major Depression according to DSM IV

- Features compatible with "Probable Vascular dementia" criteria according to NINDS-AIREN

Adapted with permission from Emre et al. [123]. © 2007 Movement Disorder Society.

Table 3. Features of PDD.

Probable PDD

1. Core features: Both must be present

2. Associated clinical features:

    - Typical profile of cognitive deficits including impairment in at least two of the four core cognitive domains (impaired attention which may fluctuate, impaired executive functions, impairment in visuo-spatial functions, and impaired free recall memory which usually improves with cueing)

    - The presence of at least one behavioral symptom (apathy, depressed or anxious mood, hallucinations, delusions, excessive daytime sleepiness) supports the diagnosis of Probable PDD, lack of behavioral symptoms, however, does not exclude the diagnosis

3. None of the group III features present

4. None of the group IV features present

Possible PDD

1. Core features: Both must be present

2. Associated clinical features:

    - Atypical profile of cognitive impairment in one or more domains, such as prominent or receptive-type (fluent) aphasia, or pure storage-failure type amnesia (memory does not improve with cueing or in recognition tasks) with preserved attention

    - Behavioral symptoms may or may not be present

    OR

3.   One or more of the group III features present

4.   None of the group IV features present

Adapted with permission from Emre et al. [123]. © 2007 Movement Disorder Society.

Table 4. Criteria for the diagnosis of probable and possible PDD.

All epidemiological studies assessing the progression to dementia in PD have observed a high frequency of cognitive defects in patients without dementia; neuropsychological defects indicative of predominant posterior cortical dysfunction have been associated to dementia [125]. Along these lines, some investigations have examined whether cognitive performance in the first stages of the disease could predict the future development of dementia. The results obtained by different authors show that memory domain performance was a significant predictor to develop PDD [87, 90, 126, 127], although other cognitive domains such as attention [87], executive [128], visuospatial [82], and language [126] have also been identified as predictors of the development of dementia. Once again, these outcomes can be considered as evidence of the neuropathological heterogeneity associated with the evolution of PD. Over time, progression of cognitive impairment in PD is explained by the deterioration of the previously affected cognitive domains, but new symptoms and new cognitive defects seem to have a special impact on the conversion to PDD. In a longitudinal study, patients who developed PDD were characterized by the presence of defects in language functions; the comparison between patients with PDD, Alzheimer's disease, and dementia with Lewy bodies showed that the three groups had the same degree of difficulty in confrontation naming [129].

On the other hand, different clinical and demographic variables have been associated with the development of PDD and the most consistently reported are older age, lower education, greater severity of motor symptoms and REM sleep behavior disorder [126, 130–133]. Visual hallucinations have also been considered as a risk factor to develop dementia. In an 8-year prospective study, the presence of visual hallucinations at baseline proved a significant predictor of PDD [134]. A recent investigation with a sample of PD-MCI patients showed that 50% of patients with visual hallucinations developed PDD, in contrast to 25% of patients without hallucinations [135].

Recent studies have demonstrated that PD-MCI diagnosis is also associated with the development of dementia. The results described by different authors showed that patients who were diagnosed with PD-MCI have an increased risk of developing PDD in the years following diagnosis. In a 3 year longitudinal study with early PD patients, significantly more patients with PD-MCI than PD patients with normal cognition progressed to dementia; among patients with PD-MCI 27% developed PDD (annual progression rate of 9%), whereas only 0.7% of patients with normal cognition developed PDD [87]. Domellöf et al. [88] conducted a 5 year longitudinal study which included 115 PD patients with neuropsychological testing. Of the 115 patients, 31 (27%) developed PDD, which corresponds to an incidence rate of 62.6 per 1000 person-years. Forty-nine (42.6%) patients were classified as having MCI according to MDS criteria, of which 25 (51%) developed PDD within 5 years, corresponding to an incidence rate of 142 per 1000 person-years. Similarly, Galtier et al. [90] showed that 42.3% of PD-MCI patients had dementia in a six to eight follow up study, whereas in the group of PD patients with normal cognition only 23.5% developed dementia during the follow up study. In addition, a 16 year longitudinal study showed that 91% of PD-MCI patients had progressed to PDD [93]. Santangelo et al. [136] examined 76 patients who underwent neuropsychological testing at baseline (Hoehn and Yahr stage 1–2), and at 2 and 4 years; 32.9% of PD patients had developed PD-MCI at baseline (level 2). No patient went from PD-MCI to dementia after 2 years, while 5.5% developed dementia after 4 years. The percentage of conversion to PDD is lower than that reported in previous studies. The authors considered that a possible explanation for this discrepancy might be found in the characteristics of our patients, who were relatively young and had mild disease severity compared to other studies stated above.

6. Conclusions

In summary, the study of cognitive functions in PD has awakened much scientific and research interest during the last 60 years. PD patients may even show cognitive deficits in the early stages of the pathology, as has been confirmed in studies with newly diagnosed patients. Cognitive impairment in PD is associated with alterations in different cognitive domains including deficits in attention, executive, memory, visuospatial and language functions. However, the heterogeneity in the manifestations and progression of these deficits is a characteristic of the pathology. In addition, different clinical and demographic variables have been linked to the evolution of cognitive impairment, with some of the most relevant being neurological impairment, disease duration, older age and educational level. Diagnostic criteria for PD-MCI and PDD have recently been developed and provide a uniform method to characterize the evolution of cognitive impairment in PD and advance the understanding of this pathology. The results demonstrate that PD-MCI is common in PD patients affecting around 25% in the first stages and increasing to over 50% according to the progression of the disease. Moreover, PD-MCI is considered a risk factor in the development of PDD, with a high conversion rate to dementia in the years following the PD-MCI diagnosis.

Author details

Ivan Galtier*, Antonieta Nieto and Jose Barroso

*Address all correspondence to: igaltier@ull.edu.es

School of Psychology, University of La Laguna, Tenerife, Spain

References

[1] Parkinson J. An Essay on the Shaking Palsy. London: Sherwood, Neely and Jones; 1817. 88 p.

[2] Charcot JM. [Lectures on the diseases of the nervous system]. 2° Edition. Paris: Delahaye et Lecrosnier; 1875.

[3] Reitan RM, Boll TJ. Intellectual and cognitive functions in Parkinson's disease. J Consult Clin Psychol. 1971;37(3):364–9.

[4] Cummings JL, Benson DF. Subcortical dementia. Review of an emerging concept. Arch Neurol. 1984;41(8):874–9.

[5] Huber SJ, Shuttleworth EC, Paulson GW. Dementia in Parkinson's disease. Arch Neurol. 1986;43(10):987–90.

[6] Levin BE, Llabre MM, Weiner WJ. Cognitive impairments associated with early Parkinson's disease. Neurology. 1989;39(4):557–61.

[7] Matthews CG, Haaland KY. The effect of symptom duration on cognitive and motor performance in parkinsonism. Neurology. 1979;29(7):951–6.

[8] Huber SJ, Freidenberg DL, Shuttleworth EC, Paulson GW, Christy JA. Neuropsychological impairments associated with severity of Parkinson's disease. J Neuropsychiatry Clin Neurosci. 1989;1(2):154–8.

[9] Pillon B, Dubois B, Lhermitte F, Agid Y. Heterogeneity of cognitive impairment in progressive supranuclear palsy, Parkinson's disease, and Alzheimer's disease. Neurology. 1986;36(9):1179–85.

[10] Pillon B, Dubois B, Bonnet AM, Esteguy M, Guimaraes J, Vigouret JM, et al. Cognitive slowing in Parkinson's disease fails to respond to levodopa treatment: the 15-objects test. Neurology. 1989;39(6):762–8.

[11] Starkstein SE, Bolduc PL, Preziosi TJ, Robinson RG. Cognitive impairments in different stages of Parkinson's disease. J Neuropsychiatry Clin Neurosci. 1989;1(3):243–8.

[12] Lees AJ, Smith E. Cognitive deficits in the early stages of Parkinson's disease. Brain. 1983;106 (Pt 2):257–70.

[13] Akamatsu T, Fukuyama H, Kawamata T. The effects of visual, auditory, and mixed cues on choice reaction in Parkinson's disease. J Neurol Sci. 2008;269(1–2):118–25.

[14] Dubois B, Pillon B, Legault F, Agid Y, Lhermitte F. Slowing of cognitive processing in progressive supranuclear palsy. A comparison with Parkinson's disease. Arch Neurol. 1988;45(11):1194–9.

[15] Hietanen M, Teräväinen H. Cognitive performance in early Parkinson's disease. Acta Neurol Scand. 1986;73(2):151–9.

[16] Jahanshahi M, Brown RG, Marsden CD. Simple and choice reaction time and the use of advance information for motor preparation in Parkinson's disease. Brain. 1992;115 (Pt 2:539–64.

[17] Jordan N, Sagar HJ, Cooper JA. Cognitive components of reaction time in Parkinson's disease. J Neurol Neurosurg Psychiatry. 1992;55(8):658–64.

[18] Kutukcu Y, Marks WJ, Goodin DS, Aminoff MJ. Simple and choice reaction time in Parkinson's disease. Brain Res. 1999 9;815(2):367–72.

[19] Camicioli RM, Wieler M, de Frias CM, Martin WRW. Early, untreated Parkinson's disease patients show reaction time variability. Neurosci Lett. 2008;441(1):77–80.

[20] de Frias CM, Dixon RA, Fisher N, Camicioli R. Intraindividual variability in neuro-cognitive speed: a comparison of Parkinson's disease and normal older adults. Neuropsychologia. 2007;45(11):2499–507.

[21] Gauntlett-Gilbert J, Brown VJ. Reaction time deficits and Parkinson's disease. Neurosci Biobehav Rev. 1998;22(6):865–81.

[22] Dujardin K, Denève C, Ronval M, Krystkowiak P, Humez C, Destée A, et al. Is the paced auditory serial addition test (PASAT) a valid means of assessing executive function in Parkinson's disease? Cortex. 2007;43(5):601–6.

[23] Galtier I, Nieto A, Barroso J, Lorenzo N. [Visuospatial learning impairment in Parkinson Disease]. Psicothema. 2009;21:21–6.

[24] Kemps E, Szmalec A, Vandierendonck A, Crevits L. Visuo-spatial processing in Parkinson's disease: evidence for diminished visuo-spatial sketch pad and central executive resources. Parkinsonism Relat Disord. 2005;11(3):181–6.

[25] Siegert RJ, Weatherall M, Taylor KD, Abernethy DA. A meta-analysis of performance on simple span and more complex working memory tasks in Parkinson's disease. Neuropsychology. 2008;22(4):450–61.

[26] Beato R, Levy R, Pillon B, Vidal C, du Montcel ST, Deweer B, et al. Working memory in Parkinson's disease patients: clinical features and response to levodopa. Arq Neuropsiquiatr. 2008;66(2A):147–51.

[27] Uc EY, Rizzo M, Anderson SW, Qian S, Rodnitzky RL, Dawson JD. Visual dysfunction in Parkinson disease without dementia. Neurology. 2005;65(12):1907–13.

[28] Bruna O, Roig C, Junqué C, Vendrell P. [Relationship between visuospatial impairment and oculomotor parameters in Parkinson's disease]. Psicothema. 2000;12:187–91.

[29] Sanchez Rodriguez JL. [Neuropsychological deficit in Parkinson's disease. Its relation with clinical variables]. Rev Neurol. 2002;35(4):310–7.

[30] Witt K, Nuhsman A, Deuschl G. Dissociation of habit-learning in Parkinson's and cerebellar disease. J Cogn Neurosci. 2002;14(3):493–9.

[31] Lezak MD. Neuropsychological Assessment. 3rd edition. New York: Oxford University Press; 1995.

[32] Liozidou A, Potagas C, Papageorgiou SG, Zalonis I. The role of working memory and information processing speed on Wisconsin card sorting test performance in Parkinson disease without dementia. J Geriatr Psychiatry Neurol. 2012;25(4):215–21.

[33] Paolo AM, Axelrod BN, Tröster AI, Blackwell KT, Koller WC. Utility of a Wisconsin card sorting test short form in persons with Alzheimer's and Parkinson's disease. J Clin Exp Neuropsychol. 1996;18(6):892–7.

[34] Henry JD, Crawford JR. A meta-analytic review of verbal fluency performance following focal cortical lesions. Neuropsychology. 2004;18(2):284–95.

[35] Bouquet CA, Bonnaud V, Gil R. Investigation of supervisory attentional system functions in patients with Parkinson's disease using the Hayling task. J Clin Exp Neuropsychol. 2003;25(6):751–60.

[36] Mimura M, Oeda R, Kawamura M. Impaired decision-making in Parkinson's disease. Parkinsonism Relat Disord. 2006;12(3):169–75.

[37] Muslimovic D, Post B, Speelman JD, Schmand B. Motor procedural learning in Parkinson's disease. Brain. 2007;130(Pt 11):2887–97.

[38] Brand M, Labudda K, Kalbe E, Hilker R, Emmans D, Fuchs G, et al. Decision-making impairments in patients with Parkinson's disease. Behav Neurol. 2004;15(3–4):77–85.

[39] Schneider JS. Behavioral persistence deficit in Parkinson's disease patients. Eur J Neurol. 2007;14(3):300–4.

[40] Troyer AK, Moscovitch M, Winocur G, Leach L, Freedman M. Clustering and switching on verbal fluency tests in Alzheimer's and Parkinson's disease. J Int Neuropsychol Soc. 1998;4(2):137–43.

[41] Henry JD, Crawford JR. Verbal fluency deficits in Parkinson's disease: a meta-analysis. J Int Neuropsychol Soc. 2004;10(4):608–22.

[42] Signorini M, Volpato C. Action fluency in Parkinson's disease: a follow-up study. Mov Disord. 2006;21(4):467–72.

[43] Hsieh Y-H, Chen K-J, Wang C-C, Lai C-L. Cognitive and motor components of response speed in the stroop test in Parkinson's disease patients. Kaohsiung J Med Sci. 2008;24(4):197–203.

[44] el-Awar M, Becker JT, Hammond KM, Nebes RD, Boller F. Learning deficit in Parkinson's disease. Comparison with Alzheimer's disease and normal aging. Arch Neurol. 1987;44(2):180–4.

[45] Revonsuo A, Portin R, Koivikko L, Rinne JO, Rinne UK. Slowing of information processing in Parkinson's disease. Brain Cogn. 1993;21(1):87–110.

[46] Stefanova ED, Kostic VS, Ziropadja LJ, Ocic GG, Markovic M. Declarative memory in early Parkinson's disease: serial position learning effects. J Clin Exp Neuropsychol. 2001;23(5):581–91.

[47] Galtier I, Nieto A, Lorenzo JN, Barroso J. Cognitive impairment in Parkinson's disease: more than a frontostriatal dysfunction. Span J Psychol. 2014;17:1–8.

[48] Higginson CI, Wheelock VL, Carroll KE, Sigvardt KA. Recognition memory in Parkinson's disease with and without dementia: evidence inconsistent with the retrieval deficit hypothesis. J Clin Exp Neuropsychol. 2005;27(4):516–28.

[49] Kelly SW, Jahanshahi M, Dirnberger G. Learning of ambiguous versus hybrid sequences by patients with Parkinson's disease. Neuropsychologia. 2004;42(10):1350–7.

[50] Vingerhoets G, Vermeule E, Santens P. Impaired intentional content learning but spared incidental retention of contextual information in non-demented patients with Parkinson's disease. Neuropsychologia. 2005;43(5):675–81.

[51] Whittington CJ, Podd J, Kan MM. Recognition memory impairment in Parkinson's disease: power and meta-analyses. Neuropsychology. 2000;14(2):233–46.

[52] Uekermann J, Daum I, Peters S, Wiebel B, Przuntek H, Müller T. Depressed mood and executive dysfunction in early Parkinson's disease. Acta Neurol Scand. 2003;107(5): 341–8.

[53] Pillon B, Ertle S, Deweer B, Sarazin M, Agid Y, Dubois B. Memory for spatial location is affected in Parkinson's disease. Neuropsychologia. 1996;34(1):77–85.

[54] Pillon B, Deweer B, Vidailhet M, Bonnet AM, Hahn-Barma V, Dubois B. Is impaired memory for spatial location in Parkinson's disease domain specific or dependent on "strategic" processes? Neuropsychologia. 1998;36(1):1–9.

[55] Critchley EM. Speech disorders of Parkinsonism: a review. J Neurol Neurosurg Psychiatry. 1981;44(9):751–8.

[56] Ho AK, Iansek R, Bradshaw JL. The effect of a concurrent task on Parkinsonian speech. J Clin Exp Neuropsychol. 2002;24(1):36–47.

[57] Lloyd AJ. Comprehension of prosody in Parkinson's disease. Cortex. 1999;35(3):389–402.

[58] Cummings JL, Darkins A, Mendez M, Hill MA, Benson DF. Alzheimer's disease and Parkinson's disease: comparison of speech and language alterations. Neurology. 1988;38(5):680–4.

[59] Illes J, Metter EJ, Hanson WR, Iritani S. Language production in Parkinson's disease: acoustic and linguistic considerations. Brain Lang. 1988;33(1):146–60.

[60] Murray LL. Spoken language production in Huntington's and Parkinson's diseases. J Speech Lang Hear Res. 2000;43(6):1350–66.

[61] Goldman WP, Baty JD, Buckles VD, Sahrmann S, Morris JC. Cognitive and motor functioning in Parkinson disease: subjects with and without questionable dementia. Arch Neurol. 1998;55(5):674–80.

[62] Skeel RL, Crosson B, Nadeau SE, Algina J, Bauer RM, Fennell EB. Basal ganglia dysfunction, working memory, and sentence comprehension in patients with Parkinson's disease. Neuropsychologia. 2001;39(9):962–71.

[63] Bertella L, Albani G, Greco E, Priano L, Mauro A, Marchi S, et al. Noun verb dissociation in Parkinson's disease. Brain Cogn. 2002;48(2–3):277–80.

[64] Cotelli M, Borroni B, Manenti R, Zanetti M, Arévalo A, Cappa SF, et al. Action and object naming in Parkinson's disease without dementia. Eur J Neurol. 2007;14(6):632–7.

[65] Rodríguez-Ferreiro J, Menéndez M, Ribacoba R, Cuetos F. Action naming is impaired in Parkinson disease patients. Neuropsychologia. 2009;47(14):3271–4.

[66] Grossman M. Sentence processing in Parkinson's disease. Brain Cogn. 1999;40(2):387–413.

[67] Grossman M, Carvell S, Stern MB, Gollomp S, Hurtig HI. Sentence comprehension in Parkinson's disease: the role of attention and memory. Brain Lang. 1992;42(4):347–84.

[68] Grossman M, Kalmanson J, Bernhardt N, Morris J, Stern MB, Hurtig HI. Cognitive resource limitations during sentence comprehension in Parkinson's disease. Brain Lang. 2000;73(1):1–16.

[69] Grossman M, Zurif E, Lee C, Prather P, Kalmanson J, Stern MB, et al. Information processing speed and sentence comprehension in Parkinson's disease. Neuropsychology. 2002;16(2):174–81.

[70] Lee C, Grossman M, Morris J, Stern MB, Hurtig HI. Attentional resource and processing speed limitations during sentence processing in Parkinson's disease. Brain Lang. 2003;85(3):347–56.

[71] Reisberg B, Ferris SH, de Leon MJ, Crook T. The Global Deterioration Scale for assessment of primary degenerative dementia. Am J Psychiatry. 1982;139(9):1136–9.

[72] Reisberg B, Ferris SH, de Leon MJ, Franssen ESE, Kluger A, Mir P, et al. Stage-specific behavioral, cognitive, and in vivo changes in community residing subjects with age-associated memory impairment and primary degenerative dementia of the Alzheimer type. Drug Dev Res. 1988;15(2–3):101–14.

[73] Petersen RC, Stevens JC, Ganguli M, Tangalos EG, Cummings JL, DeKosky ST. Practice parameter: early detection of dementia: mild cognitive impairment (an evidence-based review). Report of the Quality Standards Subcommittee of the American Academy of Neurology. Neurology. 2001;56(9):1133–42.

[74] Winblad B, Palmer K, Kivipelto M, Jelic V, Fratiglioni L, Wahlund L-O, et al. Mild cognitive impairment—beyond controversies, towards a consensus: report of the

International Working Group on Mild Cognitive Impairment. J Intern Med. 2004;256(3): 240–6.

[75] Janvin C, Aarsland D, Larsen JP, Hugdahl K. Neuropsychological profile of patients with Parkinson's disease without dementia. Dement Geriatr Cogn Disord. 2003;15(3): 126–31.

[76] Litvan I, Aarsland D, Adler CH, Goldman JG, Kulisevsky J, Mollenhauer B, et al. MDS Task Force on mild cognitive impairment in Parkinson's disease: critical review of PD-MCI. Mov Disord. 2011;26(10):1814–24.

[77] Caviness JN, Driver-Dunckley E, Connor DJ, Sabbagh MN, Hentz JG, Noble B, et al. Defining mild cognitive impairment in Parkinson's disease. Mov Disord. 2007;22(9): 1272–7.

[78] Sollinger AB, Goldstein FC, Lah JJ, Levey AI, Factor S a. Mild cognitive impairment in Parkinson's disease: subtypes and motor characteristics. Parkinsonism Relat Disord. Elsevier Ltd; 2010;16(3):177–80.

[79] Foltynie T, Brayne CEG, Robbins TW, Barker R a. The cognitive ability of an incident cohort of Parkinson's patients in the UK. The CamPaIGN study. Brain. 2004;127(Pt 3): 550–60.

[80] Janvin CC, Larsen JP, Salmon DP, Galasko D, Hugdahl K, Aarsland D. Cognitive profiles of individual patients with Parkinson's disease and dementia: comparison with dementia with Lewy bodies and Alzheimer's disease. Mov Disord. 2006;21(3):337–42.

[81] Muslimovic D, Post B, Speelman JD, Schmand B. Cognitive profile of patients with newly diagnosed Parkinson disease. Neurology. 2005;65(8):1239–45.

[82] Williams-Gray CH, Foltynie T, Brayne CEG, Robbins TW, Barker R a. Evolution of cognitive dysfunction in an incident Parkinson's disease cohort. Brain. 2007;130(Pt 7): 1787–98.

[83] Hoops S, Nazem S, Siderowf AD, Duda JE, Xie SX, Stern MB, et al. Validity of the MoCA and MMSE in the detection of MCI and dementia in Parkinson disease. Neurology. 2009;73(21):1738–45.

[84] Litvan I, Goldman JG, Tröster AI, Schmand BA, Weintraub D, Petersen RC, et al. Diagnostic criteria for mild cognitive impairment in Parkinson's disease: Movement Disorder Society Task Force guidelines. Mov Disord. 2012;27(3):349–56.

[85] Broeders M, de Bie RMA, Velseboer DC, Speelman JD, Muslimovic D, Schmand B. Evolution of mild cognitive impairment in Parkinson disease. Neurology. 2013;81(4): 346–52.

[86] Stefanova E, Žiropadja L, Stojković T, Stanković I, Tomić A, Ječmenica-Lukić M, et al. Mild Cognitive Impairment in Early Parkinson's Disease Using the Movement

Disorder Society Task Force Criteria: Cross-Sectional Study in Hoehn and Yahr Stage 1. Dement Geriatr Cogn Disord. 2015;40(3–4):199–209.

[87] Pedersen KF, Larsen JP, Tysnes O-B, Alves G. Prognosis of mild cognitive impairment in early parkinson disease: the Norwegian ParkWest Study. JAMA Neurol. 2013;70(5):580–6.

[88] Domellöf ME, Ekman U, Forsgren L, Elgh E. Cognitive function in the early phase of Parkinson's disease, a five-year follow-up. Acta Neurol Scand. 2015;132(2):79–88.

[89] Marras C, Armstrong MJ, Meaney C a., Fox S, Rothberg B, Reginold W, et al. Measuring mild cognitive impairment in patients with Parkinson's disease. Mov Disord. 2013;28(5):626–33.

[90] Galtier I, Nieto A, Lorenzo JN, Barroso J. Mild cognitive impairment in Parkinson's disease: diagnosis and progression to dementia. J Clin Exp Neuropsychol. 2016;38(1): 40–50.

[91] Goldman JG, Holden S, Bernard B, Ouyang B, Goetz CG, Stebbins GT. Defining optimal cutoff scores for cognitive impairment using movement disorder society task force criteria for mild cognitive impairment in Parkinson's disease. Mov Disord. 2013;28(14): 1972–9.

[92] Goldman JG, Holden S, Ouyang B, Bernard B, Goetz CG, Stebbins GT. Diagnosing PD-MCI by MDS Task Force criteria: how many and which neuropsychological tests? Mov Disord. 2015;30(3):402–6.

[93] Hobson P, Meara J. Mild cognitive impairment in Parkinson's disease and its progression onto dementia: a 16-year outcome evaluation of the Denbighshire cohort. Int J Geriatr Psychiatry. 2015;30(10):1048–55.

[94] Alegret M, Junqué C, Pueyo R, Valldeoriola F, Vendrell P, Tolosa E, et al. MRI atrophy parameters related to cognitive and motor impairment in Parkinson's disease. Neurol (Barcelona, Spain). 2001;16(2):63–9.

[95] Deroost N, Kerckhofs E, Coene M, Wijnants G, Soetens E. Learning sequence movements in a homogenous sample of patients with Parkinson's disease. Neuropsychologia. 2006;44(10):1653–62.

[96] Alevriadou A, Katsarou Z, Bostantjopoulou S, Kiosseoglou G, Mentenopoulos G. Wisconsin card sorting test variables in relation to motor symptoms in Parkinson's disease. Percept Mot Skills. 1999;89(3 Pt 1):824–30.

[97] Pereira JB, Junqué C, Martí MJ, Ramirez-Ruiz B, Bartrés-Faz D, Tolosa E. Structural brain correlates of verbal fluency in Parkinson's disease. Neuroreport. 2009;20(8):741–4.

[98]   Morris RG, Downes JJ, Sahakian BJ, Evenden JL, Heald A, Robbins TW. Planning and spatial working memory in Parkinson's disease. J Neurol Neurosurg Psychiatry. 1988;51(6):757–66.

[99]   Crucian GP, Barrett AM, Schwartz RL, Bowers D, Triggs WJ, Friedman W, et al. Cognitive and vestibulo-proprioceptive components of spatial ability in Parkinson's disease. Neuropsychologia. 2000;38(6):757–67.

[100] Vakil E, Herishanu-Naaman S. Declarative and procedural learning in Parkinson's disease patients having tremor or bradykinesia as the predominant symptom. Cortex. 1998;34(4):611–20.

[101] Sommer M, Grafman J, Clark K, Hallett M. Learning in Parkinson's disease: eyeblink conditioning, declarative learning, and procedural learning. J Neurol Neurosurg Psychiatry. 1999;67(1):27–34.

[102] Dalrymple-Alford JC, Kalders AS, Jones RD, Watson RW. A central executive deficit in patients with Parkinson's disease. J Neurol Neurosurg Psychiatry. 1994;57(3):360–7.

[103] Colman KSF, Koerts J, van Beilen M, Leenders KL, Post WJ, Bastiaanse R. The impact of executive functions on verb production in patients with Parkinson's disease. Cortex. 2009;45(8):930–42.

[104] Crescentini C, Mondolo F, Biasutti E, Shallice T. Supervisory and routine processes in noun and verb generation in nondemented patients with Parkinson's disease. Neuropsychologia. 2008;46(2):434–47.

[105] Péran P, Rascol O, Démonet J-F, Celsis P, Nespoulous J-L, Dubois B, et al. Deficit of verb generation in nondemented patients with Parkinson's disease. Mov Disord. 2003;18(2):150–6.

[106] Whittington CJ, Podd J, Stewart-Williams S. Memory deficits in Parkinson's disease. J Clin Exp Neuropsychol. 2006;28(5):738–54.

[107] Girotti F, Soliveri P, Carella F, Geminiani G, Aiello G, Caraceni T. Role of motor performance in cognitive processes of Parkinsonian patients. Neurology. 1988;38(4): 537–40.

[108] Natsopoulos D, Grouios G, Bostantzopoulou S, Mentenopoulos G, Katsarou Z, Logothetis J. Algorithmic and heuristic strategies in comprehension of complement clauses by patients with Parkinson's disease. Neuropsychologia. 1993;31(9):951–64.

[109] Natsopoulos D, Katsarou Z, Alevriadou A, Grouios G, Bostantzopoulou S, Menteno-poulos G. Deductive and inductive reasoning in Parkinson's disease patients and normal controls: review and experimental evidence. Cortex. 1997;33(3):463–81.

[110] Flowers KA, Pearce I, Pearce JM. Recognition memory in Parkinson's disease. J Neurol Neurosurg Psychiatry. 1984;47(11):1174–81.

[111] Aarsland D, Andersen K, Larsen JP, Perry R, Wentzel-Larsen T, Lolk A, et al. The rate of cognitive decline in Parkinson disease. Arch Neurol. 2004;61(12):1906–11.

[112] Dubois B, Pillon B, Sternic N, Lhermitte F, Agid Y. Age-induced cognitive disturbances in Parkinson's disease. Neurology. 1990;40(1):38–41.

[113] Locascio JJ, Corkin S, Growdon JH. Relation between clinical characteristics of Parkinson's disease and cognitive decline. J Clin Exp Neuropsychol. 2003;25(1):94–109.

[114] Cummings JL. Depression and Parkinson's disease: a review. Am J Psychiatry. 1992;149(4):443–54.

[115] Shulman LM, Taback RL, Bean J, Weiner WJ. Comorbidity of the nonmotor symptoms of Parkinson's disease. Mov Disord. 2001;16(3):507–10.

[116] Rojo A, Aguilar M, Garolera MT, Cubo E, Navas I, Quintana S. Depression in Parkinson's disease: clinical correlates and outcome. Parkinsonism Relat Disord. 2003;10(1):23–8.

[117] Starkstein SE, Bolduc PL, Mayberg HS, Preziosi TJ, Robinson RG. Cognitive impairments and depression in Parkinson's disease: a follow up study. J Neurol Neurosurg Psychiatry. 1990;53(7):597–602.

[118] Cubo E, Bernard B, Leurgans S, Raman R. Cognitive and motor function in patients with Parkinson's disease with and without depression. Clin Neuropharmacol. 2000;23(6):331–4.

[119] Tröster AI, Stalp LD, Paolo AM, Fields JA, Koller WC. Neuropsychological impairment in Parkinson's disease with and without depression. Arch Neurol. 1995;52(12): 1164–9.

[120] Ng A, Chander RJ, Tan LCS, Kandiah N. Influence of depression in mild Parkinson's disease on longitudinal motor and cognitive function. Parkinsonism Relat Disord. 2015;21(9):1056–60.

[121] Aarsland D, Zaccai J, Brayne C. A systematic review of prevalence studies of dementia in Parkinson's disease. Mov Disord. 2005;20(10):1255–63.

[122] Hely MA, Reid WGJ, Adena MA, Halliday GM, Morris JGL. The Sydney multicenter study of Parkinson's disease: the inevitability of dementia at 20 years. Mov Disord. 2008;23(6):837–44.

[123] Emre M, Aarsland D, Brown R, Burn DJ, Duyckaerts C, Mizuno Y, et al. Clinical diagnostic criteria for dementia associated with Parkinson's disease. Mov Disord. 2007;22(12):1689–707; quiz 1837.

[124] Hughes AJ, Daniel SE, Kilford L, Lees AJ. Accuracy of clinical diagnosis of idiopathic Parkinson's disease: a clinico-pathological study of 100 cases. J Neurol Neurosurg Psychiatry. 1992;55(3):181–4.

[125] Williams-Gray CH, Evans JR, Goris A, Foltynie T, Ban M, Robbins TW, et al. The distinct cognitive syndromes of Parkinson's disease: 5 year follow-up of the CamPaIGN cohort. Brain. 2009;132(Pt 11):2958–69.

[126] Hobson P, Meara J. Risk and incidence of dementia in a cohort of older subjects with Parkinson's disease in the United Kingdom. Mov Disord. 2004;19(9):1043–9.

[127] Levy G, Jacobs DM, Tang M-X, Côté LJ, Louis ED, Alfaro B, et al. Memory and executive function impairment predict dementia in Parkinson's disease. Mov Disord. 2002;17(6):1221–6.

[128] Woods SP, Tröster AI. Prodromal frontal/executive dysfunction predicts incident dementia in Parkinson's disease. J Int Neuropsychol Soc. 2003;9(1):17–24.

[129] Noe E, Marder K, Bell KL, Jacobs DM, Manly JJ, Stern Y. Comparison of dementia with Lewy bodies to Alzheimer's disease and Parkinson's disease with dementia. Mov Disord. 2004;19(1):60–7.

[130] Gjerstad MD, Aarsland D, Larsen JP. Development of daytime somnolence over time in Parkinson's disease. Neurology. 2002;58(10):1544–6.

[131] Hughes TA, Ross HF, Musa S, Bhattacherjee S, Nathan RN, Mindham RH, et al. A 10-year study of the incidence of and factors predicting dementia in Parkinson's disease. Neurology. 2000;54(8):1596–602.

[132] Levy G, Schupf N, Tang M-X, Cote LJ, Louis ED, Mejia H, et al. Combined effect of age and severity on the risk of dementia in Parkinson's disease. Ann Neurol. 2002;51(6):722–9.

[133] Mahieux F, Fénelon G, Flahault A, Manifacier MJ, Michelet D, Boller F. Neuropsychological prediction of dementia in Parkinson's disease. J Neurol Neurosurg Psychiatry. 1998;64(2):178–83.

[134] Aarsland D, Andersen K, Larsen JP, Lolk A, Kragh-Sørensen P. Prevalence and characteristics of dementia in Parkinson disease: an 8-year prospective study. Arch Neurol. 2003;60(3):387–92.

[135] Gasca-Salas C, Clavero P, García-García D, Obeso JA, Rodríguez-Oroz MC. Significance of visual hallucinations and cerebral hypometabolism in the risk of dementia in Parkinson's disease patients with mild cognitive impairment. Hum Brain Mapp. 2016;37(3):968–77.

[136] Santangelo G, Vitale C, Picillo M, Moccia M, Cuoco S, Longo K, et al. Mild cognitive impairment in newly diagnosed Parkinson's disease: a longitudinal prospective study. Parkinsonism Relat Disord. 2015;21(10):1219–26.

8

The Role of Nurses in Parkinson's Disease

Michelle Hyczy de Siqueira Tosin and
Beatriz Guitton Renaud Baptista de Oliveira

Abstract

Background: The complexity of motor and nonmotor symptoms in patients with Parkinson's disease (PD) requires multidisciplinary health actions.

Objective: To describe the role of nurses as members of multidisciplinary teams tasked with treatment of motor and nonmotor symptoms and provide nursing protocols for the care of patients with Parkinson's disease.

Methods: Analysis of the main diagnoses, outcomes, and ICNP® interventions identified by cross-mapping empirical evidence described in 2123 nursing documents and data from medical records of patients with Parkinson's disease in the specialized rehabilitation program at the Sarah Network of Rehabilitation Hospitals in Brazil. The protocols were based on scientific evidence and international recommendations.

Results: Clinical nursing protocols were developed based on a standardized nursing language of diagnoses, outcomes, and interventions focused on motor and nonmotor symptoms and principles of rehabilitation.

Conclusion: These protocols are expected to guide the clinical reasoning of nurses for comprehensive care of patients with Parkinson's disease and their families.

Keywords: Parkinson's disease, nursing role, specialist nurses, rehabilitation nurses, multidisciplinary teams

1. Introduction

Parkinson's disease (PD) affects approximately 1% of women and men worldwide, especially those over the age of 60 [1]. It is a multisystem and neurodegenerative disease with genetic and environmental factors that result in deficits in the production of neurotransmitters, including dopamine [2].

PD is diagnosed through a clinical evaluation of motor symptoms; the presence of nonmotor symptoms combined with the current lack of cure reflects the complexity of health care, which aims to control symptoms in order to maintain the quality of life of the patient and family [3–5].

Currently, health system remodelling is observed for the development of guidelines with multidisciplinary actions that address the complexity of care [6, 7].

Enabling health professionals with specific areas of knowledge allows standardization of behaviors that will minimize the challenges of interprofessional collaboration.

In this context, nursing care of patients with PD must focus on the biopsychosocial context and must be based on ethical, legal, operational, and theoretical assumptions of the profession for health promotion, prevention of complications, treatment, and rehabilitation [8].

Thus, the clinical reasoning of nurses should be based on the pathophysiology of the disease as well as the nursing process and should be structured in a standardized language for communication with other professionals on the team. Standardization of the nursing language enables communication and comparison of data between different contexts, countries, and languages, and maximizes dissemination of knowledge from clinical data [9, 10].

Among existing nursing terminologies is the International Classification for Nursing Practice (ICNP®), which was developed by the International Council of Nurses and is integrated into the family of international classifications of the World Health Organization [9]. This terminology allows development of terminological subsets of diagnoses, outcomes, and interventions targeted to specific areas of clinical nursing practice.

2. The role of nurses in Parkinson's disease

Research has shown increasing specialization among nurses who care for patients with PD [11–13]; thus, knowledge of the pathophysiology of this disease is arguably an important starting point for vocational training [14]. Based on this, we sought to hierarchically organize the major motor and nonmotor symptoms of PD using evidence gathered from the literature (**Figure 1**).

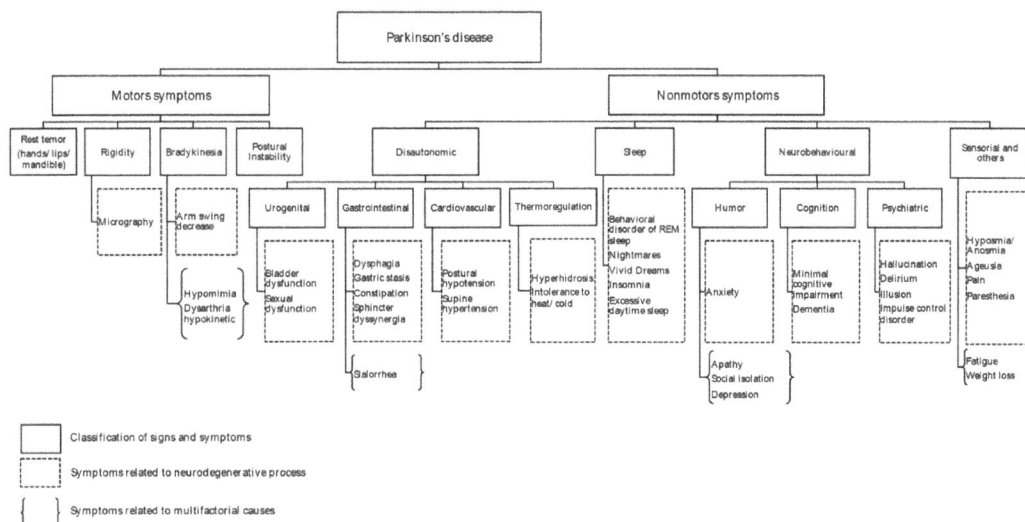

Figure 1. Classification of the main motor and nonmotor symptoms in Parkinson's disease.

The symptoms of PD are divided into motor and nonmotor; each of these classifications contains various other signs and symptoms related to both the neurodegenerative disease process itself as well as multifactorial causes. Thus, hierarchical organization of symptoms is not an easy task, and various descriptions have been proposed to facilitate understanding of the pathophysiology of the disease [15–18]; however, none of them have structured the symptoms into an organizational chart.

Our research on nursing diagnoses, outcomes, and interventions was based on this chart.

2.1. Nursing diagnoses/outcomes and interventions of ICNP® for patients with Parkinson's disease in rehabilitation

We analyzed 2123 nursing documentations from 352 medical records of patients with PD who participated in a rehabilitation program at a specialized centre in Rio de Janeiro, Brazil, from May 2009 to March 2014. From these documents, empirical evidence regarding nursing diagnoses, outcomes, and interventions was extracted. These dates were cross-mapped with ICNP® 2013 and validated by judges (nurses) to build a terminological subset of ICNP® for patients with PD in rehabilitation [19].

The diagnoses, outcomes, and interventions were divided into categories including motor symptoms, nonmotor symptoms, and principles of rehabilitation, as shown in **Figure 2**.

Greater variability was observed in nursing diagnoses, outcomes, and interventions related to nonmotor symptoms of Parkinson's disease; in general, it appears that nurses work in a comprehensive and communicative manner with other professionals on multidisciplinary teams.

Diagnoses and Outcomes ICNP® 2013 release	Interventions ICNP® 2013 release
Motor symptoms and Self Care and Safety	
Tremor	Teaching the Patient to Self Care
Hypoactivity	Teaching about Feeding Device
Impaired Ability To Communicate By Talking, Impaired Ability To Transfer, Impaired Bed Mobility, Impaired Mobility, Impaired Psychomotor Activity, Slurred Speech	Teaching Adaptation for Communication
	Teaching the Patient a to Applying Safety Device to Self Care
Self Care Deficit	Teaching the Family to Obtaining a Caregiver
Impaired Ability To Bath, Impaired Ability To Dress, Impaired Ability to Feed Self, Impaired Ability To Groom, Impaired Ability To Perform Hygiene	Teaching the Patient About House Safety
	Teaching The Family About Fall Prevention
	Teaching about Transfer Technique
Impaired House Safety	Referring To Physical Therapy
Risk For Fall, Risk for Fall Injury	Teaching the Patient About Rehabilitation
Impaired Walking	Teaching the Group About Disease and About Rehabilitation
Wheelchair Mobility	Teaching About Health Seeking Behaviour
Lack Of Knowledge Of Disease	Referring the Patient and Family to the Group to Teaching About Disease and Teaching About Rehabilitation
Non-motor Symptoms - Disautonomic - Urogenital	
Impaired Urinary System Process	Teaching Patient about the Urinary System Process, Evaluating Genitourinary Status, Assessing Bowel Status, Measuring Fluid Intake, Measuring Fluid Output, Assessing Urinary Retention Using Ultrasound, Teaching for Urination Controlling, Teaching Self Catheterisation, Referring to Interprofessional Team, Catheterising Bladder to Collecting Specimen of Urine, Collecting Specimen of Urine
Enuresis, Stress Incontinence, Impaired Urine, Urge Incontinence, Urinary Incontinence	
Risk For Urine Infection, Urinary Tract Infection	
Impotence	
Non-motor Symptoms - Disautonomic - Gastrointestinal	
Impaired Gastrointestinal System Process	Teaching the Group About Eating Pattern, Teaching the Patient About Eating Pattern, Collecting Specimen of Faeces, Teaching the Group About Fluid Intake, Teaching the Patient About Fluid Intake, Teaching the Group about Gastrointestinal System Process, Teaching the Patient about Gastrointestinal System Process
Constipation, Impaired Swallowing, Nausea, Perceived Constipation, Bowel Incontinence, Abnormal Salivation	
Non-motor Symptoms - Disautonomic - Cardiovascular	
Hypotension	Measuring Blood Pressure, Teaching Measuring Blood Pressure, Teaching About Disease, Referring to Interprofessional Team
Peripheral Oedema	
Non-motor Symptoms - Sleep Disorders	
Impaired Sleep	Referring to Interprofessional Team
Nightmare, Somnolence	Teaching About Sleep, Teaching About Disease
Non-motor Symptoms - Neuro Behavioral	
Impaired Mood Equilibrium	Facilitating the Family Ability to Participate in Care Planning
Anxiety, Depression, Chronic Sadness, Impaired Adaptation, Impaired Coping	Referring to Interprofessional Team
	Teaching Family Support
Impaired Cognition	Teaching About Disease
Impaired Memory, Disorientation, Delirium, Hallucination, Agitation, Fear, Craving, Impaired Behaviour, Low Initiative	
Non-motor Symptoms - Sensory	
Altered Perception	Referring to Interprofessional Team, Teaching About Managing Withdrawal Symptoms, Teaching the Patient About Disease, Teaching the Patient About Eating Pattern
Dizziness, Fatigue, Pain, Weakness	
Body Weight Problem	

Principles of Rehabilitation - Medication Regime	
Impaired Ability To Manage Medication Regime	Assessing Risk for Negative Response to Medication, Referring for the Group to Teaching About Treatment Regime, Teaching About Medication Handling, Teaching the Group About Medication,, Teaching the Patient About Medication, Teaching the Group About Treatment Regime
Lack Of Knowledge Of Medication Regime	
Medication Supply Deficit	
Negative Response to Medication	
Principles of Rehabilitation - Quality of life	
Caregiver Stress, Inadequate Routine, Impaired Socialisation, Impaired Quality of Life	Promoting Socialisation, Teaching the Adaptation of the Routine, Teaching the Patient to Contacting the Health Care Facility, Encouraging Positive Affirmations, Contracting for Adherence

Figure 2. The main Nursing Diagnoses/Outcomes and Interventions of Parkinson's disease mapped according to ICNP®.

2.1.1. Nursing diagnoses and outcomes related to motor symptoms, self-care, and safety

The motor symptoms of PD include resting tremor, muscle rigidity, bradykinesia, and postural instability. These symptoms were described in 1817 in a monograph by James Parkinson and are currently considered the cardinal signs for clinical diagnosis of the disease [20]. In the ICNP®, these symptoms are represented by the diagnoses and outcomes *tremor, hypoactivity,* and *risk for fall.*

2.1.1.1. Tremor

Resting tremor affects up to 75% of the patients with PD. It is characterized by involuntary tremors of the hands, lips, and jaw 4–6 Hz in intensity. They occur at rest but may worsen in stressful situations or while walking and stopping when actions are performed by the affected limb [21].

2.1.1.2. Hypoactivity

Muscle rigidity and bradykinesia are represented in the ICNP® by the term *hypoactivity*. This is a broad term that can be considered a syndrome that encompasses several specific terms corresponding to this diagnosis.

Muscle rigidity is characterized by disharmony of the flexor and extensor muscles, compromising joint mobility by making them rigid. Rigidity may lead to motor symptoms, among other problems, evidenced by reduced handwriting capacity, which is referred to as a micrograph in PD and is represented in the ICNP® by the term *impaired psychomotor activity*. Its prevalence in this population ranges from 10 to 63.2% [22].

Bradykinesia is defined as difficulty and slowness in initiating movement. It may affect the ability to perform simultaneous tasks and slow reaction times [14] and is associated with other disorders, such as decreased arm balance, hypomimia, and hypokinetic dysarthria, which are encompassed by the ICNP® terms *slurred speech* and *impaired ability to communicate by talking*.

Decreased arm balance occurs asymmetrically in the early stages of PD [3]. Hypomimia is defined as the reduction of voluntary orofacial movements that result in reduced facial expression in patients with PD. These symptoms may be related to bradykinesia [3], as well as other cognitive disorders that impair emotional recognition of facial expression [23].

Lack of motor control speech, called hypokinetic dysarthria, affects about 90% of patients with PD. It is characterized by deficits in vocalization related to the variation in the height and intensity during speech [24–26]. Its pathophysiological mechanisms have been studied, and there is empirical evidence that in addition to motor mechanisms associated with bradykinesia, cognitive mechanisms of self-perception, and self-monitoring of speech are involved [24, 25].

2.1.1.3. Risk for fall

Postural instability is related to the loss of postural reflexes, which occurs in the later stages of PD. Instability is measured by retropulsion or propulsion tests. Postural instability is defined as more than two steps backward or forward, or when there is an absence of postural response. This symptom is the most common cause of falls and contributes significantly to the risk of fractures [17].

2.1.1.4. Lack of knowledge of disease or self-care deficit

Knowledge about the disease and its symptoms promotes better patient and family management of limitations. The role of the family, both to encourage maximum independence in the patient's activities of daily living and to provide compensatory care for the deficits, is not an easy task. Thus, identification of these diagnoses is considered the starting point of the rehabilitation program.

2.1.2. Nursing diagnoses and outcomes related to nonmotor symptoms

The hierarchical organization of nonmotor symptoms includes disautonomic (urogenital, gastrointestinal, cardiovascular, and thermoregulation), sleep, neurobehavioral (mood, cognition, and psychiatric), sensory, and other subdivisions. In the ICNP®, these symptoms are represented by diagnoses and results, including impaired urinary system process, impotence, impaired gastrointestinal system process, hypotension, impaired sleep, impaired mood equilibrium, impaired cognition, and altered perception.

2.1.2.1. Impaired urinary system process

Bladder urogenital symptoms may be present in up to 96% of the patients with PD; they are characterized as storage symptoms (urgency, urge incontinence, increased daytime urinary frequency above eight micturitions, and two or more nocturnal micturitions) and emptying symptoms (hesitancy, decreased, or intermittent urine stream, sensation of incomplete emptying, and urinary retention) [27, 28].

2.1.2.2. Impotence

Sexual dysfunctions are the result of neurodegeneration and include difficulty with erection, loss of libido, and lack of orgasm. However, patients may also experience the opposite symptoms, mainly related to dopamine agonist therapy, which are characterized by obsessions or compulsions related to sex [15, 16].

2.1.2.3. Impaired gastrointestinal system process

In the ICNP® the diagnosis or outcome *impaired gastrointestinal system process* is also considered a broad term that may include specific diagnoses related to the same problem.

In PD, degenerative impairment of the vagus nerve, which is responsible for nervous control of the esophagus, stomach, and intestine via the parasympathetic and spinal cord system, causes dysfunction of the motility of the entire gastrointestinal tract, resulting in the following symptoms: oropharyngeal dysphagia (*impaired swallowing*), gastric stasis, constipation or slow motility (*constipation*), and sphincter dyssynergism and drooling (*abnormal salivation*) related to the decrease or absence of the swallowing reflex, which leads to the accumulation of saliva in the mouth [29, 30]. A review study also revealed that drooling may be related to both increased saliva production and slowed orofacial movements [31].

2.1.2.4. Hypotension

Orthostatic hypotension can result in dizziness during position changes (particularly to a standing position), fatigue, and even fainting and falls. This symptom may be subtle in early PD and does not necessarily worsen with disease progression [15, 16]. It affects about 40–60% of patients with PD, but only 20% may be symptomatic [32]. Supine hypertension, described in the organizational chart, is a sign recently debated among scientists who are in the early stages of studies on the pathophysiological mechanisms [33]. What we do know is that this symptom usually coexists with hypotension, both related to changes in the circadian rhythms of blood pressure [34].

2.1.2.5. Impaired sleep

Sleep disorders are very prevalent in patients with PD and have been studied extensively by scientists. Their pathophysiology is complex and results in overall impairment of the sleep–wake cycle [35, 36]. These disorders may negatively affect many biological functions and enhance associated symptoms such as cognitive, neuropsychiatric, and fatigue and affect quality of life of the patient/family [37].

2.1.2.6. Impaired mood equilibrium

Among neurobehavioral symptoms, mood disorders are present in 40–70% of patients with PD. The pathophysiological mechanisms of neurotransmitter regulation are demonstrably involved in the causes of depression (*depression*), apathy (*low initiative*), and social isolation (*impaired socialisation*) [16, 38, 39]. However, it is important to consider the impact of other symptoms, including motor symptoms, on the mood of patients with this disease [39].

2.1.2.7. Impaired cognition

The cognitive (minimum cognitive impairment and dementia) and neuropsychiatric (hallucination, delusion, illusion, and impulses control disorder) impairments associated with PD also have a complex pathophysiology; the manifestations vary in severity, tending to worsen with disease progression [39]. They deserve special attention from multidisciplinary health teams as they may endanger patient's health and overwhelm patient's families and caregivers [40].

2.1.2.8. Altered perception

Sensory symptoms directly related to the pathophysiology of PD include hyposmia and anosmia, ageusia, pain, and paresthesia [15, 16, 39, 41]. Fatigue has also been recently studied as an additional symptom. The prevalence of altered perception ranges from 33 to 58% and may be related to depression and apathy, sleep changes, cardiovascular dysfunction, motor symptoms, drug use, or insufficient blood flow in the frontal lobe [41].

2.1.2.9. Body weight problem

One review study described weight loss as a very common symptom in patients with PD, who have low body mass indexes compared with those of healthy controls matched by sex and age. The etiology has been described as multifactorial, related to motor symptoms, changes in eating habits, and medication use (especially levodopa) in addition to being potentially related to physiological changes in the neurodegenerative process [39].

2.1.3. Nursing diagnoses related to the principles of rehabilitation

Most of the symptoms of Parkinson's disease can be controlled by drugs, which make it necessary to assess patient adherence to treatment.

Drug treatment regimens for PD are complex since the variability in symptoms denotes the necessity of drug combination subdivided into smaller doses over 24 hours [42]. While the indication and prescription of drugs are obviously performed by physicians, nurses play an important role in treatment adherence.

There are several reasons why patients may not adhere to drug treatment, which are classified as intentional and unintentional [43].

2.1.3.1. Lack of knowledge of medication regime and negative response to medication

One of the unintentional reasons for compromised treatment adherence is a lack of patient's understanding on the importance of treatment. Patients often believe that drug therapy will cure their symptoms, not realizing that the therapy is aimed at reducing their severity in order to promote better quality of life. Moreover, the presence of motor fluctuations and complications of the therapy itself promotes disbelief regarding the effectiveness of treatment, which in turn contributes to nonadherence.

2.1.3.2. Medication supply deficit and impaired ability to manage medication regime

The factors associated with unintentional nonadherence are often a result of poor access to treatment because of the high cost of medications. Likewise, unintentional nonadherence may result from the patient's inability to self-manage their medications. This inability may result from cognitive deficits, education level, and cultural, religious, and behavioral factors.

Thus, accurate assessment of the causes of nonadherence to drug therapy in patients with PD underscores the importance of the nursing care plan, which therefore will complement multiprofessional health actions focused on the patient, promoting improvement of their quality of life through better control of their symptoms.

2.1.3.3. Impaired quality of life and socialisation, inadequate routine, and caregiver stress

The impact of the disease on routine activities, socialization, and quality of life of patients who are affected by the symptoms of PD may compromise their independence in performing the activities of daily life as well as their professional lives. In a ripple effect, these problems will results in individual, family, and social losses [13, 44, 45].

2.1.4. Nursing interventions related to nonmotor and motor symptoms and principles of rehabilitation

2.1.4.1. "Teaching" interventions

Among the main nursing interventions mapped, those related to educational practice and used by nurses as the main tool for health promotion were of particular importance.

Health education is considered a change of strategy in care models and is an alternative used to improve the quality of health and life of the population through increased understanding of health and disease [46].

Health promotion actions in neurological rehabilitation facilitate recovery and adaptation to the limitations imposed by disabilities on individual and contextualized bases. These actions mainly focus on functional, motor, psychosocial, and spiritual aspects [46].

Therefore, it is imperative for nurses to establish bonds with patients and their families when providing orientations in order to promote facilitation and implementation of learning. In this coparticipatory relationship, the focus is on personal autonomy for affirmation of the principles of citizenship and democracy, with the aim to improve health status [46].

2.1.4.2. "Referring" interventions

We highlight the interventions that reveal the important role played by interprofessional nurses, which are based on the best evidence to identify symptoms and collaborate with the team through discussion and referral of patients for evaluation. These interventions show that nurses are often the connection point with other members of the professional team in order to provide holistic care [47].

2.2. Nursing protocols for patients with Parkinson's disease

Accurate identification of nursing diagnoses is essential for clinical practice since it enables proper planning of care, implementation of interventions, and efficient evaluation of the results.

Therefore, it is necessary to use diagnostic support tools prepared in accordance with institutional settings and the complexity of patient's conditions. These tools should still be based on the best clinical evidence and recommendations described in the scientific literature.

This subchapter presents several nursing assessment protocols in the context of the activities of daily living, gastrointestinal and genitourinary function, sleep disorders, hypotension, and medication adherence.

Nursing assessment for daily life activities in patients with Parkinson's disease

Date: _____/_____/_____

Personal data
Name: _____ Age: ___ Sex: ( ) Female ( ) Male Family/Caregiver:_____
Date of onset of symptoms of Parkinson's disease: _____
Concomitant diseases: _____ Daily medications: _____
Housing conditions and family support
( ) Own residence ( ) Rented residence ( ) Residence of relatives/friends ( ) Institutionalized
( ) House with a single level ( ) House with multiple levels ( ) Stairs with unilateral handrail ( ) Stairs with bilateral handrail ( ) Stairs without handrail ( ) No stairs ( ) Apartment with elevator ( ) Apartment with no elevator
Adaptation at residence? ( ) yes ( ) no Where?_____
( ) Live alone ( ) Live with whom? _____ Family/caregiver support? ( ) Yes ( ) No
Routine
Describe your routine before the Parkinson's disease diagnosis:_____
_____
Describe your current routine:_____
_____
Schwab and England activities of daily living [48]
100%-Completely independent. Able to do all chores without slowness, difficulty, or impairment. Essentially normal. Unaware of any difficulty.

90%-Completely independent. Able to do all chores with some degree of slowness, difficulty, and impairment. Might take twice as long. Beginning to be aware of difficulty.

80%-Completely independent in most chores. Takes twice as long. Conscious of difficulty and slowness.

70%-Not completely independent. More difficulty with some chores. Three to four times as long in some. Must spend a large part of the day with chores.

60%-Some dependency. Can do most chores but exceedingly slowly and with much effort. Errors; some impossible.

50%-More dependent. Help with half, slower, et cetera. Difficulty with everything.

40%-Very dependent. Can assist with all chores, but few alone.

30%-With effort, now and then does a few chores alone or begins alone. Much help needed.

20%-Nothing alone. Can be a slight help with some chores. Severe invalid.

10%-Total dependent, helpless. Complete invalid.

0%-Vegetative functions such as swallowing, bladder, and bowel functions are not functioning. Bed-ridden.

MDS-UPDRS Part II scale can be applied

Nursing diagnoses	Nursing interventions

Evaluation of patient's ability to perform activities of daily life is complex because it involves environmental aspects (usually related to the accessibility of the house), family support or caregivers, and commitment to the routine. The assessment should be based on standardized scales, such as the Unified Parkinson's Disease Rating Scale (UPDRS) Part II and the Schwab and England activities of daily living scales widely used in research and clinical practice [48–50].

Nursing assessment of bowel status in patients with Parkinson's disease

Date: _____/_____/_____

Personal data

Name: _____ Age: ____ Sex: ( ) Female ( ) Male Family/Caregiver:_____

Onset date of symptoms of PD: _____

Concomitant diseases: _____

Daily medications:_____

Digestive system function

Main complaint: _____

Onset of symptoms: _____ Presence of symptoms before PD: ( ) Yes ( ) No How many years? _____

Background surgical gastrointestinal tract: ( ) Yes ( ) No What: _____

Regular monitoring by gastroenterologist: ( ) Yes ( ) No

Feel the urge for bowel movement? ( ) Several times/day ( ) Daily ( ) Every 1-2 days ( ) Every 1-_ days

Flatulence? ( ) Never ( ) Sometimes ( ) Often ( ) Always

Fecal Incontinence? ( ) Never ( ) Sometimes ( ) Often ( ) Always

When does fecal incontinence occur? (You can mark more than one answer)

( ) During a diarrheal episode ( ) Every time because of the urgency ( ) When coughing and rising ( ) Unexpectedly

Rome III Criteria [51]

Must include two or more of the following:

( ) Straining during at least 25% of defecations

( ) Lumpy or hard stools in at least 25% of defecations

( ) Sensation of incomplete evacuation for at least 25% of defecations

( ) Sensation of anorectal obstruction/blockage for at least 25% of defecations

( ) Manual maneuvers to facilitate at least 25% of defecations (e.g., digital evacuation)

( ) Fewer than three defecations per week

* Criteria fulfilled for the last three months with symptom onset at least six months prior to diagnosis

Bristol scale

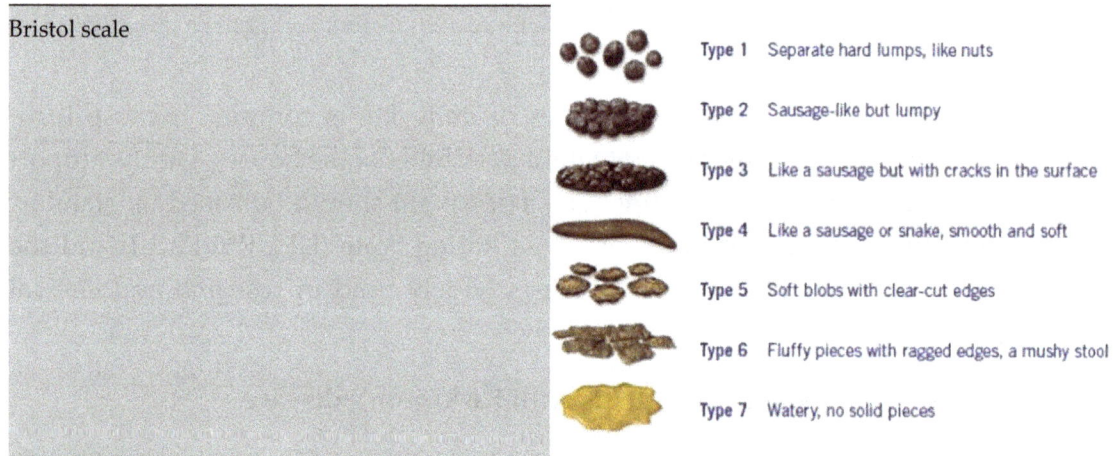

Type 1   Separate hard lumps, like nuts

Type 2   Sausage-like but lumpy

Type 3   Like a sausage but with cracks in the surface

Type 4   Like a sausage or snake, smooth and soft

Type 5   Soft blobs with clear-cut edges

Type 6   Fluffy pieces with ragged edges, a mushy stool

Type 7   Watery, no solid pieces

In most evacuations, what is the characteristic of the feces? _____

Devices for evacuation	Complications
( ) External device for evacuation ( ) Toilet	( ) Diverticulitis
( ) Diapers	( ) Hernia
( ) Have you ever undergone intestinal cleansing	( ) Volvulus
( ) Laxatives/or antigas medication Which?_____	( ) Other: _____
How often do you use laxative or antigas medication? ( ) > 1×/month ( ) > 1×/week ( ) > 1×/day	

Mobility

Are you dependent on others for evacuation: ( ) Yes ( ) No

Transfer to lavatory seat: ( ) Independent ( ) Dependent

Locomotion: ( ) Without assistance and without support ( ) Locomotion assistance

Self-care

Dependant on others to eat and/or drink ( ) Yes ( ) No Why?_____ Daily water intake _____

Low tolerance for liquids? ( ) Yes ( ) No Do you have adipsia? ( ) Yes ( ) No

( ) Dysphagia for liquids ( ) Dysphagia for solids ( ) Need to change food consistency

Food routine:

Breakfast: _____

Snack: _____

Lunch: _____

Snack: _____

Dinner: _____

Supper: _____

Mental function

Dependant on others? ( ) Yes ( ) No Why?_____

Cognitive disorders? ( ) Yes ( ) No What: _____

Behavioral disorders? ( ) Yes ( ) No What: _____

Housing conditions

Easy access to the bathroom: ( ) Yes ( ) No

Modifications made to bathroom/home: ( ) Yes ( ) No What? _____

Modifications to the bathroom/home are required: ( ) Yes ( ) No What? _____

Community, social, and civic life

Impact on labour activities related to constipation ( ) Yes ( ) No ( ) Not applicable

Impact on leisure activities related to constipation ( ) Yes ( ) No

Impact on quality of life related to constipation ( ) Yes ( ) No

Have financial resources for modifications, medicines, and intestinal devices? ( ) Yes ( ) No

Physical examination

Inspection:

- Skin: _____

- Contour: ( ) Plan ( ) Excavated ( ) Globular

- Symmetry: _____

Abdominal auscultation (Intestinal noises): ( ) 2 to 5/min ( ) < 2 to 5/min ( ) > than 2 to 5/min

Percussion: ( ) Tympanic ( ) Hypertympanic ( )Massive Quadrant:_____

Abdominal palpation: _____

Nursing diagnoses	Nursing interventions

Evaluation of intestinal symptoms in patients with PD focuses on constipation, which is the main problem. However, it is important to assess other symptoms such as fecal incontinence and related factors that enhance intestinal symptoms such as changes in mobility/accessibility, swallowing, and cognitive function, among others. The Rome III criteria and the Bristol Stool Scale are recommended tools for evaluation of constipation [51, 52].

Genitourinary nursing assessment in patients with Parkinson's disease

Date: _____/_____/_____

Personal data

Name: _____ Age: ___ Sex: ( ) Female ( ) Male Family/Caregiver:_____

Date of onset of symptoms of Parkinson's disease: _____

Concomitant diseases: _____

Daily medications: _____

Genitourinary, reproductive, and bowel functions

Number of pregnancies and births: _____ ( ) Vaginal birth ( ) Caesarean ( ) Abortions: _____

Main complaint: _____

Onset of symptoms: _____ Presence of symptoms before PD: ( ) Yes ( ) No

History of uro/gynaecology surgery: ( ) Yes ( ) No Which: _____

Regular monitoring by urologist/gynaecologist: ( ) Yes ( ) No

Sensation of bladder fullness ( ) Yes ( ) No

Bladder control ( ) Yes ( ) No Urinary Urgency ( ) Yes ( ) No Urinary Loss ( ) Yes ( ) No

Intestinal function: ( ) Regular ( ) Irregular Frequency:_____

Do the bladder symptoms impact sexual capacity ( ) Yes ( ) No How? _____

Storage symptoms

( ) Urinary Urgency ( ) Urge Incontinence

( ) Stress incontinence ( ) Enuresis

( ) Increased frequency of diurnal urinary

( ) Nocturia. How many times?_____

Voiding symptoms

( )Decreased urinary stream( )Hesitation

( )Urinary flow intermittent ( )Voiding Effort

( )Sensation of incomplete emptying ( )Dysuria

( )Dripping ( )Initial Dripping ( )Terminal Dripping

Urinary devices

( ) Toilet ( ) urinals bedpans

( ) Indwelling catheter

( ) Diapers

( ) Absorbent intimate feminine

( ) Catheterization intermittent bladder

( ) External condom collecting device

Complications of urinary tract

( ) Urethral fistula

( ) Cystocele

( ) Prostatic hyperplasia

( ) Urethral Stenosis

( )Hydronephrosis D/E

( ) Urethral diverticulum

( ) Lithiasis vescial

( ) Renal lithiasis

( ) Renal failure

( ) Lesion of penis

( ) Urinary tract infection

Self-care

Daily water intake _____ Appropriate division of ingestion ( ) Yes ( ) No

Liquid dysphagia ( ) Yes ( ) No Low tolerance for liquids ( ) Yes ( ) No

Dependant on others for toileting ( ) Yes ( ) No

Do you require instruction on how to use the urinary device? ( ) Yes ( ) No

Mobility

Dependant on others ( ) Yes ( ) No Why?_____

Impairment: ( ) Bradykinesia ( ) Tremor ( ) Postural instability ( ) Motor complications

Locomotion: ( ) Without Assistance and without support ( ) Locomotion with assistance Which?_____

Falls: ( ) Yes ( ) No ( ) Falls between bed- and bathroom: ( ) Yes ( ) No Risk of falls: ( ) Yes ( ) No Why?

_____

Mental function

Cognitive/behavioral disorders: ( ) Yes ( ) No Which: _____

Sleep

Dependent on medication: ( ) Yes ( ) No Wakes from sleep by urinary desire: ( ) Yes ( ) No

Sleep disorders: ( ) Yes ( ) No

Housing conditions

Live alone ( ) Yes ( ) No Accessible bathroom ( ) Yes ( ) No

It is able to maintain a safe environment without help? ( ) Yes ( ) No

Has made modification to the bathroom ( ) Yes ( ) No What? _____

Needs to modify the bathroom/home ( ) Yes ( ) No What?_____

Community, social, and civic life

Impact on labor activities related to genitourinary disorders ( ) Yes ( ) No ( ) Not applicable

Impact on leisure activities related to genitourinary disorders ( ) Yes ( ) No

Impact on quality of life related to genitourinary disorders ( ) Yes ( ) No

Have financial resources for modifications, medicines, and urinary devices? ( ) Yes ( ) No

Nursing diagnoses	Nursing interventions

Evaluation of bladder symptoms in patients with PD is complex because it involves investigation of urinary, gynecological/urological, cognitive/behavioral, and sleep symptoms, as well as mobility/accessibility and quality of life. Thus, nurse evaluations should focus on several aspects that may contribute to these changes in order to propose appropriate interventions. Some measurement scales may be used, including the Overactive Bladder questionnaire (OAB-q) [53], Questionnaire on Pelvic Organ Function [54], and the Scale for Outcomes in Parkinson's disease (SCOPA-AUT) [55].

Nursing assessment for sleep disorders in patients with Parkinson's disease

Date: _____/_____/_____

Personal data	
Name: _____ Age: ___ Sex: ( ) Female ( ) Male Family/Caregiver:_____	
Date of onset of symptoms of Parkinson's disease: _____	
Concomitant diseases: _____	
Daily medications: _____	
Sleep assessment	
Complaint: _____ Onset of symptoms of sleep disorder: _____	
Use medication to sleep? ( ) yes ( ) no Impact on quality of life of the patient: ( ) yes ( ) no	
Has sleep routine? ( ) yes ( ) no Impact on quality of life of the family: ( ) yes ( ) no	
Sleep disorders related to motor symptoms	
Difficulty with movement in bed: ( ) Yes ( ) No	Morning dystonia: ( ) Yes ( ) No
Tremors that compromise the quality of sleep: ( ) Yes ( ) No	Restless leg syndrome: ( ) Yes ( ) No
Sleep disorders related to nonmotor symptoms	
Hallucinations: ( ) Yes ( ) No	Mental confusion: ( ) Yes ( ) No
Sleep apnoea/difficulty breathing: ( ) Yes ( ) No	Pain: ( ) Yes ( ) No
Nocturia: ( ) Yes ( ) No	
Specific symptoms of sleep disorders	
Initial insomnia: ( ) Yes ( ) No	Sleep-talking: ( ) Yes ( ) No
Terminal insomnia: ( ) Yes ( ) No	Nightmares: ( ) Yes ( ) No
Nonrestorative sleep: ( ) Yes ( ) No	Vivid dreams: ( ) Yes ( ) No
Specific symptoms of daytime sleep disorders	
Sleeping unexpectedly during the day: ( ) Yes ( ) No	Sleep while talking: ( ) Yes ( ) No
Sleeping while watching TV: ( ) Yes ( ) No	Sleep while sitting: ( ) Yes ( ) No
Difficulty staying awake during the day: ( ) Yes ( ) No	

Nursing diagnoses	Nursing interventions

Evaluations of symptoms that cause sleep disorders should be approached with care and cover various related aspects, including motor/nonmotor function and night/day sleep disorders. Measurement scales can be used for this assessment and may include those recommended by the Movement Disorders Society Task Force: the PD sleep scale (PDSS), Pittsburgh sleep quality index (PSQI), SCOPA-sleep (SCOPA), and the Epworth sleepiness scale (ESS) [56]. We also emphasize that the PDSS scale has been revised and the PDSS-2 version has been validated [57].

Nursing assessment for orthostatic hypotension in patients with Parkinson's disease

Date: _____/_____/_____

Personal data
Name: _____ Age: ___ Sex: ( ) Female ( ) Male Family/Caregiver:_____
Date of onset of symptoms of Parkinson's disease: _____
Concomitant diseases: _____
Daily medications: _____

Autonomic scale for outcomes in Parkinson's disease (SCOPA-AUT): Hypotension section
In the past month, when standing up, have you had the feeling of either becoming light-headed, not seeing properly, or not thinking clearly?
( ) Never ( ) Sometimes ( ) Regularly ( ) Often
In the past month, did you become light-headed after standing for sometime?
( ) Never ( ) Sometimes ( ) Regularly ( ) Often
Have you fainted in the past six months?
( ) Never ( ) Sometimes ( ) Regularly ( ) Often

Composite Autonomic Symptom Scale (COMPASS 31): Hypotension section [59]
1. In the past year, have you ever felt faint, dizzy, "goofy", or had difficulty thinking soon after standing up from a sitting or lying position? (1) Yes (2) No
2. When standing up, how frequently do you get these feelings or symptoms?
(1) Rarely (2) Occasionally (3) Frequently (4) Almost Always
3. How would you rate the severity of these feelings or symptoms?
(1) Mild (2) Moderate (3) Severe
4. In the past year, have these feelings or symptoms that you have experienced:
(1) Gotten much worse (2) Gotten somewhat worse (3) Stayed about the same
(4) Gotten somewhat better (5) Gotten much better (6) Completely gone

Physical Examination	
Blood pressure (BP) lying:_____X_____mmHg	Cardiac frequency (CF) lying:___hpm
BP in orthostasis:____X___mmHg (immediately)	CF in orthostasis:___hpm (immediately)

BP in orthostasis: ___X___mmHg (after 3min)   CF in orthostasis:___hpm (after 3min)

*Criteria for orthostatic hypotension: when a person moves from a supine to a sitting or a standing position occurs a decline of >20 mmHg in systolic blood pressure or a decline of >10 mmHg in diastolic blood pressure. The decrease must be present within 3 minutes after the postural change [60].

Nursing diagnoses	Nursing interventions

Evaluation of orthostatic hypotension in patients with PD should be part of nursing protocol. Different measurement scales can be used, including those recommended by the Movement Disorders Society Task Force [58]: SCOPA-AUT and the Composite Autonomic Symptom Scale (COMPASS) [59]. Nursing care can be based on "Clinical Practice Guidelines: Patient Self-Management of BP Instability in Multiple System Atrophy, Parkinson's Disease and Other Neurological Disorders" [60].

Nursing assessment for medication adherence in patients with Parkinson's disease

Date: _____/_____/_____

Personal Data
Name: _____ Age: ___ Sex: ( ) Female ( ) Male Family/Caregiver:_____
Date of onset of symptoms of Parkinson's disease: _____

Daily medication		
Number of pills/time of ingestion Number of pills/time of ingestion		Medication action/Side effects
		Time-action:_____
		( ) dyskinesia ( ) wearing-off
		( ) ON/OFF ( ) nausea/vomiting
		( ) No side effect ( ) Other:
		( ) take the pills with food/protein

Morisky Medication Adherence Scale: High adherence (8 points), medium (6 to < 8 points) and low adherence (<6 points) [61]	
1) Do you sometimes forget to take your pills for PD?	(0) Yes (1) No
2) People sometimes miss taking their medications for reasons other than forgetting. Thinking over the past two weeks, were there any days when you did not take your medicine?	(0) Yes (1) No
3) Have you ever cut back or stopped taking your medicine without telling your doctor because you felt worse when you took it?	(0) Yes (1) No
4) When you travel or leave home, do you sometimes forget to bring along your medicine?	(0) Yes (1) No
5) Did you take all your medicine yesterday?	(0) Yes (1) No
6) When you feel like your symptoms are under control, do you sometimes stop taking your medicine?	(0) Yes (1) No

7) Taking medicine every day is a real inconvenience for some people. Do (0) Yes (1) No
you ever feel hassled about sticking to your treatment plan?

8) How often do you have difficulty remembering to take all your medicine?	( )Never/rarely ( )Once in a while ( )Sometimes ( )Usually ( )All the time

Self-care

Dependent on others for management of medications? ( ) yes ( ) no

( )Dysphagia for liquids ( )Dysphagia for solids: capsules/tablets ( )Change the consistency of medications

Mental function

Cognitive disorders: ( ) Yes ( ) No What: _____

Neuropsychiatric disorders: ( ) No ( ) Visual hallucinations ( ) Auditory hallucinations ( ) Impulsivity

( ) Hypersexuality ( ) Anxiety

Housing conditions

Live alone ( ) Yes ( ) No Easy access to where medications are stored ( ) Yes ( ) No

Community, social, and civic life

Impact on labor activities related to drug use? ( ) Yes ( ) No ( ) Not applicable

Impact on leisure activities related to drug use? ( ) Yes ( ) No

Impact on quality of life related to drug use? ( ) Yes ( ) No

Have financial resources to purchase medicines? ( ) Yes ( ) No

Support and relationships

Requires support of family/caregiver for management of medicines? ( ) Yes ( ) No

Resources to remember to take medication (box organizer, alarms, cellular)? ( )Yes ( ) No

Have financial resources to purchase medicines? ( ) Yes ( ) No

Acquires the medications by the public health system? ( ) Yes ( ) No

Suffers consequences of insufficient supply of medicines? ( ) Yes ( ) No ( ) Public services ( ) Private service

Nursing diagnoses	Nursing interventions

Evaluation of medication adherence should consider aspects related to medication (expected, adverse, and side effects; action time; costs; etc.), other symptoms of PD (dysphagia, cognitive/neuropsychiatric disorders), impact on the quality of life, and family support/ caregiver for management of treatment. The scale most commonly used in research and clinical practice is the Morisky Medical Adherence Scale (MMAS) [62–64].

3. Conclusion

The important role of nurses in the multidisciplinary care of patients with PD is obvious, and training of increasing numbers of professionals to meet the growing demand is an absolutely plausible goal.

Health actions based on comprehensive care centered on patients and their families, based on ethical, legal, operational, and theoretical premises of the profession and grounded in the concepts of prevention, promotion, treatment, and rehabilitation, provide quality and scientific rigor for patient care. These actions may help to improve the quality of life of individuals with neurodegenerative diseases that are multisystem, incurable, and often disabling.

Development of an organizational chart of the motor and nonmotor symptoms of PD and a survey of the main diagnoses/outcomes and nursing interventions based on a standardized language can direct clinical reasoning of professionals who care for these patients. Moreover, these tools may enable the development and/or improvement of clinical protocols that underlie the systematization of nursing care.

Author details

Michelle Hyczy de Siqueira Tosin[1*] and Beatriz Guitton Renaud Baptista de Oliveira[2]

*Address all correspondence to: michellehyczy@gmail.com

1 Sarah Network of Rehabilitation Hospitals, Rio de Janeiro, RJ, Brazil

2 School of Nursing, Federal Fluminense University, Niterói, RJ, Brazil

References

[1] Martinez-Martin P, Jeukens-Visser M, Lyons KE, Rodriguez-Blazquez C, Selai C, Siderowf A, et al. Health-related quality-of-life scales in Parkinson's disease: critique and recommendations. Mov Disord. 2011;26(13):2371–80.

[2] Nalls MA, McLean CY, Rick J, Eberly S, Hutten SJ, Gwinn K, et al. Diagnosis of Parkinson's disease on the basis of clinical and genetic classification: a population-based modelling study. Lancet Neurol. 2015;14(10):1002–9.

[3] Postuma RB, Berg D, Stern M, Poewe W, Olanow CW, Oertel W, et al. MDS clinical diagnostic criteria for Parkinson's disease. Mov Disord. 2015;30(12):1591–601.

[4] Martinez-Martin P, Rodriguez-Blazquez C, Paz S, Forjaz MJ, Frades-Payo B, Cubo E, et al. Parkinson symptoms and health related quality of life as predictors of costs: a

longitudinal observational study with linear mixed model analysis. PLoS One. 2015;10(12):e0145310.

[5]   Skelly R, Lindop F, Johnson C. Multidisciplinary care of patients with Parkinson's disease. Prog Neurol Psychiatry. 2012;16(2):10–4.

[6]   Cohen EV, Hagestuen R, Gonzalez-Ramos G, Cohen HW, Bassich C, Book E, et al. Interprofessional education increases knowledge, promotes team building, and changes practice in the care of Parkinson's disease. Parkinsonism Relat Disord. 2016;22:21–7.

[7]   Noorden RV. Interdisciplinary research by the numbers. Nature. 2015;525:306–7.

[8]   Tosin MH, Campos DM, Blanco L, Santana RF, Oliveira BG. Mapping nursing language terms of Parkinson's disease. Rev Esc Enferm USP. 2015;49(3):409–16.

[9]   Kim TY, Hardiker N, Coenen A. Inter-terminology mapping of nursing problems. J Biomed Inform. 2014;49:213–20.

[10] Tosin MH, Mecone CA, Oliveira BG. International Classification for Nursing Practice —ICNP(R): application to the Brazilian reality. Rev Bras Enferm. 2015;68(4):730–1.

[11] Cotton P, Heisters D. How to care for people with Parkinson's disease. Nurs Times. 2012;108(16):12–3.

[12] Campos DbM, Tosin MHdS, Blanco L, Santana RF, Oliveira BGRBd. Nursing diagnoses for urinary disorders in patients with Parkinson's disease. Acta Paul Enferm. 2015;28(2):190–5.

[13] Beaudet L, Ducharme F. Living with moderate-stage Parkinson disease: intervention needs and preferences of elderly couples. J Neurosci Nurs. 2013;45(2):88–95.

[14] Gopalakrishna A, Alexander SA. Understanding Parkinson disease: a complex and multifaceted illness. J Neurosci Nurs. 2015;47(6):320–6.

[15] Chen W, Xu ZM, Wang G, Chen SD. Non-motor symptoms of Parkinson's disease in China: a review of the literature. Parkinsonism Relat Disord. 2012;18(5):446–52.

[16] Hou J-GG, Lai EC. Nonmotor symptoms of Parkinson's disease. Int J Gerontol. 2007;1(2):53.

[17] Jankovic J. Parkinson's disease: clinical features and diagnosis. J Neurol Neurosurg Psychiatry. 2008;79(4):368–76.

[18] Vernon GM. Parkinson disease and the nurse practitioner: diagnostic and management challenges. J Nurse Pract. 2009;5(3):195–206.

[19] Tosin, MHS. Subconjunto terminológico da CIPE® para pacientes com doença de Parkinson em reabilitação. 2016. 193 f. Dissertação (Mestrado Profissional em Enfermagem Assistencial) - Escola de Enfermagem Aurora de Afonso Costa, Niterói, 2016 URL: http://www.repositorio.uff.br/jspui/handle/1/1775

[20] Kurtis MM, Rodriguez-Blazquez C, Martinez-Martin P, Group E. Relationship between sleep disorders and other non-motor symptoms in Parkinson's disease. Parkinsonism Relat Disord. 2013;19(12):1152–5.

[21] Behari M, Bhattacharyya KB, Borgohain R, Das SK, Ghosh B, Kishore A, et al. Parkinson's disease. Ann Indian Acad Neurol. 2011;14(Suppl 1):S2–6.

[22] Letanneux A, Danna J, Velay JL, Viallet F, Pinto S. From micrographia to Parkinson's disease dysgraphia. Mov Disord. 2014;29(12):1467–75.

[23] Ricciardi L, Bologna M, Morgante F, Ricciardi D, Morabito B, Volpe D, et al. Reduced facial expressiveness in Parkinson's disease: A pure motor disorder? J Neurol Sci. 2015;358(1–2):125–30.

[24] New AB, Robin DA, Parkinson AL, Eickhoff CR, Reetz K, Hoffstaedter F, et al. The intrinsic resting state voice network in Parkinson's disease. Hum Brain Mapp. 2015;36(5):1951–62.

[25] Kwan LC, Whitehill TL. Perception of speech by individuals with Parkinson's disease: a review. Parkinsons Dis. 2011;2011:389767.

[26] Ramig LO, Fox C, Sapir S. Speech treatment for Parkinson's disease. Expert Rev Neurother 2008;8(2):299–311.

[27] Uchiyama T, Sakakibara R, Yamamoto T, Ito T, Yamaguchi C, Awa Y, et al. Urinary dysfunction in early and untreated Parkinson's disease. J Neurol Neurosurg Psychiatry. 2011;82(12):1382–6.

[28] Xue Peng WT, Zong Huantao and Zhang Yong. Urodynamic analysis and treatment of male Parkinson's disease. Chin Med J. 2014;127(5):878–81.

[29] Jost WII. Gastrointestinal dysfunction in Parkinson's Disease. J Neurol Sci. 2010;289(1–2):69–73.

[30] Sung H-Y, Park J-W, Kim J-S. The frequency and severity of gastrointestinal symptoms in patients with early Parkinson's disease. Mov Disord. 2014;7(1):7–12.

[31] Zlotnik Y, Balash Y, Korczyn AD, Giladi N, Gurevich T. Disorders of the oral cavity in Parkinson's disease and parkinsonian syndromes. Parkinsons Dis. 2015;2015:379482.

[32] Isaacson SH, Skettini J. Neurogenic orthostatic hypotension in Parkinson's disease: evaluation, management, and emerging role of droxidopa. Vasc Health Risk Manag. 2014;10:169–76.

[33] Mazza A, Ravenni R, Antonini A, Casiglia E, Rubello D, Pauletto P. Arterial hypertension, a tricky side of Parkinson's disease: physiopathology and therapeutic features. Neurol Sci. 2013;34(5):621–7.

[34] Berganzo K, Díez-Arrola B, Tijero B, Somme J, Lezcano E, Llorens V, et al. Nocturnal hypertension and dysautonomia in patients with Parkinson's disease: are they related? J Neurol. 2013;260(7):1752–6.

[35] Postuma RB, Adler CH, Dugger BN, Hentz JG, Shill HA, Driver-Dunckley E, et al. REM sleep behavior disorder and neuropathology in Parkinson's disease. Mov Disord. 2015;30(10):1413–7.

[36] Boeve BF. Idiopathic REM sleep behaviour disorder in the development of Parkinson's disease. Lancet Neurol. 2013;12(5):469–82.

[37] Maass A, Reichmann H. Sleep and non-motor symptoms in Parkinson's disease. J Neural Transm. 2013;120(4):565–9.

[38] Robert G, Le Jeune F, Lozachmeur C, Drapier S, Dondaine T, Peron J, et al. Apathy in patients with Parkinson disease without dementia or depression: a PET study. Neurology. 2012;79(11):1155–60.

[39] Munhoz RP, Moro A, Silveira-Moriyama L, Teive HA. Non-motor signs in Parkinson's disease: a review. Arq Neuropsiquiatr. 2015;73(5):454–62.

[40] Martinez-Martin P, Rodriguez-Blazquez C, Forjaz MJ, Frades-Payo B, Agüera-Ortiz L, Weintraub D, et al. Neuropsychiatric symptoms and caregiver's burden in Parkinson's disease. Parkinsonism Relat Disord. 2015;21(6):629–34.

[41] Berardelli A, Conte A, Fabbrini G, Bologna M, Latorre A, Rocchi L, et al. Pathophysiology of pain and fatigue in Parkinson's disease. Parkinsonism Relat Disord. 2012;18:S226–S8.

[42] Connolly BS, Lang AE. Pharmacological treatment of Parkinson disease: a review. JAMA. 2014;311(16):1670–83.

[43] Shin JY, Habermann B, Pretzer-Aboff I. Challenges and strategies of medication adherence in Parkinson's disease: a qualitative study. Geriatr Nurs. 2015;36(3):192–6.

[44] Starhof C, Anker N, Henriksen T, Lassen CF. Dependency and transfer incomes in idiopathic Parkinson's disease. Dan Med J. 2014;61(10):1–5.

[45] Young-Mason J. The fine art of caring: people with Parkinson disease and their care partners. Clin Nurse Spec. 2015;29(2):121–2.

[46] Silva KnLd, Sena RRnd, Grillo MJC, Horta NldCs, Prado PMC. Nursing education and the challenges for health promotion. Rev Bras Enferm. 2009;62(1):86–91.

[47] Vaughn S, Mauk KL, Jacelon CS, Larsen PD, Rye J, Wintersgill W, et al. The competency model for professional rehabilitation nursing. Rehabil Nurs. 2015;0:1–12.

[48] Rehabilitation Measures Database [Internet]. Available from: http://www.rehabmeasures.org/Lists/RehabMeasures/DispForm.aspx?ID=1012. [Accessed: 2016-03-13].

[49] Lawrence BJ, Gasson N, Kane R, Bucks RS, Loftus AM. Activities of daily living, depression, and quality of life in Parkinson's disease. PLoS One. 2014;9(7):e102294.

[50] Martinez-Martin P, Prieto L, Forjaz MJo. Longitudinal metric properties of disability rating scales for Parkinson's disease. Value Health. 2006;9(6):386–93.

[51] Guidelines WGOG. Constipation: a global perspective; 2010.

[52] Evatt ML, Chaudhuri KR, Chou KL, Cubo E, Hinson V, Kompoliti K, et al. Dysautonomia rating scales in Parkinson's disease: sialorrhea, dysphagia, and constipation—critique and recommendations by movement disorders task force on rating scales for Parkinson's disease. Mov Disord. 2009;24(5):635–46.

[53] Iacovelli E, Gilio F, Meco G, Fattapposta F, Vanacore N, Brusa L, et al. Bladder symptoms assessed with overactive bladder questionnaire in Parkinson's disease. Mov Disord. 2010;25(9):1203–9.

[54] Sakakibara R, Shinotoh H, Uchiyama T, Sakuma M, Kashiwado M, Yoshiyama M, et al. Questionnaire-based assessment of pelvic organ dysfunction in Parkinson's disease. Auton Neurosci. 2001(92):76–85.

[55] Visser M, Marinus J, Stiggelbout AM, Van Hilten JJ. Assessment of autonomic dysfunction in Parkinson's disease: the SCOPA-AUT. Mov Disord. 2004;19(11):1306–12.

[56] Hogl B, Arnulf I, Comella C, Ferreira J, Iranzo A, Tilley B, et al. Scales to assess sleep impairment in Parkinson's disease: critique and recommendations. Mov Disord. 2010;25(16):2704–16.

[57] Trenkwalder C, Kohnen R, Hogl B, Metta V, Sixel-Doring F, Frauscher B, et al. Parkinson's disease sleep scale—validation of the revised version PDSS-2. Mov Disord. 2011;26(4):644–52.

[58] Pavy-Le Traon A, Amarenco G, Duerr S, Kaufmann H, Lahrmann H, Shaftman SR, et al. The movement disorders task force review of dysautonomia rating scales in Parkinson's disease with regard to symptoms of orthostatic hypotension. Mov Disord. 2011;26(11):1985–92.

[59] Sletten DM, Suarez GA, Low PA, Mandrekar J, Singer W. COMPASS 31: a refined and abbreviated Composite Autonomic Symptom Score. Mayo Clin Proc. 2012;87(12):1196–201.

[60] Viscomi P, Jeffrey J. Development of clinical practice guidelines or patient management of blood pressure in stability in multiple system atrophy, Parkinson's disease, and other neurological disorders. Can J Neurosci Nurs. 2010;32(2):6–19.

[61] Morisky Medication Adherence Scales: MMAS-4 and MMAS-8 [Internet]. https://www.mainequalitycounts.org/image_upload/5_Morisky_Medication_Adherence.pdf. [Accessed: 2016-03-13].

[62] Fabbrini G, Abbruzzese G, Barone P, Antonini A, Tinazzi M, Castegnaro G, et al. Adherence to anti-Parkinson drug therapy in the "REASON" sample of Italian patients with Parkinson's disease: the linguistic validation of the Italian version of the "Morisky Medical Adherence Scale-8 items." Neurol Sci. 2013;34(11):2015–22.

[63] Lakshminarayana R, Wang D, Burn D, Chaudhuri KR, Cummins G, Galtrey C, et al. Smartphone- and Internet-assisted self-management and adherence tools to manage Parkinson's disease (SMART-PD): study protocol for a randomised controlled trial. Trials. 2014;7(15).

[64] Santos-García D, Prieto-Formoso M, Fuente-Fernández Rdl. Levodopa dosage determines adherence to long-acting dopamine agonists in Parkinson's disease. Neurol Sci. 2012;318(1–2):90–3.

9

Mechanisms for Neuronal Cell Death in Parkinson's Disease: Pathological Cross Talks Between Epigenetics and Various Signalling Pathways

S Meenalochani, ST Dheen and SSW Tay

Abstract

Parkinson's disease (PD) is an incapacitating neurodegenerative disorder affecting the population over the age of 65 years. Clinically, most patients present with the symptoms of bradykinesia, resting tremor, rigidity, and postural instability. A number of patients also suffer from autonomic, cognitive, and psychiatric disturbances. The symptoms of PD result from the selective loss of dopaminergic (DA) neurons in the substantia nigra (SNc) pars compacta. However, the exact molecular mechanism that causes this cell death still remains elusive. The cross talk between various molecular signals facilitates the cell to undergo developmental and differentiation programs with such tantalizing accuracy. In recent years, epigenetic mechanisms have advanced as a regulatory driver of processes such as signal transduction, cell cycle control, and stress response. These include DNA methylation, histone modifications, and small RNA-mediated mechanisms. Increasing evidence suggests that epigenetic mechanisms play a major role in the pathogenesis of PD. Researchers are now working to comprehend the therapeutic promises of epigenetic molecules to offset age-related neurodegenerative diseases. In this chapter, we focus on some examples of the cross talk between epigenetic processes and various signal transduction pathways that underlie the pathogenesis of PD.

Keywords: Parkinson's disease, epigenetics, DNA methylation, histone modifications, non-coding RNAs

1. Introduction

Parkinson's disease (PD) is a devastating disorder of the brain characterized by continuous deterioration of motor functions owing to the loss of dopaminergic neurons in the substantia nigra of the mid brain. It is the second most common neurodegenerative disorder after Alzheimer's disease. The first clear medical explanation about PD was written in 1817 by an English physician James Parkinson in his work titled *An Essay on the Shaking Palsy* [1]. The SNc of the midbrain contains the DA neurons which produce dopamine. Dopamine is a neurotransmitter responsible for coordinating movements. Although few in number, these DA neurons play a vital role in controlling multiple brain functions including voluntary movement and a broad array of behavioural processes [2]. In PD, there is a severe depletion in the levels of dopamine due to the degeneration of DA neurons. This results in the lack of control over body movements [2]. Nevertheless, the precise cause of this neuronal cell death still remains an enigma.

The signs and symptoms of PD may vary from person to person. The symptoms have a gradual onset and usually advance simultaneously with the progression of the disease. Early signs may be mild and may go unnoticed and later tend to worsen over time. If left untreated, it may lead to disability with associated immobility. The early classic symptoms of PD include motor symptoms such as postural instability, resting tremor, bradykinesia, and rigidity [3]. These symptoms are linked to the progressive loss of dopamine and are usually improved by treatment with levodopa or dopamine agonists [4]. Nevertheless, as the disease progresses, symptoms that fail to respond to levodopa develop [5]. These symptoms include flexed posture, freezing phenomenon, and loss of postural stability [6]. Although the motor symptoms lead the clinical picture of PD, some patients are also associated with a range of nonmotor symptoms such as sleep, sensation, autonomic, mood disturbances as well as cognitive disturbances such as dementia [7].

The diagnosis of PD is extremely complicated, mainly during its early stages. This is due to the fact that as the disease advances, the symptoms might mimic other ailments. Moreover, at present, there is no specific lab test available to diagnose the disease. In most cases, physical examination of the patient forms the basis for the diagnosis of PD. Levodopa continues to be the most effective treatment for PD [8]. Another feasible option is deep brain stimulation, although some patients encounter the necessity for surgery. New treatments that offer better control over the symptoms stay on developmental demand.

2. Possible pathways involved in the pathogenesis of PD

Several enthralling theories have shown that different molecular pathways are involved in the propagation of PD pathogenesis. Accumulating evidence has confirmed that mitochondrial dysfunction, impairment of the ubiquitin proteasome system (UPS), and oxidative stress may perhaps represent the prime molecular pathways that generally mitigate the pathogenesis of both sporadic and familial forms of PD [9]. In addition to these, inflammation and loss of neurotrophic factors have also been shown to play a major role in the progress of PD [9].

3. Potential risk factors in PD

Age is one of the prominent risk factors in PD [10, 11]. Studies have shown that dopaminergic neuronal populations appear selectively susceptible to loss with ageing compared to many other brain regions and those related to other neurodegenerative disorders [12]. Furthermore, studies have also shown that the dopaminergic neurons are particularly vulnerable to the mitochondrial dysfunction with advancing age [13, 14].

4. Genetic factors in PD

Although PD was long considered to be sporadic in origin, monogenic Parkinsonism disorders are gaining growing importance in recent years. Genetic factors appear to be the main cause in about 5–10% of the PD patients [15]. However, in both cases, the degeneration of nigrostriatal DA neurons remains a general overlapping characteristic [16]. Studies have shown that around 13 genetic loci are involved in the rare forms of PD [17]. Out of the 13, around 6 PARK loci genes have been identified and have been reported to carry mutations that are related to relatives who are affected by PD. Out of the six genes, four have similarly been shown to be involved in sporadic PD [17].

There is considerable evidence that, in addition to well-defined genetic mechanisms, environmental factors play a crucial role in PD pathogenesis. Nevertheless, the exact mechanism by which the environment could affect the genetic factors and contribute to PD development remains obscure. In recent years, epigenetic mechanisms such as DNA methylation, chromatin remodelling, and alterations in gene expression via non-coding RNAs (ncRNAs) are surging in importance as potential factors in the pathogenesis of PD.

5. Epigenetics

Epigenetics refers to mechanisms which can alter the expression of genes without modifying the actual DNA sequence and are heritable [18]. Epigenetic modulation exists throughout life, beginning in prenatal stages, is dependent on the lifestyle, environmental exposure, and genetic makeup of an individual and may serve as a missing link between PD risk factors and development of the disease [18].

At the molecular level, epigenetic mechanisms influence protein expression through post-translational modifications of histones (e.g. acetylation, methylation, phosphorylation, and ubiquitination), the methylation of cytosine bases and positioning of nucleosome, and by activation/deactivation of microRNAs (miRNAs). These processes act as a switch for the fate of the cell through regulating gene and miRNA expression, as well as through parental imprinting, X chromosome inactivation, suppressing transposons, and regulating developmental processes [19]. The epigenome offers the flexibility to address a fluctuating environment above the relatively rigid architecture of DNA sequence information and thus influences the formation of a phenotype without altering the genotype. The three distinct mechanisms of epigenetic regulation that are complex and interrelated are DNA methylation, histone modification, and RNA-based mechanisms.

5.1. Epigenetic mechanisms in PD

In spite of having a familial aspect, PD does not show a clear Mendelian pattern of inheritance, making it difficult to correlate the genetic variations with the disease state. In this case, an epigenetic framework would be most useful in understanding the age dependence (which is not clearly explained by the accumulation of genetic mutations) and the environmental impact on genetic predisposition to the disease. A better understanding of the complex interplay of genetic and epigenetic factors can help in improving the existing knowledge on disease mechanisms and therapeutic strategies. In diseases where age and environment play an important role, the identification of epigenetic variations contributing to the age- and environment-mediated control of disease mechanism will simplify the disease diagnosis [20]. Studying epigenetic mechanisms involved in PD can hence be a major milestone in the pursuit of understanding the disease better. In recent years, the impact of epigenetic mechanisms in PD has been increasingly studied [21]. DNA methylation, histone tail modifications, and microRNA-mediated pathways are considered to play a role in the pathogenesis of PD based on recent evidence ([22–26]).

6. DNA methylation

6.1. Principle of DNA methylation

DNA methylation is one such epigenetic modification that has been studied extensively for the past several decades since its discovery in cancer in 1983 [27]. DNA methylation involves the transfer of a methyl group to the 5′ position of a cytosine residue. This dinucleotide unit is always written as CpG (representing a cytosine followed by guanine and a phosphate group between them). Regions that are enriched with CpGs are called CpG islands. These CpG islands are usually located in the promoter region of genes. CpG islands are usually non-methylated, except in some rare cases where methylation of CPG islands is required. On the contrary, CpGs outside CpG islands are usually methylated [28, 29]. Methylation of CpG sequences can modify gene expression levels by inducing conformational changes in the chromatin. This impedes the availability of the gene promoter region for the transcriptional machinery [30]. Therefore, it is obvious that promoter hyper-methylation leads to gene silencing while hypo-methylation will augment gene expression. CpG methylation within promoter and intragenic sites has been extensively studied, and moreover, there has been surging interest regarding non-CpG methylation. This denotes the methylation that occurs at cytosine of non-CpG dinucleotides, such as CA, CT, or CC. DNA methylation works in congruence with histone modification (such as histone acetylation) to control memory formation and synaptic plasticity [31], and it also has a possible impact on genetic and neuronal function affecting behaviours [32]. Moreover, the association between DNA methylation, chromatin structure, and gene silencing has been extensively studied for many years, and gene silencing is thought to be an epigenetic intervention on neurodegenerative diseases like Alzheimer's disease (AD) [33]. Therefore, it seems justified to suggest that there is a very strong potential link between DNA methylation and neurodegenerative diseases.

6.1.1. DNA methylation in PD

Methylation can be instigated by a variety of factors, which can be the cause of many serious diseases including PD. Ageing has been shown to decrease global DNA methylation [34], while it increases methylation in specific promoters. This could be a contributing factor in PD as it is an age-related disorder.

Although there have not been many reports, there are indications of impaired methylation in PD patients [25]. DNA methylation has been widely studied in the SNCA gene. Methylation of intron 1 of the SNCA gene is associated with decreased transcription [35]. Decreased methylation of the SNCA gene and of the SNCA intron 1 has been observed in the SNc of clinical PD cases [36]. It is obvious from these results that the increased α-synuclein production (that is associated with PD) is caused by the increased SNCA gene expression, as a result of a decreased methylation state of the SNCA gene. Furthermore, it has been demonstrated that α-synuclein could sequester DNA methyltransferase 1 (which maintains DNA methylation) in the cytoplasm. DNA methyltransferase 1 is an important enzyme which is expressed copiously in the brain and maintains DNA methylation in the cytoplasm. Sequestering DNMT1 leads to global DNA hypo-methylation in PD patients with dementia and presence of neuronal Lewy body (DLB) [37]. A GWAS on methylation of candidate genes identified changes in methylation status of proximal DNA CpG sites of other genes such as PARK16/1q32, glycoprotein (transmembrane) nmb (GPNMB), and syntaxin 1b (STX1B), ARK16. This is indicative of the fact that other PD-related genes may possibly be susceptible to these methylation changes (International Parkinson's Disease Genomics and Welcome Trust Case Control, 2011). Nevertheless, the clear undeviating link between DNA methylation and PD still remains obscure. The epigenetic regulation of SNCA gene has also been reported in an A53T-linked familial case of PD. A recent methylation study on brain and blood samples from PD patients has revealed that there is differential methylation of CpG sites [25]. Of these, over 80% of the sites were hypo-methylated in both blood and brain. The same study has reported that genes such as major histocompatibility complex, class II (MHC II), dq alpha 1 (HLA-DQA1), glutamine-fructose-6-phosphate transaminase 2 (GFPT2), MAPT, and vault RNA2-1 (VTRNA2-1) are highly associated with PD being similarly methylated in brain and blood samples from clinical PD cases [25].

The number of methylated sites in DNA has been reported to increase with ageing [34] which is a major risk factor for PD. Results from the GWAS have already provided many novel and important perceptions for molecular mechanisms underlying the pathogenesis of complex diseases such as PD. Nevertheless, it is probable that understanding exact epigenetic modifications might be significantly assisted by knowledge of genetic susceptibility loci determined from GWAS.

7. Histone modifications

7.1. Principle behind histone modification and the different types of histone modifications

Histones are proteins that pack and order DNA into nucleosomes. Each nucleosome contains two subunits each of histones H2A, H2B, H3, and H4, known as the core histones (octomers). A 147-bp segment of DNA wrapped around the histone octamer and neighbouring nucleosomes are separated by, on average, 50 bp of free DNA. Histone H1 is termed the linker histone, and it does not form the integral part of the nucleosome. However, it binds to the linker DNA (that is, the DNA separating two histone complexes), sealing off the nucleosome at the location where DNA enters and leaves.

Histones play a crucial role in epigenetics. All histones are subject to several post-transcriptional modifications such as acetylation, methylation, phosphorylation, ubiquitination, SUMOylation, and ADP-ribosylation, among others [38]. These post-translational modifications made to histone tails can influence gene expression by altering the structure of chromatin or using histone modifiers. Histone protein modifications can alter the availability of transcriptional machinery to specific promoters leading to gene activation or silencing [39]. Histone modifications have vital roles in transcriptional regulation, DNA repair, DNA replication, alternative splicing [40], and chromosome condensation [41]. With respect to its transcriptional state, the human genome can be roughly divided into actively transcribed euchromatin and transcriptionally inactive heterochromatin. Euchromatin is characterized by high levels of histone modifications such as acetylation and trimethylated H3K4, H3K36, and H3K79. On the contrary, heterochromatin is characterized by low levels of acetylation and high levels of H3K9, H3K27, and H4K20 methylation [42]. Recent studies have demonstrated that actively transcribed genes are characterized by high levels of H3K4me3, H3K27ac, H2BK5ac, and H4K20me1 in the promoter and H3K79me1 and H4K20me1 in the gene body [43].

7.1.1. Histone acetylation/deacetylation

Histone modifications such as acetylation and deacetylation play important roles in gene regulation. These are associated with transcriptional activation and repression respectively [41]. Histone acetylation is a reversible process. Acetylation is catalysed by histone acetyltransferases (HATs), which are categorized into three families (GNAT, MYST, and CBP/p300) [44]. HATs catalyse acetylation via the transfer of an acetyl group from acetyl-coenzyme A to the ε-amino group of lysine side chains on the N-terminal tails of H2A, H2B, H3, and H4 [44]. It has recently been shown that HATs can catalyse acetylation at lysine 56 (K56) within the core domain of H3 [41]. Histone deacetylation is performed by a class of enzymes known as histone deacetylases (HDACs). These HDACs remove the acetyl groups from the ε-amino group of lysines. HDACs are classified into four classes based upon sequence homology and cofactor dependencies.

7.1.2. Histone methylation/demethylation

Histone methylation involves the transfer of methyl groups from S-adenosyl-L-methionine to lysine or arginine residues of histone proteins by histone methyltransferases (HMTs). As described earlier, DNA methylation and histone modifications work in association with each other. HMTs control DNA methylation through transcriptional repression or activation which is chromatin dependent. Several different histone methyltransferases exist, and each of them is specific for the lysine or arginine residue they modify. For example, on histone H3, SET1, SET7/9, Ash1, ALL-1, MLL, ALR, Trx, and SMYD3 are the histone methyltransferases that catalyse methylation of histone H3 at lysine 4 (H3-K4) in mammalian cells [45]. ESET, SUV39-h1, SUV39-h2, SETDB1, Dim-5, and Eu-HMTase are histone methyltransferases that catalyse methylation of histone H3 at lysine 9 (H3-K9) in mammalian cells [45]. G9a and polycomb group enzymes such as EZH2 are histone methyltransferases that catalyse methylation of histone H3 at lysine 27 (H3-K27) in mammalian cells [46]. Arginine methylation of histones H3 and H4 promotes transcriptional activation and is mediated by a family of protein arginine methyltransferases (PRMTs) [47]. Based on the position to which the methyl groups are added, PRMTs are classified into type I (CARM1, PRMT1, PRMT2, PRMT3, PRMT6, and PRMT8) and type II (PRMT5 and PRMT7) [47].

7.2. Histone modifications in PD

The precise role of histone modifications in the pathogenesis of PD still remains indefinable, and most of the data are obtained from experimental cell cultures and animal models of PD.

α-synuclein, the major protein involved in PD pathogenesis, is known to interact with histones and inhibit histone deacetylation [48]. Several histone deacetylase inhibitors have been reported to protect against α-synuclein-mediated toxicity in PD models [48]. Inhibition of the histone deacetylase sirtuin-2 is known to decrease α-synuclein-mediated toxicity and protect against dopaminergic neuronal death [49]. When mouse nigral neurons were treated with the herbicide paraquat, alpha-synuclein translocated into the nucleus and was able to interact directly with histones [50]. Another study in Drosophila model of PD has demonstrated that alpha-synuclein interacts directly with histones by inhibiting histone acetylation. This neurotoxic effect of alpha-synuclein was counteracted by the administration of HDAC inhibitors [51]. Together with alpha-synuclein, HDAC6 and HDAC4 are the chief components of Lewy bodies in PD [52]. It is interesting to note that HDAC6 protects dopaminergic neurons from alpha-synuclein toxicity by promoting inclusion formation [53]. This has been confirmed by various other reports on neuronal cell lines expressing mutant alpha-synuclein wherein they have reported that the neurons are rescued from alpha-synuclein toxicity by HDAC6. In PD, histones seem to be more involved in aggregate formation, than in epigenetic dysregulation of gene expression. It has also been demonstrated that α-synuclein, interact with histone H1, which is localized in the cytoplasm of neurons and astrocytes from affected brain areas in PD. This has been shown to play a role in fibril formation [54]. Although not directly linked to histone acetylation, alpha-synuclein overexpression can downregulate the expression of histone genes. Previous reports on *C. elegans* model have demonstrated that overexpressing human alpha-synuclein leads to downregulation of nine genes coding for histones H1, H2B, and H4 [55]. It is clear from these studies that most of histone PTM evidence in PD is derived from the effects of alpha-synuclein. Moreover, few other genes associated with PD pathogenesis have been linked to HDAC function. Mutations in parkin cause early onset of familial PD (AR-JP) [56]. Parkin has been shown to promote mitophagy by catalysing mitochondrial ubiquitination, which in turn employs ubiquitin-binding autophagic components, such as HDAC6 [56]. The treatment of a dopaminergic cell line with the HDAC inhibitor phenylbutyrate resulted in increased levels of DJ-1 which protected these cells from mutant alpha-synuclein toxicity. An increase in DJ-1 expression was also observed in mice treated with phenylbutyrate and protected MPP^+-challenged dopaminergic neurons [57]. In addition, PINK-1 is also affected by HDAC activity. Transgenic expression of sirtuin 2 in PINK-1 Drosophila mutants rescued mitochondrial defects and spared dopaminergic neurons [58]. This suggests that depending on the PD model, HDACs may have a neuroprotective role. Levodopa remains as the most effective and extensively used therapy in the treatment of PD although it is tied with some serious side effects. Prolonged treatment with levodopa leads to the development of abnormal involuntary movements, termed levodopa-induced dyskinesia (LDID). Interestingly, histone PTMs have been shown to play a role in LDID. Previous reports on primate model have demonstrated that LDID is associated with marked deacetylation of histone H4, hyperacetylation, and dephosphorylation of histone H3 in the striatum [59]. In mouse models of LDID, histone H3 exhibited decreased trimethylation [59]. Histone H3 phosphorylation changes have also been demonstrated in striatonigral medium spiny neurons, thereby linking ERK-dependent histone phosphorylation in striatal plasticity leading to dyskinesia [60]. Future studies are warranted in order to understand the underlying molecular mechanism and the direct link between histone modifications in PD. This will enhance our knowledge and light up new avenues for the identification of epigenetics-based therapeutics for the better treatment of PD.

8. Non-coding RNAs

8.1. What are microRNAs?

miRNAs are critical regulators of gene expression. Their discovery adds a new facet to our understanding of intricate gene regulatory networks. These are a family of small, ncRNAs that regulate gene expression in a sequence-specific manner. They were first identified in *Caenorhabditis elegans* as genes that were responsible for the regulation of developmental events. Since then, hundreds of microRNAs have been identified in almost all species [61]. MicroRNAs have diverse expression patterns and play a vital role in various developmental and physiological processes. These small ncRNAs are transcribed by RNA polymerase II (RNA Pol II) from two primary genomic loci: miRNA genes and intronic sequences. In the canonical biogenesis pathway, pri-miRNAs are transcribed from miRNA genes [62]. These are processed in the nucleus by the Drosha/DGCR8 microprocessor complex to produce pre-miRNAs. The processed pre-miRNAs are then exported to the cytoplasm by Exportin-5. In the cytoplasm, these pre-miRNAs are further cleaved by the RNase III enzyme Dicer to yield a mature miRNA duplex. The mature strand also termed the guide strand is 20–22 nucleotides in length and associates with Argonaute proteins, AGO 1–4, to form a functional RNA-induced silencing complex (RISC) [62]. The antisense strand, denoted by miRNA*, was previously thought to be degraded; recent evidence suggests that some of these may have biological activity. The mature miRNA functions by aligning the RISC to target mRNA by binding at complementary seed sequences in the 3'UTR. This association of target mRNA with the miRNA-containing RISC results in silencing the gene expression by translational repression and recruitment of protein complexes causing deadenylation and degradation of target mRNA [63].

9. Interaction between miRNAs and PD-related genes

Overproduction of a gene product is one of the cardinal mechanisms by which the gene contributes to PD pathogenesis (a best known example is α-synuclein). There is a strong association that miRNA-mediated gene suppression could hold prospective approaches to improve the disease phenotype.

On this ground, miR-7 was first discovered as a regulator of α-synuclein expression [64, 65]. Junn et al. [64] demonstrated that miR-7 level is 40 times higher in neurons than in other cells. Further miR-7 is higher in the substantia nigra and striatum of mice, compared to cerebral cortex and cerebellum. This provides support for endogenous miR-7 regulation of α-synuclein levels in neurons. To further this study and to understand the clear mechanistic underpinnings of miR-7 in PD, the same group investigated miR-7 levels in MPP+-treated SH-SY5Y cells, and MPTP-intoxicated mice [65]. From this study, it was demonstrated that overexpressing miR-7 reduces endogenous α-synuclein levels. Hence it seems justified to suggest that a reduction in miR-7 might be a major contributor to nigrostriatal degeneration. In addition to miR-7, Doxakis [65] described the role of miR-153. In the regulation of α-synuclein, overexpression of miR-153 in cultured cortical neurons has been shown to reduce endogenous α-synuclein levels to around 30–40%. These results advocate the potential role of miR-7 and miR-153 as promising therapeutic targets to promote neuroprotection in patients with known α-synuclein gene multiplications. Another major gene involved in the PD pathogenesis is LRRK2 gene. Although the function of the leucine-rich repeat kinase 2 (LRRK2 gene) still remains largely unknown, some recent evidence suggests that this gene could be involved in membrane trafficking [66]. Mutation in the LRRK2 gene has been implicated as a risk factor for both familial and sporadic PD [67]. Reports have demonstrated that LRRK2 gene inhibition blocks neurotoxicity *in vitro* and *in vivo* [68]. These reports provide further support for its role in PD [69]. Cho et al. [70] have demonstrated that normal LRRK2 gene levels are higher in the frontal cortex of sporadic PD and PD with dementia (PDD) patients compared to controls (NPC) . Interestingly, MiR-205 has been identified as a putative regulator of LRRK2 gene. In addition, further investigations revealed significantly lower levels of miR-205 in the frontal cortex and striatum of PD patients, compared to NPC. Inhibition of miR-205 is associated with upregulation of the LRRK2 gene protein and vice versa. DA neurons in rodent brain displayed a high level of miR-205. Reports on transgenic mice overexpressing mutant LRRK2 gene, miR-205 treatment rescued impairment of neurite outgrowth. Like miR-7 and miR153, miR 205 is a potential target for therapeutic intervention, particularly for sporadic cases in which LRRK2 gene levels were found to be elevated, and miR-205 levels were found to be low [70]. DJ1 and parkin are other genes that are regulated by miR34b and miR34c, respectively. Miñones-Moyano et al. [71] first discovered a dysregulation of miR-34b and miR-34c in the post-mortem brains of clinical PD cases. Their study demonstrated that miR-34 reduction compromises neuronal viability by mitochondrial dysfunction and production of reactive oxygen species in an SH-SY5Y neuroblastoma culture model. They further characterized that the miR-34b/c reduction is correlated with decreased expression of DJ1 and Parkin, noting that these proteins were indeed downregulated in PD brain tissue as well [71]. This provides evidence that miR-34b/c downregulation may involve DJ1 and Parkin; however, the exact molecular mechanism by which this interaction occurs remains unclear. Previous work from our group has demonstrated that downregulation of MiR124 in the MPTP-induced mouse model of PD modulates the expression of Calpain/CDK5 pathway proteins [72]. This study proves that miRNAs can serve as a powerful tool to gain in-depth knowledge about the underlying mechanism that leads to the pathogenesis of the disease, and miRNA-based therapies can be used to validate drug targets for PD.

10. Examples of cross talks between epigenetics and signalling pathways underlying PD pathogenesis

MAPK pathway has been reported to cause neurodegeneration in PD. In addition, it has also been demonstrated that cocaine induces the MAPK pathway and through MSK1 phosphorylates histone H3 at Ser10 [73]. In addition, DNA methylation has been shown to affect the stimulation of aurora-B kinase which has been reported to phosphorylate H3S10 [74]. Casein kinase II (CKII) which is a serine/threonine kinase has been reported to phosphorylate histone H4 serine 1 in response to DNA damage [75]. CKII can also phosphorylate synphilin-1, reducing its interaction with α-synuclein and formation of inclusion bodies [76]. In addition, CKII phosphorylates Ser-129 of α-synuclein in human brain and inhibits Cdk5 [77]. It is well known that α-synuclein by the activation of nitric oxide synthase (NOS) and releasing NO considerably reduces PARP-1 [78]. Activation of PARP-1 in response to DNA damage inhibits aurora-B kinase, which is required for H3S10 phosphorylation [79]. Reports on miRNAs have shed light on the fact that miRNAs regulate various signalling pathways such as checkpoint transduction cascades or transcriptional repression that are associated with PD pathogenesis [80]. An interesting study in human H4 neuroglioma cells identified a large set of putative α-synuclein target (interacting) genes which are widely used as a model for studying the molecular basis of PD, providing the first insight into the interaction of endogenous α-synuclein. Their study identified several primary targets of α-synuclein, with the glycosphingolipid biosynthesis and the protein ubiquitination pathways being common to miRNome IPA analysis. In addition, they have also shown that miR-30b, miR-30c, and miR-26a which are among the most abundant miRNAs in primary human neuronal and glial cells and are reported to be involved in the regulation of α-synuclein [81] emerged as the main modulators of these two pathways. Taken together, these reports highlight a few examples on the role of epigenetic mechanism that may act as modulators of cellular mechanisms leading to PD.

11. Conclusion

Evidence has shed light on the role of epigenetics in PD and has increased our understanding of the genetics of PD since the first report. The studies described in this chapter provide evidence that targeting the epigenome, with small drugs such as HDAC inhibitors that are able to cross the blood-brain barrier, can be one of the potential candidates to delay the onset and progression of the symptoms in animal models of PD. Further studies aiming at understanding the complex interplay between genetic and epigenetic biomarkers, lifestyles, and environmental factors are warranted in order to completely counter the progression of PD in the near future.

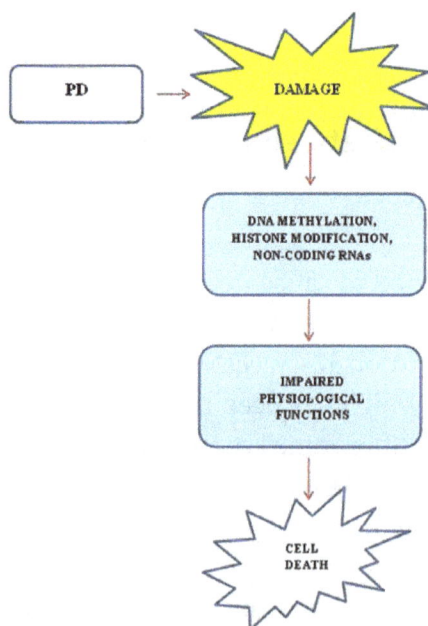

Figure 1. Epigenetics and cell death in PD.

Author details

S Meenalochani, ST Dheen and SSW Tay*

*Address all correspondence to: anttaysw@nus.edu.sg

Department of Anatomy, Yong Loo Lin school of Medicine, National University Health System, National University of Singapore, Singapore

References

[1] Parkinson, J., *An essay on the shaking palsy. 1817*. J Neuropsychiatry Clin Neurosci, 2002. 14(2): pp. 223–36; discussion 222.

[2] Chinta, S.J. and J.K. Andersen, *Dopaminergic neurons*. Int J Biochem Cell Biol, 2005. 37(5): pp. 942–946.

[3] Jankovic, J., *Parkinson's disease: clinical features and diagnosis*. J Neurol Neurosurg Psychiatry, 2008. 79(4): pp. 368–376.

[4] Katzenschlager, R. and A.J. Lees, *Treatment of Parkinson's disease: levodopa as the first choice*. J Neurol, 2002. 249 Suppl 2: pp. Ii19–24.

[5] Thanvi, B., N. Lo, and T. Robinson, *Levodopa-induced dyskinesia in Parkinson's disease: clinical features, pathogenesis, prevention and treatment*. Postgrad Med J, 2007. 83(980): pp. 384–388.

[6] Davie, C.A., *A review of Parkinson's disease*. Br Med Bull, 2008. 86: pp. 109–27.

[7] Shulman, L.M., et al., *Non-recognition of depression and other non-motor symptoms in Parkinson's disease*. Parkinsonism Rel Disord, 2002. 8(3): pp. 193–197.

[8] Gelb, D.J., E. Oliver, and S. Gilman, *Diagnostic criteria for Parkinson disease*. Arch Neurol, 1999. 56(1): pp. 33–39.

[9] Dawson, T.M. and V.L. Dawson, *Molecular Pathways of Neurodegeneration in Parkinson's disease*. Science, 2003. 302(5646): pp. 819–822.

[10] Schapira, A.H. and P. Jenner, *Etiology and pathogenesis of Parkinson's disease*. Mov Disorders, 2011. 26(6): pp. 1049–1055.

[11] Reeve, A., E. Simcox, and D. Turnbull, *Ageing and Parkinson's disease: why is advancing age the biggest risk factor?* Ageing Res Rev, 2014. 14(0): pp. 19–30.

[12] Hirsch, E.C., et al., *Neuronal loss in the pedunculopontine tegmental nucleus in Parkinson disease and in progressive supranuclear palsy*. Proc Natl Acad Sci, 1987. 84(16): pp. 5976–5980.

[13] Bender, A., et al., *High levels of mitochondrial DNA deletions in substantia nigra neurons in aging and Parkinson disease*. Nature Genet, 2006. 38(5): pp. 515–517.

[14] Kraytsberg, Y., et al., *Mitochondrial DNA deletions are abundant and cause functional impairment in aged human substantia nigra neurons*. Nature Genet, 2006. 38(5): pp. 518–520.

[15] Lesage, S. and A. Brice, *Parkinson's disease: from monogenic forms to genetic susceptibility factors.* Hum Mol Gen, 2009. 18(R1): pp. R48–R59.

[16] Hardy, J., M.R. Cookson, and A. Singleton, *Genes and parkinsonism.* Lancet Neurol, 2003. 2(4): pp. 221–8.

[17] Farrer, M.J., *Genetics of Parkinson disease: paradigm shifts and future prospects.* Nat Rev Genet, 2006. 7(4): pp. 306–18.

[18] Egger, G., et al., *Epigenetics in human disease and prospects for epigenetic therapy.* Nature, 2004. 429(6990): pp. 457–463.

[19] Ammal Kaidery, N., S. Tarannum, and B. Thomas, *Epigenetic landscape of Parkinson's disease: emerging role in disease mechanisms and therapeutic modalities.* Neurotherapeutics, 2013. 10(4): pp. 698–708.

[20] Bjornsson, H.T., M. Daniele Fallin, and A.P. Feinberg, *An integrated epigenetic and genetic approach to common human disease.* Trends Genetics, 2004. 20(8): pp. 350–358.

[21] Coppedè, F., *Genetics and epigenetics of Parkinson's disease.* Sci World J, 2012. 2012.

[22] Filatova, E., et al., *MicroRNAs: possible role in pathogenesis of Parkinson's disease.* Biochemistry (Moscow), 2012. 77(8): pp. 813–819.

[23] Kaut, O., I. Schmitt, and U. Wüllner, *Genome-scale methylation analysis of Parkinson's disease patients' brains reveals DNA hypomethylation and increased mRNA expression of cytochrome P450 2E1.* Neurogenetics, 2012. 13(1): pp. 87–91.

[24] Mouradian, M.M., *MicroRNAs in Parkinson's disease.* Neurobiol Dis, 2012. 46(2): pp. 279–84.

[25] Masliah, E., et al., *Distinctive patterns of DNA methylation associated with Parkinson disease: identification of concordant epigenetic changes in brain and peripheral blood leukocytes.* Epigenetics, 2013. 8(10): pp. 1030–8.

[26] Pena-Altamira, L.E., E. Polazzi, and B. Monti, *Histone post-translational modifications in Huntington's and Parkinson's diseases.* Curr Pharm Des, 2013. 19(28): pp. 5085–92.

[27] Weinhold, B., *Epigenetics: the science of change.* Environ Health Perspect, 2006. 114(3): pp. A160–7.

[28] Reik, W., et al., *Age at onset in Huntington's disease and methylation at D4S95.* J Med Genet, 1993. 30(3): pp. 185–8.

[29] Bird, A., *DNA methylation patterns and epigenetic memory.* Genes Dev, 2002. 16(1): pp. 6–21.

[30] Curradi, M., et al., *Molecular mechanisms of gene silencing mediated by DNA methylation.* Mol Cell Biol, 2002. 22(9): pp. 3157–73.

[31] Miller, C.A., S.L. Campbell, and J.D. Sweatt, *DNA methylation and histone acetylation work in concert to regulate memory formation and synaptic plasticity.* Neurobiol Learn Mem, 2008. 89(4): pp. 599–603.

[32] Day, J.J. and J.D. Sweatt, *DNA methylation and memory formation.* Nat Neurosci, 2010. 13(11): pp. 1319–23.

[33] Scarpa, S., et al., *Gene silencing through methylation: an epigenetic intervention on Alzheimer disease.* J Alzheimers Dis, 2006. 9(4): pp. 407–14.

[34] Hernandez, D.G., et al., *Distinct DNA methylation changes highly correlated with chronological age in the human brain.* Hum Mol Genet, 2011. 20(6): pp. 1164–72.

[35] Jowaed, A., et al., *Methylation regulates alpha-synuclein expression and is decreased in Parkinson's disease patients' brains.* J Neurosci, 2010. 30(18): pp. 6355–9.

[36] Matsumoto, L., et al., *CpG demethylation enhances alpha-synuclein expression and affects the pathogenesis of Parkinson's disease.* PLoS One, 2010. 5(11): pp. e15522.

[37] Desplats, P., et al., *Alpha-synuclein sequesters Dnmt1 from the nucleus: a novel mechanism for epigenetic alterations in Lewy body diseases.* J Biol Chem, 2011. 286(11): pp. 9031–7.

[38] Maze, I., K.M. Noh, and C.D. Allis, *Histone regulation in the CNS: basic principles of epigenetic plasticity.* Neuropsychopharmacology, 2013. 38(1): pp. 3–22.

[39] Cheung, P., et al., *Synergistic coupling of histone H3 phosphorylation and acetylation in response to epidermal growth factor stimulation.* Mol Cell, 2000. 5(6): pp. 905–15.

[40] Luco, R.F., et al., *Regulation of alternative splicing by histone modifications.* Science, 2010. 327(5968): pp. 996–1000.

[41] Kouzarides, T., *Chromatin modifications and their function.* Cell, 2007. 128(4): pp. 693–705.

[42] Li, B., M. Carey, and J.L. Workman, *The Role of Chromatin during Transcription.* Cell, 2007. 128(4): pp. 707–719.

[43] Karlić, R., et al., *Histone modification levels are predictive for gene expression.* Proc Natl Acad Sci, 2010. 107(7): pp. 2926–2931.

[44] Roth, S.Y., J.M. Denu, and C.D. Allis, *Histone acetyltransferases.* Annu Rev Biochem, 2001. 70: pp. 81–120.

[45] Trievel, R.C., *Structure and function of histone methyltransferases.* Crit Rev Eukaryot Gene Expr, 2004. 14(3): pp. 147–69.

[46] Greer, E.L. and Y. Shi, *Histone methylation: a dynamic mark in health, disease and inheritance.* Nat Rev Genet, 2012. 13(5): pp. 343–357.

[47] Morales, Y., et al., *Biochemistry and regulation of the protein arginine methyltransferases (PRMTs).* Arch Biochem Biophys, 2015. 590: pp. 138–152.

[48] Kontopoulos, E., J.D. Parvin, and M.B. Feany, *Alpha-synuclein acts in the nucleus to inhibit histone acetylation and promote neurotoxicity.* Hum Mol Genet, 2006. 15(20): pp. 3012–23.

[49] Outeiro, T.F., et al., *Sirtuin 2 inhibitors rescue alpha-synuclein-mediated toxicity in models of Parkinson's disease.* Science, 2007. 317(5837): pp. 516–9.

[50] Goers, J., et al., *Nuclear localization of alpha-synuclein and its interaction with histones.* Biochemistry, 2003. 42(28): pp. 8465–71.

[51] Abel, T. and R.S. Zukin, *Epigenetic targets of HDAC inhibition in neurodegenerative and psychiatric disorders.* Curr Opin Pharmacol, 2008. 8(1): pp. 57–64.

[52] Simoes-Pires, C., et al., *HDAC6 as a target for neurodegenerative diseases: what makes it different from the other HDACs?* Mol Neurodegener, 2013. 8(1): p. 7.

[53] Du, G., et al., *Drosophila histone deacetylase 6 protects dopaminergic neurons against {alpha}-synuclein toxicity by promoting inclusion formation.* Mol Biol Cell, 2010. 21(13): pp. 2128–37.

[54] Duce, J.A., et al., *Linker histone H1 binds to disease associated amyloid-like fibrils.* J Mol Biol, 2006. 361(3): pp. 493–505.

[55] Vartiainen, S., et al., *Identification of gene expression changes in transgenic* C. elegans *overexpressing human alpha-synuclein.* Neurobiol Dis, 2006. 22(3): pp. 477–86.

[56] Lee, J.Y., et al., *Disease-causing mutations in parkin impair mitochondrial ubiquitination, aggregation, and HDAC6-dependent mitophagy.* J Cell Biol, 2010. 189(4): pp. 671–9.

[57] Sharma, S. and R. Taliyan, *Targeting histone deacetylases: a novel approach in Parkinson's disease.* Parkinson's Disease, 2015. 2015: p. 11.

[58] Koh, H., et al., *Silent information regulator 2 (Sir2) and Forkhead box O (FOXO) complement mitochondrial dysfunction and dopaminergic neuron loss in Drosophila PTEN-induced kinase 1 (PINK1) null mutant.* J Biol Chem, 2012. 287(16): pp. 12750–8.

[59] Nicholas, A.P., et al., *Striatal histone modifications in models of levodopa-induced dyskinesia.* J Neurochem, 2008. 106(1): pp. 486–94.

[60] Santini, E., et al., *L-DOPA activates ERK signaling and phosphorylates histone H3 in the striatonigral medium spiny neurons of hemiparkinsonian mice.* J Neurochem, 2009. 108(3): pp. 621–33.

[61] Almeida, M.I., R.M. Reis, and G.A. Calin, *MicroRNA history: Discovery, recent applications, and next frontiers.* Mut Res/Fund Mol Mech Mut, 2011. 717(1–2): pp. 1–8.

[62] Ha, M. and V.N. Kim, *Regulation of microRNA biogenesis.* Nat Rev Mol Cell Biol, 2014. 15(8): pp. 509–524.

[63] Wahid, F., et al., *MicroRNAs: Synthesis, mechanism, function, and recent clinical trials.* Biochimica et Biophysica Acta (BBA) - Molecular Cell Research, 2010. 1803(11): pp. 1231–1243.

[64] Junn, E., et al., *Repression of alpha-synuclein expression and toxicity by microRNA-7.* Proc Natl Acad Sci U S A, 2009. 106(31): pp. 13052–7.

[65] Doxakis, E., *Post-transcriptional regulation of alpha-synuclein expression by mir-7 and mir-153.* J Biol Chem, 2010. 285(17): pp. 12726–34.

[66] Gandhi, P.N., S.G. Chen, and A.L. Wilson-Delfosse, *Leucine-rich repeat kinase 2 (LRRK2): a key player in the pathogenesis of Parkinson's disease.* J Neurosci Res, 2009. 87(6): pp. 1283–1295.

[67] Kett, L.R., et al., *LRRK2 Parkinson disease mutations enhance its microtubule association.* Hum Mol Gen, 2012. 21(4): pp. 890–899.

[68] Martin, I., et al., *LRRK2 Pathobiology in Parkinson's Disease.* J Neurochem, 2014. 131(5): pp. 554–565.

[69] Skibinski, G., et al., *Mutant LRRK2 Toxicity in Neurons Depends on LRRK2 Levels and Synuclein But Not Kinase Activity or Inclusion Bodies.* J Neurosci, 2014. 34(2): pp. 418–433.

[70] Cho, H.J., et al., *MicroRNA-205 regulates the expression of Parkinson's disease-related leucine-rich repeat kinase 2 protein.* Hum Mol Genet, 2013. 22(3): pp. 608–20.

[71] Minones-Moyano, E., et al., *MicroRNA profiling of Parkinson's disease brains identifies early downregulation of miR-34b/c which modulate mitochondrial function.* Hum Mol Genet, 2011. 20(15): pp. 3067–78.

[72] Kanagaraj, N., et al., *Downregulation of miR-124 in MPTP-treated mouse model of Parkinson's disease and MPP iodide-treated MN9D cells modulates the expression of the calpain/cdk5 pathway proteins.* Neuroscience, 2014. 272: pp. 167–179.

[73] Renthal, W. and E.J. Nestler, *Chromatin regulation in drug addiction and depression.* Dialogues in Clinical Neuroscience, 2009. 11(3): pp. 257–268.

[74] Latham, J.A. and S.Y. Dent, *Cross-regulation of histone modifications.* Nat Struct Mol Biol, 2007. 14(11): pp. 1017–24.

[75] Cheung, W.L., et al., *Phosphorylation of histone H4 serine 1 during DNA damage requires casein kinase II in S. cerevisiae.* Curr Biol, 2005. 15(7): pp. 656–60.

[76] Lee, G., et al., *Casein kinase II-mediated phosphorylation regulates alpha-synuclein/synphilin-1 interaction and inclusion body formation.* J Biol Chem, 2004. 279(8): pp. 6834–9.

[77] Cavallarin, N., M. Vicario, and A. Negro, *The role of phosphorylation in synucleinopathies: focus on Parkinson's disease.* CNS Neurol Disord-Dr Targets (Formerly Current Drug Targets-CNS & Neurological Disorders), 2010. 9(4): pp. 471–481.

[78] Adamczyk, A. and A. Kazmierczak, *Alpha-synuclein inhibits poly (ADP-ribose) polymerase-1 (PARP-1) activity via NO-dependent pathway.* Folia Neuropathol, 2009. 47(3): pp. 247–51.

[79] Monaco, L., et al., *Inhibition of Aurora-B kinase activity by poly(ADP-ribosyl)ation in response to DNA damage.* Proc Natl Acad Sci U S A, 2005. 102(40): pp. 14244–8.

[80] Saijo, K., et al., *A Nurr1/CoREST pathway in microglia and astrocytes protects dopaminergic neurons from inflammation-induced death.* Cell, 2009. 137(1): pp. 47–59.

[81] Sethi, P. and W.J. Lukiw, *Micro-RNA abundance and stability in human brain: specific alterations in Alzheimer's disease temporal lobe neocortex.* Neurosci Lett, 2009. 459(2): pp. 100–104.

10

Chronic Inflammation Connects the Development of Parkinson's Disease and Cancer

Zhiming Li and Chi-Meng Tzeng

Abstract

Increasing number of genetic studies suggest that the pathogenesis of Parkinson's disease (PD) and cancer may involve similar genes, pathways, and mechanisms. The differences in the pathological and cellular mechanisms, and the associated genetic mutations, may result in two such divergent diseases. However, the links between the molecular mechanisms that cause PD and cancer remain to be elucidated. This article appraises the overlapping molecular features of these diseases and discusses the implications for prevention and treatment. We propose that chronic inflammation (CI) in neurons and tumors contributes to a microenvironment that favors the amassing of DNA mutations and facilitating disease formation. CI may therefore play a key role in the development of PD and cancer, and provide a link between these two diseases.

Keywords: Parkinson's disease, cancer, chronic inflammation, neurodegenerative disease, genetic mutation

1. Introduction

Parkinson's disease (PD) is the second most common neurodegenerative disease, after Alzheimer's disease [1]. Typical symptoms include static tremors, muscle rigidity, and bradykinesia. These are caused by the premature death of dopaminergic neurons in the midbrain. The motor symptoms can be treated with dopaminergic drugs; however, the effectiveness diminishes as the severity of the clinical symptoms increases due to the development of the primary neuro-degeneration [2]. In contrast, cancer is a type of selectively advantageous cells with clonal proliferation. Although the two may appear distinctive, early epidemiological surveys have shown a connection between them. In 1954, Doshay [3] reported that the cancer incidence rate was lower among PD patients, but the reason for this was undistinguishable. Later, several epidemiological studies of cancer showed that the incidence of cancer was generally low among PD patients, regardless of whether they smoke or not [4]. However, the incidence of thyroid cancer, breast cancer, and melanoma was relatively high [5]. A recent study covering 219,194 people with PD displayed that the rate ratio (RR) for all subsequent primary malignant cancers combined was 0.92 [95% confidence interval (CI): 0.91–0.93], including increased RRs (p < 0.05) of breast cancer and melanoma cancer, and decreased RRs of 11 cancers [6]. This has been the most commanding epidemiological evidence for a connection between PD and cancer. Surely, there is a difference between association and causality, and it has been proposed that the association between PD and skin cancer could be linked to the way of therapy, such as Levodopa treatment, rather than with the disease itself. However, some observations did not support the causality [7, 8]. Moreover, some people thought that the low incidence of cancer in PD patients comes from the negative relationship between PD and smoking [4]. This may widely explain the decrease of smoking-related cancers, but the reduction of non-smoking-related cancers cannot be resolved.

The unusual epidemiological relation between PD and cancer has drawn the attention of many investigators. The genetic assessment encouraged an additional understanding: most of these familial PD genes had been found and summarized to be associated with cancer (**Table 1**). Mutations found in *parkin* (*PARK2*), *PINK1* (*PARK6*), *DJ-1* (*PARK7*), and *LRRK2* (*PARK8*) might cause distinctive significances and consequences of PD and cancer, respectively, in different types of cells [9]. PD and cancer have been discovered to share a PI3K/AKT/mTOR pathway, which is a central mechanism of cell growth and proliferation that mainly functions through modulating protein synthesis and responding both intrinsic and environmental stress promptly [10]. Currently, more than 12 loci were found to be related to familial PD [11]. Among these, six genes have been cloned. The monogenic forms of PD display both autosomal dominant and recessive modes of inheritance, and account for 1–3% of late-onset disease and approximately 20% of young-onset disease [1, 12]. PD-related genes are involved in a series of cellular mechanisms including misfolding and degradation of proteins, mitochondrial damage, oxidative stress response, cell cycle control, and DNA repair. These all play a vital role in both PD and cancer. Understanding of the functions of these genes in cell survival and cell death might help to reveal the connection between the two diseases.

Gene	PD locus	Chromosome location	Inheritance in PD*	Expression in cancer	Proliferation in Cancer†	Cancer
α-Synuclein	PARK1/ PARK4	4q21–q23	AD	Overexpressed (not express in normal tissue)	+	Brain tumors [74] Melanoma [75] Ovary cancer [76]
Parkin	PARK2	6q25.2–q27	AR	Decreased§	–	Glioblastoma [9] Colon cancer [9] Lung cancer [9]
UCHL1	PARK5	4p14	AD	Silenced	–	Nasopharyngeal carcinoma [77]

Gene	PD locus	Chromosome location	Inheritance in PD*	Expression in cancer	Proliferation in Cancer†	Cancer
				(via CpG methylation)		Colorectal cancer [78]
PINK1	PARK6	1p35–p36	AR	Decreased§	–	Breast cancer [79]
DJ-1	PARK7	1p36	AR	Overexpressed	+	Non-small-cell lung cancer [80]
LRRK2	PARK8	12p11.2–q13.1	AD	Overexpressed	+	Papillary renal cell carcinoma [64], Thyroid cancer [64]

*AD, autosomal dominant; AR, autosomal recessive
§The telomeric end of chromosome 1p is subject to frequent deletion and rearrangement in many cancers
† +/– denotes proliferation and antipoliferation.

Table 1. Parkinson's disease involved genes identified in cancer.

If genetic defect was "the match that lights the fire" of PD and cancer, chronic inflammation (CI) might supply "the fuel that feeds the flames." Over the past decades, the insight on cytokine and chemokine network has contributed to invention of a series of cytokine/chemokine antagonists used for inflammatory diseases. The first clinic practice, tumor necrosis factor antagonists, has shown encouraging efficacy [13]. CI is considered as a driving force behind many chronic diseases including cancerization and neurodegeneration. In PD, there are many activated microglia surrounding the lost neuron, and experiments have shown that inflammatory reaction does help killing neurons [14]. Epidemiological surveys have shown that taking non-steroidal anti-inflammatory drugs (NSAIDs) can reduce the risk of PD development. CI has long been known to mediate a wide variety of illnesses, including neurodegenerative disease and malignant tumors [15]. In 1863, Rudolf Virchow noticed leucocytes in neoplastic tissues and proposed a connection between inflammation and cancer. The role for inflammation in tumorigenesis is now mostly accepted, and it has become an evident that an inflammatory microenvironment is an essential piece for most tumors [16]. Inflammatory mediators in the microenvironment of CI not only benefit cancer cells proliferation and escape from immunological surveillance but also cause a large number of random mutations [17]. Amassing research evidence supports the view that inflammatory mediators, some of that are direct mutagens, directly or indirectly downregulate DNA repair pathways and cell cycle checkpoints, consequently destabilizing cell genome and contributing to the accumulation of random genetic alterations. Thus, inflammation is considered as the seventh most important sign of cancer [18].

The cellular pathways and its associated mechanisms (**Figure 1**) that involve genes common to PD and cancer have been discussed in our previous paper [19]. In this manuscript, we further explain the environmental factors that cause PD and cancer from the perspective of CI and related genes to provide a better understanding and treatment options of these two diseases.

To emphasize the multiple pathological functions of these gene mutations, they are discussed separately.

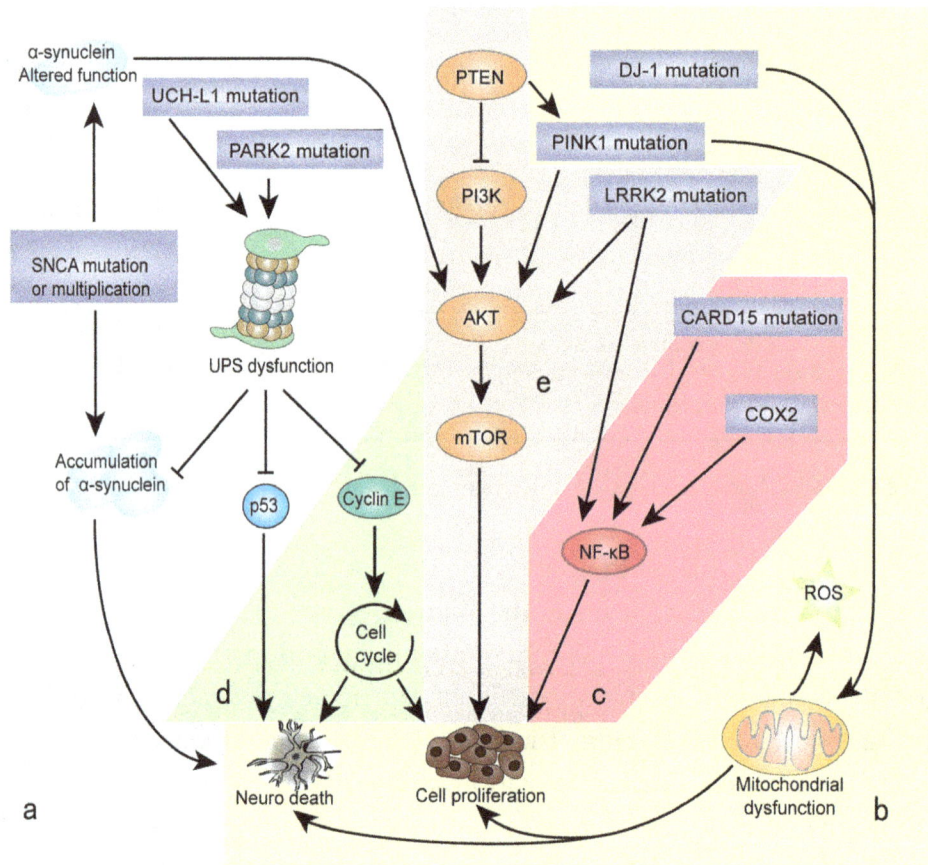

Figure 1. Overlapping genes and cellular pathways between PD and cancer. The biological connection of PD and cancer mainly includes five fields: (a) misfolding and degradation of proteins, (b) mitochondrial damage and oxidative stress response, (c) CI, (d) cell cycle control and DNA repair, and (e) PI3K/AKT/mTOR pathway regulation. The α-synuclein polymer attributed to *SNCA* multiplication is the main component of LBs. *SNCA* mutations alter the normal function of α-synuclein, which activates the PI3K/AKT/mTOR pathway and promotes cell proliferation. Under the cascade of phosphorylating AKT, PINK1, and LRRK2 can also activate mTOR. *PARK2* and *UCH-L1* mutations disrupt the degradation function of ubiquitin proteasome system (UPS) for the misfolded and aggregated α-synuclein, cyclin E, and p53. *PINK1* and *DJ-1* mutations result in the overproduction of ROS and oxidative stress in mitochondria, damaging neurons, and stimulating cell proliferation. *COX2* and *CARD15* mutations activate the NF-kB pathway and induce CI, leading to genetic mutations and oxidative stress. The different cellular backgrounds of cancer cells and neurons (mitotic vs. post-mitotic cells) bring completely distinct reactions to external stimuli and internal changes: some undergo cell proliferation and others neuron death. The final results are two serious diseases: cancer and Parkinson's disease.

2. Chronic inflammation

The blood–brain barrier (BBB) prevents the lymphatic infiltration and neurotoxins diffusion from the blood to the CNS. Conventionally, the CNS was regarded as the immunological restriction due to its limited inflammatory reaction and lymphatic infiltration. Nonetheless, accumulating evidence indicates that the CNS actually is the immunological specialization by the resident innate immune cell in the brain: microglia. Activated microglia could prevent the CNS injury from pathogenic factors (physiological disrupt and toxic insult) through releasing a number of cytokines and chemokines [20]. These inflammatory mediators could trigger or modulate the remove of neurotoxins and inhibit their detrimental effects. Thus, acute inflammatory responses are consider to be beneficial, but long-term, high-level CI can severely damage the body. Two of the pathological characteristics of PD are loss of dopaminergic neurons and accumulation of LBs in the nigrostriata of the midbrain. LBs are abnormal intracytoplasmic filamentous aggregates of α-synuclein present, respectively, in neurons and axons. Recent studies have shown that neurons able to release α-synuclein oligomers, which can bind to toll-like receptors (TLR) to activate microglia, activating the nuclear factor kappa B (NF-kB) pathway, and releasing of inflammatory factors. These immune factors not only act directly on dopaminergic neurons to cause neuronal death but also aggravate the inflammatory reaction and continue to activate microglia. Activated microglia surround dead neurons in the substantia nigra pars compacta (SNc) of PD patients. Studies have shown that inhibition of microglia cascade reactions can prevent degradation of neurons [21]. Increasing studies demonstrated that there was a positive correlation between SNc cell loss and microglia activation in both animal models and PD patients. Timing analysis displayed that reduce microglial activation can rescue SNc neurons loss in animal models, suggesting an active effect of microglia in killing SNc cell following a range of stimuli. It is increasingly clear that activation of microglia is a highly localized inflammatory reaction rather than generalized. Even though the degenerating neuronal terminals of SNc cell cannot stimulate the similar response but only the dopaminergic neurons in the SNc [22]. Therefore, cell death of PD directly relates to a substantial increase of microglia activation. At the same time, overproduction of free radicals (superoxide and peroxynitrite) damages the balance of the redox potential of neurons and acts on biomacromolecules to modulate their roles, or causes lipid peroxidation leading to cell death eventually. Alternatively, microglia might kill SNc cells by producing other noxious compounds including cytokines and proinflammatory prostaglandins. Patients with PD have selective degeneration of neurons in the SNc accompanied by microglial activation and a challenged immune system.

The presence of activated microglia in PD might reflect a scavenging role in the wake of a primary pathologic process. However, evidence for a more sinister role comes from animal models of PD. MPTP, 6-OHDA, lipopolysaccharide, rotenone, viruses, and SNc extracts all can lead to degeneration of the dopaminergic neurons and loss of striatal dopamine in primates, rodents, and other species [23]. Each of them can cause an inflammatory response that associated with the enhancement of microglia activation in the SNc. The best evidence for the significance of inflammation during neoplastic progression maybe come from study of cancer risk among long-term users of aspirin and NSAIDs. A big prospective study of hospital workers indicated that the incidence of PD in chronic users of over-the-counter NSAIDs which scavenge free oxygen radicals and inhibit cyclooxygenase (COX) activity was 46% lower than that of age-matched non-users [24]. Inhibition of COX-mediated dopaminergic neurons oxidation, as well as inhibition of microglial-derived toxic mediator production, is likely to be among the mechanisms that contribute to decreased incidence of PD in chronic NSAIDs users [25]. Therapeutically, these findings raise the possibility that early involvement with NSAIDs or similar anti-inflammatory therapy may be neuroprotective and could delay or prevent onset of PD. That anti-inflammatory medications downregulate microglial responses to a toxic insult and directly reduce neuronal loss strongly, which indicates that localized inflammation is pathogenic in the SNc rather than merely a late response to neuronal death.

3. NOD2

Crohn's disease (CD), also known as regional enteritis, is a type of inflammatory bowel disease. In 2001, three laboratories found CD associate with genetic variants. Nucleotide-binding oligomerization domain protein 2 (NOD2) also known as caspase recruitment domain protein 15 (CARD15) is a protein that in humans which is encoded by the *CARD15* gene located on human chromosome 16q12 [26–28]. Approximately 40% of CD patients in the Western countries carry at least one of these three SNPs: R702W, G908R, and L1007fsinsC, and heterozygous mutation of any of these SNPs increases CD risk 2–4 times, whereas multiple-locus heterozygous mutations or homozygous mutations may lead to a CD risk higher than 20 times. However, it has been reported that none of these three SNPs was involved in CD among Chinese (Han) [29], Korean [30], and Japanese patients [31]. NOD2, encoded by *CARD15*, is the receptor of muramyl peptides (MDP), a component of bacterial peptidoglycan. Binding of MDP and NOD2 activates NF-kB, and inflammatory reaction occurs. It has also been shown that *CARD15* mutation plays a role in innate immune system and pathogen recognition in terms of other complex polygenic diseases. In 2007, Bialecka [32] showed that the three SNPs of *CARD15* (R702W, G908R, and L1007fsinsC) were significantly correlated with PD in the Polish population. Using RFLP, our group found P268S, another SNP of *CARD15*, to be a risk factor for Chinese PD. In addition, Crane et al. [33] reported that P268S was related to susceptibility of ankylosing spondylitis. Proell et al. [34] performed sequence comparison and found that NOD2 shared a high degree of similarity with apoptotic protease activating factor 1 (Apaf-1). They simulated the homologous structure of NOD2 based on Apaf-1 structure and found that P268S was located at the connexon (ligand-binding position) before the first helix of the NOD. Replacing Pro with Ser changed the conformation of the connexon and affected its binding to the substrate.

Whether the CD's-associated *CARD15* mutations lead to a loss or gain of function of the NOD2 receptor is subject to controversy, and by which mechanisms, this change in function might increase the susceptibility to CD which is still under investigation. Patients with CD are known to have an increased risk of developing colorectal cancer [35]. *CARD15* mutations may also increase the susceptibility of developing colorectal cancer in Caucasians without CD [36, 37]. These observations suggested that immune system mechanisms were involved in the pathogenesis of cell damage in CD and also provided evidence for an ongoing active pathologic process. Inflammation can be triggered by invading microbes and also be initiated from within the organism, by diseases affecting the nervous system. There are three common outcomes of inflammation. The offending agent or process is inactivated and the injury repaired. The host loses the battle and dies or suffers irreparable tissue damage. Neither the organism nor the injurious process prevails, resulting in a prolonged battle that provides fertile ground for the development of chronic inflammatory conditions. The last outcome may relate closely to neurodegenerative diseases and cancer, two of the greatest public health problems of this century [38].

4. COX2

COX is the central enzyme in prostaglandin biosynthesis. There are two different isoforms of COX: COX-1 and COX-2. Constitutive expression of COX-1 is commonly found in many tissues. Because COX-1 is responsible for the biosynthesis of prostaglandins which regulate some physiological homeostasis, including modulation of renal blood flow and preservation of the gastric mucosa. Normally, COX-2 could not be discovered in most tissues except for stimulating by some mitogenic and inflammatory mediators [39]. COX2 is not only key to the synthesis of prostaglandin in inflammatory reactions but also an important contributor to the degradation of neurons in PD. Inhibiting COX2 activity in mice and rats can alleviate neuronal death caused by MPTP [40] and 6-ODHA [41], respectively. Macrophages, neurons, and glial cells in the central nervous system can all express COX2. Unlike COX1, which is constitutively expressed, COX2 expression is induced by inflammatory conditions. The COX2 level in the dopaminergic neurons of PD patients is elevated, and prostanoid and ROS produced by COX2 can directly act on dopaminergic neurons causing cell toxicity [42]. The role of COX2 in inflammation and neuronal degradation has yet to be verified. However, it has been shown that NSAIDs nonselectively inhibit the activities of COX1 and COX2, thus reducing prostaglandin production and promoting clearance of ROS. An epidemiological survey has revealed that individuals who take NSAIDs have a lower risk of PD than those who do not [25]. However, there has not been any report on the effects of specific COX2 inhibitors on the occurrence and development of PD.

COX-2, the inducible isoform of prostaglandin H synthase, has been implicated in the growth and progression of a variety of human cancers [43]. There are many evidence support that COX-2 is involved in the development of cancer. Because the overexpression of COX-2 is commonly found in the premalignant and malignant tissues. The most powerful findings from genetic studies support the view that it exists a cause-and-effect relationship between COX-2 and tumorigenesis. Multiple lines of evidence indicate that COX-2 is a *bona fide* pharmacological target for anticancer therapy. Epidemiologic studies have shown a 40–50% reduction in mortality from colorectal cancer in individuals who take NSAIDs on a regular basis compared with those not taking these agents [44]. COX-2, an inducible enzyme with expression regulated by NF-kB, mediates tumorigenesis. COX2 can activate not only the NF-kB pathway, but also p38 and Jnk in the MAPK pathway [45]. High levels of COX2 have been found in many cancers, particularly colon cancer [46]. COX-2 is also expressed in 93% of melanomas, with a moderate-to-strong expression in 68% [47]. COX2 can decrease the level of arachidonic acid and inhibit cell apoptosis. It can also increase prostaglandin production and promote cell growth and differentiation. These phenomena were also observed in the clinical effect of selective COX2 inhibitors in the market [48, 49].

5. LRRK2

Leucine-rich-repeat kinase 2 (*LRRK2*) is a large gene, 144 kb in length, containing 51 exons and encoding a multi-domain kinase composed of 2527 amino acids. LRRK2 is expressed in many organs and tissues, including the brain. In 2004, two laboratories reported that *LRRK2* mutations were related to PD [50, 51]. More than 40 *LRRK2* mutations, almost all missense, have been found [52]. However, the nosogeneses of many mutations remain unclear. *LRRK2* mutations account for 10% of familial PD and 3.6% of sporadic PD, suggesting strong modifiers of *LRRK2* disease [53]. LRRK2 is a large protein (280KDs). It can activate AKT, an upstream element of the mTOR pathway, thus decreasing the anti-apoptosis activity mediated by AKT and promoting neuronal death [54]. Gene structure studies showed that LRRK2 protein was consist of five conserved domains, including a leucine-rich repeat (LRR) domain, a Roc GTPase domain, a C terminal of Roc (COR) domain, a MAPKKK mixed-lineage protein kinase domain, and a WD40 domain [55, 56]. LRRK2 contains multiple sets of internal repeats, each of which is predicted to adopt a distinct structure. Such repeats, which occur in 14% of all prokaryotic and eukaryotic proteins, commonly serve as platforms for protein interactions [57]. *LRRK2* gene was discovered as part of an evolutionarily conserved family of proteins marked by GTPase (Guanosine triphosphatase) domains usually encoded together with kinase domains [55]. The G2019S mutation in the *LRRK2* is the single most common autosomal dominantly inherited PD gene defect. The LRRK2 protein is a scaffolding-type protein kinase, and G2019S is thought to lead to the disease by increasing the LRRK2 kinase activity resulting in increased phosphorylation of as yet mostly hypothetical targets, although whether all mutations in LRRK2 have the same biochemical mechanism is uncertain [58]. Missense mutations in both the kinase and GTPase domain in LRRK2 cause late-onset PD with clinical and pathological phenotypes nearly indistinguishable from idiopathic disease, possibly through the upregulation of LRRK2 kinase activity [59]. Because the clinical phenotype ensuing from LRRK2 mutations resembles idiopathic PD, LRRK2 has emerged as, perhaps, the most relevant player in PD pathogenesis identified to date [60]. One of the consistent pathological features of patients with LRRK2 mutations is α-synuclein-positive LBs pathology [61]. Besides G2019S, there are only a handful of proven pathogenic mutations in LRRK2, which is rather surprising given its large size. Multiple pathogenic mutations (I1371V, R14441C, R1441G, R1441H, Y1699C, Y1699G, G2019S, and I2020T) are located within the GTPase and the kinase domains or within the COR domain. This structural feature can be used as a target in the design of drugs that treat PD [62]. Many of the LRRK2 kinase inhibitors identified to date were discovered by using libraries of defined kinase inhibitors [63]. As with any kinase inhibitor development for human use, issues related to safety will need to be carefully evaluated. This is particularly important for a chronic disease such as PD.

More directly supporting a role of LRRK2 in cancer, chromosomal amplification of the LRRK2 locus is required for oncogenic signaling in papillary renal and thyroid carcinomas [64]. Genetic studies have implicated LRRK2 in the pathogenesis of several human diseases, including cancer and CD [65–67]. In 2011, Liu et al. [68] found that LRRK2 could suppress the activity of the transcription factor Nuclear factor of activated T-cells (NFAT). Overexpression of LRRK2 led to increased retention of NFAT in the cytosol. When *LRRK2* was knocked out, NFAT in the cytosol was translocated to the nucleus and transcriptionally activated the expression of genes encoding cytokines and other key proteins involved in triggering inflammatory responses. It was firstly proposed that LRRK2 might play an important role in the signal pathway that induced CD. Liu and co-workers highlighted the possibility that the M2397T (replacement of methionine 2397 with threonine) polymorphism may alter the steady-state abundance of LRRK2, which is distributed in many tissues and brain regions, generally at low abundance. In addition, the structure of LRRK2 is similar to that of carcinogen B-RAF. Therefore, it can act on the MAPK pathway. G2019S, a common *LRRK2* mutation in PD, can increase the risk of non-skin cancer in Jews by three times [69]. A complex role for LRRK2 in multiple cellular processes is perhaps not surprising, because LRRK2 has multiple domains and is both an active kinase and a GTPase [70]. Binding the different LRRK2 domains and different ligands may have different functions, preventing them from connecting closely with PD, inflammation, or cancer. To understand the roles of LRRK2 in human disease, the best place to start is with examination of the genetics linked to these diseases. Various coding changes in the open reading frame of LRRK2 are linked to disease. In PD, these mutations result in functional changes in LRRK2, although no clear pattern to these changes has emerged. LRRK2 is involved in many diseases result from the distinct influence of genetic mutations. These variants not only change the potential of LRRK2 to interact with upstream regulators or downstream effector, but also can alter the biological functions of LRRK2. The discovery of more LRRK2 functions and a deeper understanding of its pleiotropism should provide the research community with more insight into the pathological functions of the same protein in different diseases. Every protein may have more than one function and may play completely different roles in different diseases. Targeted therapies with minimal side effects may be developed based on the functions of these proteins in different signal pathways.

6. Perspective and conclusion

Increasingly epidemiologic findings demonstrated the correlation between cancer and PD in recent years, but the conclusions were not completely consistent. This is because of the differences of study management. Our understanding of the control of signaling pathways is further advanced in cancer studies compared to neurodegeneration. As a result, many small molecule inhibitors have been approved as anticancer agents or are currently being tested in clinical trials. In 2010, Datamonitor Inc. (USA) estimated that there were over 1.5 million PD patients in the USA, Japan, France, Germany, Italy, Spain, and UK combined, one-third of them in the USA. With the increasing aging of world population, the incidence of PD is increasing yearly [71]. Medication is usually the first option in the treatment of PD. Levodopa is currently the most effective medication, but long-term use can reduce the effectiveness of treatment and cause complications such as motor dysfunction. Thus, discoveries in cancer research are likely to provide a solid base upon which scientists will study the pathophysiology of neurodegenerative diseases, especially PD.

The origins of the association and interplay between cancer and PD are still a matter of debate, but increasing epigenetic modifications such as DNA acetylation, DNA methylation, and miRNA scan conspire with genetic alterations in disease pathogenesis [72]. Recently, Gehrke et al. [73] found that *LRRK2* mutation in Drosophila model could have an antagonist effect on two miRNAs: let-7, a known tumor suppressor, and miR-184, a mediator of neurological development. This led to E2F1/DP over-expression, causing the cells to reenter the cell cycle. These will help us develop an understanding of these two diseases from opposing angles. Although, cancer and PD seem to have little in common, one due to enhanced resistance to cell death and the other due to premature cell death. However, the more we learn about the molecular genetics and cell biology of cancer and PD, the greater the overlap between these disorders appears. Both cancer and PD are thought to be the result of the interaction of genetic and environmental factors. The difference is that different reactions occur based on different cellular backgrounds: cell division and cell death. The inflammation hypothesis is considered one explanation for PD and cancer. The immune factor and ROS released from chronic inflammatory reactions not only promote the occurrence of the disease but also cause cellular DNA to accumulate mutations more easily, forming proteins with aberrant functions. In the end, interactions between genes and the environment cause the diseases. Recently, our group found that P268S in *CARD15* may be a risk factor for PD, and Liu and co-workers provide evidence that *LRRK2* also has a role in a signaling pathway linked with the pathogenesis of Crohn's disease, an inflammatory bowel disease. These findings both implied a correlation between PD and inflammation.

Most degenerative diseases of the brain are incurable and the study of tissue from the brains of people with significant neurodegeneration is difficult, so the postmortem specimen is probably the most valuable research material. However, academic and clinic of cancer research have accumulated a wide range of achievement in the past long time, and these results and experience must be important and beneficial to neurodegeneration study. Understanding the nature of their relationship must help scientist find novel and more efficacious therapeutic approaches for both diseases.

Author details

Zhiming Li[1,2,3] and Chi-Meng Tzeng[1,2,3*]

*Address all correspondence to: cmtzeng@xmu.edu.cn

1 Translational Medicine Research Center, School of Pharmaceutical Sciences, Xiamen University, Xiamen, Fujian, China

2 Key Laboratory for Cancer T-Cell Theranostics and Clinical Translation (CTCTCT), Xiamen, Fujian, China

3 INNOVA Clinics and TRANSLA Health Group University, Xiamen, Fujian, China

References

[1] Farrer MJ. Genetics of Parkinson disease: paradigm shifts and future prospects. Nat Rev Genet. 2006;7:306–318. doi:10.1038/nrg1831

[2] Schapira AH. Molecular and clinical pathways to neuroprotection of dopaminergic drugs in Parkinson disease. Neurology. 2009;72:S44–50. doi:10.1212/WNL.0b013e3181990438

[3] Doshay LJ. Problem situations in the treatment of paralysis agitans. J Am Med Assoc. 1954;156:680–684. doi:10.1001/jama.1954.02950070008003

[4] Hernan MA, Takkouche B, Caamano-Isorna F, Gestal-Otero JJ. A meta-analysis of coffee drinking, cigarette smoking, and the risk of Parkinson's disease. Ann Neurol. 2002;52:276–284. doi:10.1002/ana.10277

[5] D'Amelio M, Ragonese P, Sconzo G, Aridon P, Savettieri G. Parkinson's disease and cancer: insights for pathogenesis from epidemiology. Ann N Y Acad Sci. 2009;1155:324–334. doi:10.1111/j.1749-6632.2008.03681.x

[6] Ong EL, Goldacre R, Goldacre M. Differential risks of cancer types in people with Parkinson's disease: a national record-linkage study. Eur J Cancer. 2014;50:2456–2462. doi:10.1016/j.ejca.2014.06.018

[7] Fiala KH, Whetteckey J, Manyam BV. Malignant melanoma and levodopa in Parkinson's disease: causality or coincidence? Parkinsonism Relat Disord. 2003;9:321–327. doi: 10.1016/S1353-8020(03)00040-3

[8] Zanetti R, Loria D, Rosso S. Melanoma, Parkinson's disease and levodopa: causal or spurious link? A review of the literature. Melanoma Res. 2006;16:201–206. doi: 10.1097/01.cmr.0000215043.61306.d7

[9] Veeriah S, Taylor BS, Meng S, Fang F, Yilmaz E, Vivanco I, et al. Somatic mutations of the Parkinson's disease-associated gene PARK2 in glioblastoma and other human malignancies. Nat Genet. 2010;42:77–82. doi:10.1038/ng.491

[10] Devine MJ, Plun-Favreau H, Wood NW. Parkinson's disease and cancer: two wars, one front. Nat Rev Cancer. 2011;11:812–823. doi:10.1038/nrc3150

[11] Hardy J. Genetic analysis of pathways to Parkinson disease. Neuron. 2010;68:201–206. doi:10.1016/j.neuron.2010.10.014

[12] Tan EK, Skipper LM. Pathogenic mutations in Parkinson disease. Hum Mutat. 2007;28:641–653. doi:10.1002/humu.20507

[13] Balkwill F, Mantovani A. Inflammation and cancer: back to Virchow? Lancet. 2001;357:539–545. doi:10.1016/S0140-6736(00)04046-0

[14] Tansey MG, Goldberg MS. Neuroinflammation in Parkinson's disease: its role in neuronal death and implications for therapeutic intervention. Neurobiol Dis. 2010;37:510–518. doi:10.1016/j.nbd.2009.11.004

[15] Aggarwal BB, Shishodia S, Sandur SK, Pandey MK, Sethi G. Inflammation and cancer: how hot is the link? Biochem Pharmacol. 2006;72:1605–1621. doi:10.1016/j.bcp.2006.06.029

[16] Mantovani A, Allavena P, Sica A, Balkwill F. Cancer-related inflammation. Nature. 2008;454:436–444. doi:10.1038/nature07205

[17] Grivennikov SI, Greten FR, Karin M. Immunity, inflammation, and cancer. Cell. 2010;140:883–899. doi:10.1016/j.cell.2010.01.025

[18] Colotta F, Allavena P, Sica A, Garlanda C, Mantovani A. Cancer-related inflammation, the seventh hallmark of cancer: links to genetic instability. Carcinogenesis. 2009;30:1073–1081. doi:10.1093/carcin/bgp127

[19] Li Z, Lin Q, Huang W, Tzeng CM. Target gene capture sequencing in Chinese population of sporadic Parkinson disease. Medicine (Baltimore). 2015;94:e836. doi:10.1097/MD.0000000000000836

[20] Block ML, Zecca L, Hong JS. Microglia-mediated neurotoxicity: uncovering the molecular mechanisms. Nat Rev Neurosci. 2007;8:57–69. doi:10.1038/nrn2038

[21] Burguillos MA, Deierborg T, Kavanagh E, Persson A, Hajji N, Garcia-Quintanilla A, et al. Caspase signalling controls microglia activation and neurotoxicity. Nature. 2011;472:319–324. doi:10.1038/nature09788

[22] Mirza B, Hadberg H, Thomsen P, Moos T. The absence of reactive astrocytosis is indicative of a unique inflammatory process in Parkinson's disease. Neuroscience. 2000;95:425–432. doi: 10.1016/S0306-4522(99)00455-8

[23] Orr CF, Rowe DB, Halliday GM. An inflammatory review of Parkinson's disease. Prog Neurobiol. 2002;68:325–340. doi: 10.1016/S0301-0082(02)00127-2

[24] Chen H, Zhang SM, Hernan MA, Schwarzschild MA, Willett WC, Colditz GA, et al. Nonsteroidal anti-inflammatory drugs and the risk of Parkinson disease. Arch Neurol. 2003;60:1059–1064. doi:10.1001/archneur.60.8.1059

[25] Chen H, Jacobs E, Schwarzschild MA, McCullough ML, Calle EE, Thun MJ, et al. Nonsteroidal antiinflammatory drug use and the risk for Parkinson's disease. Ann Neurol. 2005;58:963–967. doi:10.1002/ana.20682

[26] Hugot JP, Chamaillard M, Zouali H, Lesage S, Cezard JP, Belaiche J, et al. Association of NOD2 leucine-rich repeat variants with susceptibility to Crohn's disease. Nature. 2001;411:599–603. doi:10.1038/35079107

[27] Ogura Y, Bonen DK, Inohara N, Nicolae DL, Chen FF, Ramos R, et al. A frameshift mutation in NOD2 associated with susceptibility to Crohn's disease. Nature. 2001;411:603–606. doi:10.1038/35079114

[28] Hampe J, Cuthbert A, Croucher PJ, Mirza MM, Mascheretti S, Fisher S, et al. Association between insertion mutation in NOD2 gene and Crohn's disease in German and British populations. Lancet. 2001;357:1925–1928. doi:10.1016/S0140-6736(00)05063-7

[29] Gao M, Cao Q, Luo LH, Wu ML, Hu WL, Si JM. NOD2/CARD15 gene polymorphisms and susceptibility to Crohn's disease in Chinese Han population. Zhonghua Nei Ke Za Zhi. 2005;44:210–212.

[30] Croucher PJ, Mascheretti S, Hampe J, Huse K, Frenzel H, Stoll M, et al. Haplotype structure and association to Crohn's disease of CARD15 mutations in two ethnically divergent populations. Eur J Hum Genet. 2003;11:6–16. doi:10.1038/sj.ejhg.5200897

[31] Yamazaki K, Takazoe M, Tanaka T, Kazumori T, Nakamura Y. Absence of mutation in the NOD2/CARD15 gene among 483 Japanese patients with Crohn's disease. J Hum Genet. 2002;47:469–472. doi:10.1007/s100380200067

[32] Bialecka M, Kurzawski M, Klodowska-Duda G, Opala G, Juzwiak S, Kurzawski G, et al. CARD15 variants in patients with sporadic Parkinson's disease. Neurosci Res. 2007;57:473–476. doi:10.1016/j.neures.2006.11.012

[33] Crane AM, Bradbury L, van Heel DA, McGovern DP, Brophy S, Rubin L, et al. Role of NOD2 variants in spondylarthritis. Arthritis Rheum. 2002;46:1629–1633. doi:10.1002/art.10329

[34] Proell M, Riedl SJ, Fritz JH, Rojas AM, Schwarzenbacher R. The Nod-like receptor (NLR) family: a tale of similarities and differences. Plos One. 2008;3:e2119. doi:10.1371/journal.pone.0002119

[35] Gasche C, Carethers JM. NOD2 and colorectal cancer: guilt by non-association. Cancer Res. 2004;64:5525; author reply 5525–5526. doi: 10.1158/0008-5472.CAN-03-3791

[36] Papaconstantinou I, Theodoropoulos G, Gazouli M, Panoussopoulos D, Mantzaris GJ, Felekouras E, et al. Association between mutations in the CARD15/NOD2 gene and colorectal cancer in a Greek population. Int J Cancer. 2005;114:433–435. doi:10.1002/ijc.20747

[37] Roberts RL, Gearry RB, Allington MD, Morrin HR, Robinson BA, Frizelle FA. Caspase recruitment domain-containing protein 15 mutations in patients with colorectal cancer. Cancer Res. 2006;66:2532–2535. doi:10.1158/0008-5472.CAN-05-4165

[38] Wyss-Coray T, Mucke L. Inflammation in neurodegenerative disease—a double-edged sword. Neuron. 2002;35:419–432. doi: 10.1016/S0896-6273(02)00794-8

[39] Smith WL, DeWitt DL, Garavito RM. Cyclooxygenases: structural, cellular, and molecular biology. Annu Rev Biochem. 2000;69:145–182. doi:10.1146/annurev.biochem.69.1.145

[40] Feng ZH, Wang TG, Li DD, Fung P, Wilson BC, Liu B, et al. Cyclooxygenase-2-deficient mice are resistant to 1-methyl-4-phenyl1, 2, 3, 6-tetrahydropyridine-induced damage of dopaminergic neurons in the substantia nigra. Neurosci Lett. 2002;329:354–358. doi: 10.1016/S0304-3940(02)00704-8

[41] Sanchez-Pernaute R, Ferree A, Cooper O, Yu M, Brownell AL, Isacson O. Selective COX-2 inhibition prevents progressive dopamine neuron degeneration in a rat model of Parkinson's disease. J Neuroinflammation. 2004;1:6. doi:10.1186/1742-2094-1-6

[42] Gao HM, Liu B, Zhang W, Hong JS. Novel anti-inflammatory therapy for Parkinson's disease. Trends Pharmacol Sci. 2003;24:395–401. doi: 10.1016/S0165-6147(03)00176-7

[43] Prescott SM, Fitzpatrick FA. Cyclooxygenase-2 and carcinogenesis. Biochim Biophys Acta. 2000;1470:M69–78. doi: 10.1034/j.1600-0463.2003.1111001.x

[44] Subbaramaiah K, Dannenberg AJ. Cyclooxygenase 2: a molecular target for cancer prevention and treatment. Trends Pharmacol Sci. 2003;24:96–102. doi:10.1016/S0165-6147(02)00043-3

[45] Hunot S, Vila M, Teismann P, Davis RJ, Hirsch EC, Przedborski S, et al. JNK-mediated induction of cyclooxygenase 2 is required for neurodegeneration in a mouse model of Parkinson's disease. Proc Natl Acad Sci USA. 2004;101:665–670. doi:10.1073/pnas.0307453101

[46] Liu W, Reinmuth N, Stoeltzing O, Parikh AA, Tellez C, Williams S, et al. Cyclooxygenase-2 is up-regulated by interleukin-1 beta in human colorectal cancer cells via multiple signaling pathways. Cancer Res. 2003;63:3632–3636.

[47] Denkert C, Kobel M, Berger S, Siegert A, Leclere A, Trefzer U, et al. Expression of cyclooxygenase 2 in human malignant melanoma. Cancer Res. 2001;61:303–308.

[48] Steinbach G, Lynch PM, Phillips RK, Wallace MH, Hawk E, Gordon GB, et al. The effect of celecoxib, a cyclooxygenase-2 inhibitor, in familial adenomatous polyposis. N Engl J Med. 2000;342:1946–1952. doi:10.1056/NEJM200006293422603

[49] Silverstein FE, Faich G, Goldstein JL, Simon LS, Pincus T, Whelton A, et al. Gastrointestinal toxicity with celecoxib vs nonsteroidal anti-inflammatory drugs for osteoarthritis and rheumatoid arthritis: the CLASS study: a randomized controlled trial. Celecoxib Long-term Arthritis Safety Study. JAMA. 2000;284:1247–1255. doi: 10.1001/jama.284.10.1247.

[50] Zimprich A, Biskup S, Leitner P, Lichtner P, Farrer M, Lincoln S, et al. Mutations in LRRK2 cause autosomal-dominant parkinsonism with pleomorphic pathology. Neuron. 2004;44:601–607. doi:10.1016/j.neuron.2004.11.005

[51] Paisan-Ruiz C, Jain S, Evans EW, Gilks WP, Simon J, van der Brug M, et al. Cloning of the gene containing mutations that cause PARK8-linked Parkinson's disease. Neuron. 2004;44:595–600. doi:10.1016/j.neuron.2004.10.023

[52] Lesage S, Brice A. Parkinson's disease: from monogenic forms to genetic susceptibility factors. Hum Mol Genet. 2009;18:R48–59. doi:10.1093/hmg/ddp012

[53] Berg D, Schweitzer KJ, Leitner P, Zimprich A, Lichtner P, Belcredi P, et al. Type and frequency of mutations in the LRRK2 gene in familial and sporadic Parkinson's disease. Brain. 2005;128:3000–3011. doi:10.1093/brain/awh666

[54] Ohta E, Kawakami F, Kubo M, Obata F. LRRK2 directly phosphorylates Akt1 as a possible physiological substrate: impairment of the kinase activity by Parkinson's disease-associated mutations. FEBS Lett. 2011;585:2165–2170. doi:10.1016/j.febslet.2011.05.044

[55] Bosgraaf L, Van Haastert PJ. Roc, a Ras/GTPase domain in complex proteins. Biochim Biophys Acta. 2003;1643:5–10. doi: 10.1016/j.bbamcr.2003.08.008

[56] Manning G, Whyte DB, Martinez R, Hunter T, Sudarsanam S. The protein kinase complement of the human genome. Science. 2002;298:1912–1934. doi:10.1126/science.1075762

[57] Andrade MA, Perez-Iratxeta C, Ponting CP. Protein repeats: structures, functions, and evolution. J Struct Biol. 2001;134:117–131. doi:10.1006/jsbi.2001.4392

[58] Cookson MR. The role of leucine-rich repeat kinase 2 (LRRK2) in Parkinson's disease. Nat Rev Neurosci. 2010;11:791–797. doi:10.1038/nrn2935

[59] West AB, Moore DJ, Biskup S, Bugayenko A, Smith WW, Ross CA, et al. Parkinson's disease-associated mutations in leucine-rich repeat kinase 2 augment kinase activity. Proc Natl Acad Sci USA. 2005;102:16842–16847. doi:10.1073/pnas.0507360102

[60] Aasly JO, Toft M, Fernandez-Mata I, Kachergus J, Hulihan M, White LR, et al. Clinical features of LRRK2-associated Parkinson's disease in central Norway. Ann Neurol. 2005;57:762–765. doi:10.1002/ana.20456

[61] Simon-Sanchez J, Schulte C, Bras JM, Sharma M, Gibbs JR, Berg D, et al. Genome-wide association study reveals genetic risk underlying Parkinson's disease. Nat Genet. 2009;41:1308–1312. doi:10.1038/ng.487

[62] Mata IF, Wedemeyer WJ, Farrer MJ, Taylor JP, Gallo KA. LRRK2 in Parkinson's disease: protein domains and functional insights. Trends Neurosci. 2006;29:286–293. doi: 10.1016/j.tins.2006.03.006

[63] Lee BD, Dawson VL, Dawson TM. Leucine-rich repeat kinase 2 (LRRK2) as a potential therapeutic target in Parkinson's disease. Trends Pharmacol Sci. 2012;33:365–373. doi:10.1016/j.tips.2012.04.001

[64] Looyenga BD, Furge KA, Dykema KJ, Koeman J, Swiatek PJ, Giordano TJ, et al. Chromosomal amplification of leucine-rich repeat kinase-2 (LRRK2) is required for

oncogenic MET signaling in papillary renal and thyroid carcinomas. Proc Natl Acad Sci USA. 2011;108:1439–1444. doi:10.1073/pnas.1012500108

[65]   Zhang J, Baran J, Cros A, Guberman JM, Haider S, Hsu J, et al. International Cancer Genome Consortium Data Portal—a one-stop shop for cancer genomics data. Database (Oxford). 2011;2011:bar026. doi:10.1093/database/bar026

[66]   Franke A, McGovern DP, Barrett JC, Wang K, Radford-Smith GL, Ahmad T, et al. Genome-wide meta-analysis increases to 71 the number of confirmed Crohn's disease susceptibility loci. Nat Genet. 2010;42:1118–1125. doi:10.1038/ng.717

[67]   Greenman C, Stephens P, Smith R, Dalgliesh GL, Hunter C, Bignell G, et al. Patterns of somatic mutation in human cancer genomes. Nature. 2007;446:153–158. doi:10.1038/nature05610

[68]   Liu Z, Lee J, Krummey S, Lu W, Cai H, Lenardo MJ. The kinase LRRK2 is a regulator of the transcription factor NFAT that modulates the severity of inflammatory bowel disease. Nat Immunol. 2011;12:1063–1070. doi:10.1038/ni.2113

[69]   Inzelberg R, Cohen OS, Aharon-Peretz J, Schlesinger I, Gershoni-Baruch R, Djaldetti R, et al. The LRRK2 G2019S mutation is associated with Parkinson disease and concomitant non-skin cancers. Neurology. 2012. doi:10.1212/WNL.0b013e318249f673

[70]   Lewis PA, Manzoni C. LRRK2 and human disease: a complicated question or a question of complexes? Sci Signal. 2012;5:pe2. doi:10.1126/scisignal.2002680

[71]   Huynh T. The Parkinson's disease market. Nat Rev Drug Discov. 2011;10:571–572. doi:10.1038/nrd3515

[72]   Jones PA, Baylin SB. The epigenomics of cancer. Cell. 2007;128:683–692. doi:10.1016/j.cell.2007.01.029

[73]   Gehrke S, Imai Y, Sokol N, Lu B. Pathogenic LRRK2 negatively regulates microRNA-mediated translational repression. Nature. 2010;466:637–641. doi:10.1038/nature09191

[74]   Kawashima M, Suzuki SO, Doh-ura K, Iwaki T. Alpha-synuclein is expressed in a variety of brain tumors showing neuronal differentiation. Acta Neuropathol. 2000;99:154–160. doi: 10.1007/PL00007419

[75]   Matsuo Y, Kamitani T. Parkinson's disease-related protein, alpha-synuclein, in malignant melanoma. Plos One. 2010;5:e10481. doi:10.1371/journal.pone.0010481

[76]   Bruening W, Giasson BI, Klein-Szanto AJ, Lee VM, Trojanowski JQ, Godwin AK. Synucleins are expressed in the majority of breast and ovarian carcinomas and in preneoplastic lesions of the ovary. Cancer. 2000;88:2154–2163. doi:10.1002/(SICI)1097-0142(20000501)88:9<2154::AID-CNCR23>3.0.CO;2-9

[77]   Li L, Tao Q, Jin H, van Hasselt A, Poon FF, Wang X, et al. The tumor suppressor UCHL1 forms a complex with p53/MDM2/ARF to promote p53 signaling and is frequently

silenced in nasopharyngeal carcinoma. Clin Cancer Res. 2010;16:2949–2958. doi: 10.1158/1078-0432.CCR-09-3178

[78] Okochi-Takada E, Nakazawa K, Wakabayashi M, Mori A, Ichimura S, Yasugi T, et al. Silencing of the UCHL1 gene in human colorectal and ovarian cancers. Int J Cancer. 2006;119:1338–1344. doi:10.1002/ijc.22025

[79] Berthier A, Navarro S, Jimenez-Sainz J, Rogla I, Ripoll F, Cervera J, et al. PINK1 displays tissue-specific subcellular location and regulates apoptosis and cell growth in breast cancer cells. Hum Pathol. 2011;42:75–87. doi:10.1016/j.humpath.2010.05.016

[80] MacKeigan JP, Clements CM, Lich JD, Pope RM, Hod Y, Ting JP. Proteomic profiling drug-induced apoptosis in non-small cell lung carcinoma: identification of RS/DJ-1 and RhoGDIalpha. Cancer Res. 2003;63:6928–6934.

Permissions

All chapters in this book were first published in CPD, by InTech Open; hereby published with permission under the Creative Commons Attribution License or equivalent. Every chapter published in this book has been scrutinized by our experts. Their significance has been extensively debated. The topics covered herein carry significant findings which will fuel the growth of the discipline. They may even be implemented as practical applications or may be referred to as a beginning point for another development.

The contributors of this book come from diverse backgrounds, making this book a truly international effort. This book will bring forth new frontiers with its revolutionizing research information and detailed analysis of the nascent developments around the world.

We would like to thank all the contributing authors for lending their expertise to make the book truly unique. They have played a crucial role in the development of this book. Without their invaluable contributions this book wouldn't have been possible. They have made vital efforts to compile up to date information on the varied aspects of this subject to make this book a valuable addition to the collection of many professionals and students.

This book was conceptualized with the vision of imparting up-to-date information and advanced data in this field. To ensure the same, a matchless editorial board was set up. Every individual on the board went through rigorous rounds of assessment to prove their worth. After which they invested a large part of their time researching and compiling the most relevant data for our readers.

The editorial board has been involved in producing this book since its inception. They have spent rigorous hours researching and exploring the diverse topics which have resulted in the successful publishing of this book. They have passed on their knowledge of decades through this book. To expedite this challenging task, the publisher supported the team at every step. A small team of assistant editors was also appointed to further simplify the editing procedure and attain best results for the readers.

Apart from the editorial board, the designing team has also invested a significant amount of their time in understanding the subject and creating the most relevant covers. They scrutinized every image to scout for the most suitable representation of the subject and create an appropriate cover for the book.

The publishing team has been an ardent support to the editorial, designing and production team. Their endless efforts to recruit the best for this project, has resulted in the accomplishment of this book. They are a veteran in the field of academics and their pool of knowledge is as vast as their experience in printing. Their expertise and guidance has proved useful at every step. Their uncompromising quality standards have made this book an exceptional effort. Their encouragement from time to time has been an inspiration for everyone.

The publisher and the editorial board hope that this book will prove to be a valuable piece of knowledge for researchers, students, practitioners and scholars across the globe.

List of Contributors

Unax Lertxundi
Pharmacy Service, Araba's Mental Health Network, Vitoria-Gasteiz, Spain

Rafael Hernández
Internal Medicine, Araba's Mental Health Network, Vitoria-Gasteiz, Spain

Saioa Domingo-Echaburu
Pharmacy Service, Alto Deba's Integrated Health Organization, Arrasate, Spain

Javier Peral-Aguirregoitia
Pharmacy Service, Galdakao-Usansolo Hospital, Galdakao, Spain

Juan Medrano
Psychiatry Service, Bizkaia's Mental Health Network, Portugalete, Spain

Andrea R. Di Sebastiano, Michael D. Staudt, Simon M. Benoit and Hu Xu
Clinical Neurological Sciences, Schulich School of Medicine & Dentistry, University of Western Ontario, London, ON, Canada

Matthew O. Hebb
Clinical Neurological Sciences, Schulich School of Medicine & Dentistry, University of Western Ontario, London, ON, Canada
Anatomy & Cell Biology, Schulich School of Medicine & Dentistry, University of Western Ontario, London, ON, Canada

Susanne Schmid
Anatomy & Cell Biology, Schulich School of Medicine & Dentistry, University of Western Ontario, London, ON, Canada

Rafael González Maldonado
Neuroconsulta, Granada, Spain

Fabin Han
The Institute for Tissue Engineering and Regenerative Medicine, Liaocheng University/The Liaocheng People's Hospital, Shandong, China

María Satue, Vicente Polo, Sofía Otin, Jose M. Larrosa, Javier Obis and Elena Garcia-Martin
IIS Aragon, Ophthalmology Department, Institute for Health Sciencies of Aragon (IACS), Miguel Servet University Hospital, Zaragoza, Spain

Priyanka Modi, Ayajuddin Mohamad, Limamanen Phom, Zevelou Koza, Abhik Das, Rahul Chaurasia, Saikat Samadder, Bovito Achumi, Muralidhara, Rajesh Singh Pukhrambam and Sarat Chandra Yenisetti
These authors contributed equally to this work Drosophila Neurobiology Laboratory, Department of Zoology, Nagaland University (Central), Lumami, Nagaland, India

Ivan Galtier, Antonieta Nieto and Jose Barroso
School of Psychology, University of La Laguna, Tenerife, Spain

Michelle Hyczy de Siqueira Tosin
Sarah Network of Rehabilitation Hospitals, Rio de Janeiro, RJ, Brazil

Beatriz Guitton Renaud Baptista de Oliveira
School of Nursing, Federal Fluminense University, Niterói, RJ, Brazil

S Meenalochani, ST Dheen and SSW Tay
Department of Anatomy, Yong Loo Lin school of Medicine, National University Health System, National University of Singapore, Singapore

Zhiming Li and Chi-Meng Tzeng
Translational Medicine Research Center, School of Pharmaceutical Sciences, Xiamen University, Xiamen, Fujian, China
Key Laboratory for Cancer T-Cell Theranostics and Clinical Translation (CTCTCT), Xiamen, Fujian, China
INNOVA Clinics and TRANSLA Health Group University, Xiamen, Fujian, China

Index

9 781632 427168